natural conception and
PREGNANCY

natural conception and
PREGNANCY

preparing for **parenting** the **holistic** way

anne charlish
and **kim davies**

LORENZ BOOKS

section 1

section 2

contents

Introduction

" This book will give you all you need to make your pregnancy as wonderful, natural and personal as it can be. "

There are two main aspects to pregnancy. On the one hand, there are the medical matters. Scientific know-how has made pregnancy and birth extremely safe, and a mother-to-be can very well entrust herself to the care of doctors. On the other hand, pregnancy is a major life experience where your personality, your ideas about parenting and the feelings you have about your own body are all highly significant.

This book aims to give you the best of both the medical and the natural, holistic approaches. It tells you everything you need to know about the common obstetric procedures, but also emphasizes the importance of nutrition, exercise and a host of supportive complementary therapies – from yoga and homeopathy to meditation and herbalism.

Preparing for pregnancy is vital. The first section of the book looks at how you can do this to best effect through improving diet and well-being. It explores the factors that affect conception, such as age and specific medical problems, and explains what can be done.

Partners, close friends and relatives can play a vital supportive role. Here, a woman practises using her partner for support during labour.

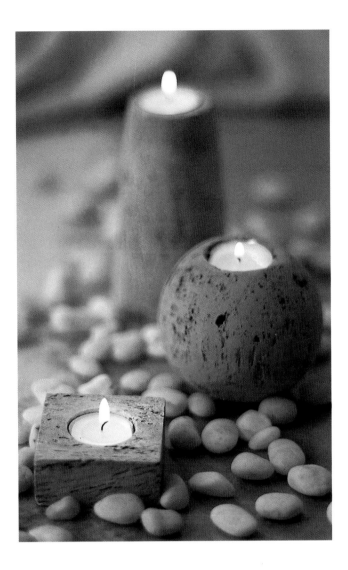

All kinds of holistic therapies can assist women through every stage of conception and pregnancy – even if it is simply burning aromatic candles to create a calm and serene atmosphere.

TAKE CARE

This book has been written with the aim of helping women who are trying to conceive or who are already pregnant. However, it is important to remember that no book can be a substitute for getting advice about your own medical circumstances. For this reason, all the suggestions in this book should be used under the guidance of your doctor and complementary practitioner.

If you are at all worried by any symptom during your pregnancy, or if you are unsure of whether or not a natural therapy is safe, do not hesitate to consult your family doctor.

You should call the emergency services and then sit down and wait for the ambulance to arrive if you notice any of the following:

- Vaginal bleeding, unless it is merely spotting.
- Severe abdominal pain, especially if you are also bleeding vaginally.
- Continuous and severe headache, with or without blurred vision and with or without swelling of the hands and ankles.
- Excessive vomiting in which you cannot keep down any food or liquid, even water.
- Breaking of the waters.
- After week 22 of your pregnancy, no fetal movements for longer than 12 hours.

Telephone your family doctor without delay if you notice any of these symptoms:

- A temperature of 38.5°C (101°F) or more.
- Sudden swelling of the hands and ankles. If you also have blurred vision and/or severe headache as well as the swelling, you should call an ambulance (see above).
- Urinating not only frequently (which is normal during pregnancy) but with pain as well when you pass water, as this usually signifies some kind of infection.

The book then takes you through each and every stage of this extraordinary life event, from the moment of conception to giving birth, and on into your new baby's first few weeks of life. It explains clearly what is happening to your body and gives you the answers to the most commonly asked questions. It also details the different choices that are available – the benefits that they can bring and the potential risks. For example, natural childbirth options are explained, but the book also advises on the drugs that are available if you decide you need them.

In the end you will decide for yourself how you deal with the ups-and-downs, the joys and pains of conception, pregnancy and childbirth. Rather than tell you what you must do, this book will give you all you need to make your pregnancy as wonderful, natural and personal as it can be.

section one

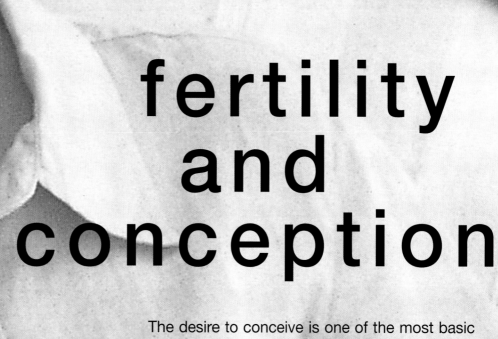

fertility and conception

The desire to conceive is one of the most basic
and powerful of human instincts, shared with all
the living things on our planet. Once you have
decided to embark upon this incredible journey,
then a whole new world opens up to you.
The key during this time is to gather as much
information as you can, and to maintain
optimum physical well-being and a healthy
mental outlook.

Preparing for pregnancy

" Enjoy all the new things that you will be discovering about yourself. "

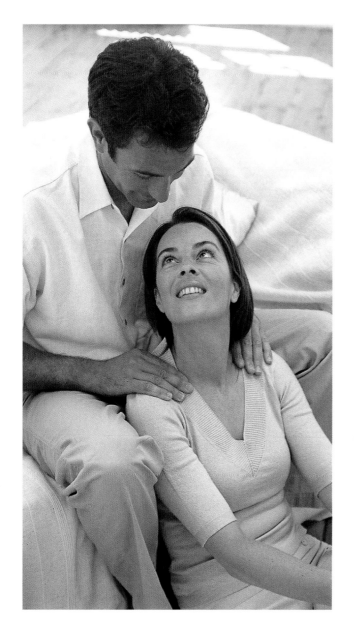

Having a child is a wonderful event, but of course it is also a life-changing one. The decision to try for a baby is one that no one else can take for you – only you know whether this is a course that you truly wish to embark on.

As you explore this exciting change in your life, consider both the emotional and practical issues. Think about the strength of the relationship with your partner, and discuss possible parenthood thoroughly with them. Weigh up your age, your current income and work prospects, your living arrangements and whether there is sufficient space for a baby. Ask yourself whether or not you really feel ready to become responsible for a new life. After all, a child will be with you for many years to come.

Find out as much as you can about pregnancy, labour, and being a parent. Talk to other parents, and spend time with people who have young children so that you get a real taste of just what it may be like.

If you have a partner, your relationship will need to be strong as you start along the road to parenthood. Many decisions lie ahead, which should be made together.

Choosing to have a child involves both instinct and reason. Don't worry if you have doubts, as no one can be totally certain of any choice that they make. We can only decide what feels right for us and then pursue our chosen goal in a positive spirit.

If you decide to go ahead, you will want to prepare as well as possible. You may need to improve your general health or fitness or lose or gain weight before trying to conceive. Look into ways of eating healthy, natural foods and find out about the wide choice of complementary therapies that will help to keep you in top mental and physical shape. Above all, enjoy all the new things that you will be discovering about yourself and the journey ahead of you.

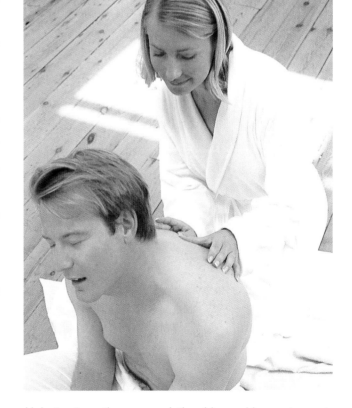

Top: Keep yourself in good physical shape, but avoid suddenly starting a tough routine that you have never tried before, and seek advice from your doctor first.

Help to strengthen your relationship, and keep stress at bay, by making time to enjoy relaxing and sensual pleasures such as a soothing massage.

Deciding to have a baby

Choosing to have a baby is without question the most momentous decision of your life. No other will have such far-reaching, and yet such potentially rewarding, implications over the years to come.

Some people feel an absolute certainty that they are ready to have a baby. Others feel more ambivalent about the effect that a child may have on their lifestyle or relationship. In addition, partners often feel differently about exactly when or if they want to become parents.

Discussing all the issues is essential. It is important that you ask yourself some searching questions before going ahead, and that you and your partner are honest about any hopes and fears that you have.

WHY YOU WANT TO HAVE A BABY

Talking about your reasons for wanting a baby can help you to pinpoint any assumptions that you have about the role a child will play in your life. For example, do you see a baby as something that will enhance an already happy life – or as a way of filling an emotional void? Are you hoping he or she will strengthen a loving partnership – or cement over the cracks in a rocky one?

It would not be wise to conceive a child in order to repair problems in your relationship or simply because you want to have someone to love. If there are tensions between you and your partner, having a baby will almost certainly exacerbate them – lack of sleep and having more to do at home soon cause tempers to fray.

Caring for a baby can be an isolating experience, especially if you do not have a loving partner to lean on. Many people bring up their children as lone parents – and

do a wonderful job. Ideally, though, you will be in a committed, loving relationship that is strong enough to withstand the challenges of bringing up a child.

PROGRESSING TO PARENTHOOD

One of the most important things for you and your partner to consider is whether or not you feel ready to welcome another person into your relationship. Are you sufficiently certain of each other's feelings for one another to be able to care for a helpless and dependent baby?

Think, too, about whether your partner is the person you want to parent your child. Do you consider him or her to be sufficiently mature, kind, compassionate, intelligent, and sensitive to be your co-parent? As a hypothetical question, would you have liked your partner as a parent yourself? Try to imagine it just for a moment.

YOUR LIFESTYLE

Before trying to conceive, discuss how you see your lives adapting to a new child. Consider some of the practical issues. Is your home a suitable place for a child, for example, or will you have to move? Is one of you planning to stay home with the baby for the first years? If so, is the other prepared to become sole breadwinner for a time?

If your career is important to you, think about whether you can take some time off without damaging your future prospects. Consider, too, how you will cope with both the costs of having a child and the likely reduction in your income as a result of working less or paying for childcare.

Take some time to think about how you see your lives in five or ten years' time. Is what you want in terms of

FERTILITY ISSUES TO CONSIDER
When considering whether or not this is the right time to try for a baby, you may need to consider biological factors. Most important of these is the age of the woman.

A woman's fertility decreases as she gets older, particularly after the age of 35. Fertility starts to decrease about ten years before a woman's periods stop, and most women start the menopause around 45-55 (though it can be much earlier). There is no way of knowing exactly when the menopause will start, so it is wise not to put off conceiving for too long, particularly if you are already in your thirties.

From a biological point of view, a woman is most likely to conceive between 20 and 25 years of age. If you delay having a child until later, be aware that you are more likely to experience delays in conception than younger women. However, age usually brings with it greater stability and maturity, which are vital factors where parenthood is concerned.

Many different factors may be involved in the timing of your pregnancy. If both you and your partner feel that you are ready to have a child together, then this is probably the right time for you to go ahead, irrespective of work, finances or any other concerns.

home and career compatible with what your partner wants? Are you agreed on how you see your future lives?

None of these issues is likely to be the deciding factor in whether or not you try to start a family. However, discussing them can help to build up a picture of how you and your partner feel about starting a family, and whether or not you need to make changes to your lifestyle first.

YOUR SUPPORT NETWORK

Family and close friends can be a vital support when you have a baby – particularly in the first few months when you are adjusting to your new lifestyle. It is a good idea to discuss with your partner the role that each of your families may play in helping you. Do you have supportive friends or relatives near to where you live at the moment? If not, would you consider moving?

Deciding whether, and when, to have a baby will probably be the biggest and most important event of your lives together – and the most exciting.

MAKING A DECISION

Ultimately, only you and your partner can know if this is the right time for you to try for a baby. Give yourselves plenty of time to make the decision, and listen carefully to what your inner voice tells you.

Listen just as carefully to what your partner says – and make sure that you hear what he or she actually says, rather than what you wish to hear. It is easy to imagine that your partner's aims are the same as yours, but this isn't always the case. Having a baby is a long-term commitment and both partners need to be sure that this is what they really want.

How pregnancy happens

For pregnancy to occur, both the man's and the woman's reproductive system must be in good working order, the couple must make love at the right time of the woman's menstrual cycle, and her body must produce a complex chain of hormones in order to keep the pregnancy going.

When a man ejaculates during sexual intercourse, millions of sperm are released into the woman's vagina. They move up the vagina and through the cervix into the uterus, propelled both by the force of ejaculation and by moving their tails like tiny fish. From there, the sperm make their way to the Fallopian tubes. This process is like a frantic race, as only one sperm among the millions can fertilize the egg. The rest fall away before they reach the goal, or else arrive too late.

If sexual intercourse has taken place without contraception, some sperm may reach the Fallopian tube and a single one may fertilize the waiting egg. The fertilized egg then makes its way towards the woman's uterus (womb), where it attaches itself to the lining. Here, it develops first into a tiny embryo, then a fetus and, eventually, into a baby.

THE WOMAN'S REPRODUCTIVE SYSTEM

A woman's reproductive system lies within her pelvis, and consists of the ovaries, the Fallopian tubes, the uterus, the cervix, the vagina and the vulva.

Baby girls are born with all their eggs in place in the ovaries – about 2-3 million of them. The ovaries are dormant during childhood and start to function only as puberty and menstruation begins. From then, women of childbearing age produce an egg every four weeks or so. This monthly timetable is called the ovulatory or menstrual cycle. About 400-500 eggs are produced during a woman's childbearing years – before ovulation ceases at menopause, usually in the woman's forties or fifties.

At the beginning of the ovulatory cycle, a number of eggs begin to grow in the ovaries. After about 14 days, one egg is mature enough to be released into the Fallopian tube. The ovulated egg enters the Fallopian tube and travels towards the uterus. It is during this journey that the egg may be fertilized. If not, some 14 days after ovulation the lining of the uterus is shed into the vagina – that is, the woman has her period. Then the entire cycle begins again.

CONCEPTION AND HORMONES

Hormones are chemicals that the body produces to regulate all kinds of natural processes. They act as messengers, telling the ovaries, for example, when to release an egg.

Two hormones play a crucial role in ovulation and pregnancy. Each month, follicle-stimulating hormone (FSH) stimulates an egg to mature, then luteinizing hormone (LH) causes the egg to be released into the Fallopian tubes, where it is ready to be fertilized. The hormones FSH and LH are produced in the brain, in an organ called the pituitary gland. The cells around the egg produce two other hormones – oestrogen and progesterone. These hormones cause the lining of the uterus to thicken – to create an environment in which an implanted, fertilized egg can thrive and grow. It is the monthly drop in the level of progesterone which, in the absence of a fertilized egg, brings on a woman's period.

The regular ebb and flow of different hormones throughout the menstrual cycle means that there are only a few days in each month when a woman is likely to conceive. This 'window of opportunity' is known as the fertile period.

FEMALE REPRODUCTIVE SYSTEM
The woman's egg is released from the ovary. It travels down the Fallopian tube to the uterus.

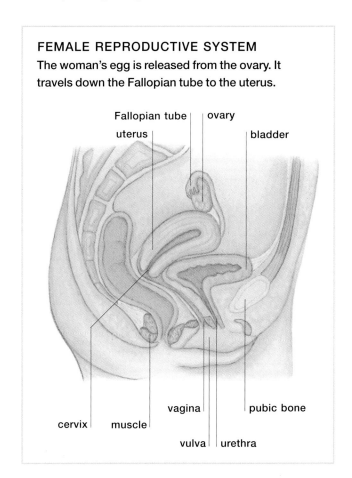

Fallopian tube | ovary
uterus | bladder
vagina | pubic bone
cervix | muscle
vulva | urethra

If the woman is menstruating but is not producing eggs for some reason, conception cannot occur. However, women can conceive even if they are not having periods – although conception is less likely.

THE MAN'S REPRODUCTIVE SYSTEM

A man's reproductive system consists of the penis, the testicles, and the various tubes that connect the two and carry sperm. Sperm is produced in the two testicles, which are contained within the scrotum. Men do not start making sperm until they reach puberty.

Thousands of microscopic tubes within the testicles connect to the two tubes – which are known as the efferent ducts. These lead into one single tube, the epididymis. The epididymis is part of the route through which sperm leaves the man's body. It is about 12 metres (40 feet) in length, and it is narrower than a fine piece of thread.

THE SPERM'S JOURNEY

Men, unlike women, are physiologically primed to reproduce at any time, and so sperm are in constant production. A series of muscular contractions in the wall of the epididymis serves to transport them along its length. During this time, the sperm are modified so that they become capable of fertilization. They also acquire their ability to move (which is known medically as motility) while they are in the epididymis. The sperm now pass

MALE REPRODUCTIVE SYSTEM
Sperm travels from the testicles through the epididymis, vas deferens and urethra to the penis.

vas deferens | bladder
urethra | seminal vesicles
epididymis | muscle
testicle
penis | scrotum | prostate gland

> **Seven days after fertilization, the egg becomes implanted in the lining of the uterus. This is the moment when conception is said to take place.**

through a tube called the vas deferens, which moves them quickly into the urethra, which passes through the penis. The urethra is the tube through which urine is passed outside the body. During sexual arousal and ejaculation, the opening between the urethra and the bladder shuts, and sperm-containing semen is rapidly transported along it.

THE RACE TO THE EGG

It takes only one sperm to fertilize an egg. When a man ejaculates during sexual intercourse, between 100 million and 300 million sperm are discharged into the woman's vagina – at about 45km (28 miles) per hour.

Each sperm is genetically unique, meaning that no two contain exactly the same set of genes. The millions of individual sperm are now in competition with each other as they race to fertilize the egg.

The route to the egg is hazardous. This is why sperm are produced in such large numbers. To stand a chance of fertilizing the egg, the sperm have to be able to withstand the environment of the woman's vagina and cervix. The acidity of this environment protects against bacteria and potentially dangerous infections, but it is also inhospitable to sperm. Weak or damaged ones will not make it.

In addition, the force of gravity means that millions of sperm simply leak out of the woman's vagina – as few as 5 per cent of them reach the cervix. Of these, only 200 or so make it as far as the woman's Fallopian tubes. Any sperm that make it this far have covered a huge distance that is, in terms of its own length, equivalent to several hundred miles.

The last few superfit sperm now proceed to the outside of the egg. Of these sperm, just one will break through the surface, leaving its tail behind. This is the moment of fertilization. In the instant that it occurs, the egg's surface becomes impenetrable to other sperm.

Fertilization of the egg may take up to 24 hours. It then undergoes a series of complex changes until eventually, seven days after fertilization, it becomes implanted in the lining of the uterus. This is the moment when conception is said to take place.

Sperm can survive for quite a long time inside the woman's body – perhaps up to 48 hours – so fertilization can still take place even if the egg is not ready when they first reach the Fallopian tube.

Aiding conception

A baby can be conceived only around the time of ovulation, during the woman's fertile period. The egg is usually fertilized by the man's sperm within 48 hours of being released by the ovary. There are various ways in which a woman can judge when she is ovulating. By identifying this fertile period a couple can make a point of having intercourse and maximize the chance of conceiving.

WHEN DO I OVULATE?

Women ovulate about 14 days before the start of their next period. This is not the same as saying that ovulation takes place 14 days after the last period because the length of the menstrual cycle varies. Women may have a cycle as short as 21 days or as long as 38 days rather than the standard 28-day cycle.

There are various methods that you can use to calculate when ovulation is likely to occur. However, bear in mind that these serve as a rough guide only. Many experts and researchers in the field of infertility are sceptical about the effectiveness of the methods used. Even if you are certain that you know when you are ovulating, you should continue to make love at other times if you want to get pregnant.

Your menstrual cycle

If you have a regular monthly cycle, you will know when the next period is likely to start. Count back 14 days from that date – this is the day on which you are likely to ovulate.

YOUR CHANCES OF CONCEIVING

Conception is more likely to take place if:
- The woman is between the ages of 20 and 34; the ideal age is 20-25.
- The man produces healthy sperm.
- Intercourse takes place at the right time in the woman's menstrual cycle.
- Both partners are fit and well, and are following a healthy lifestyle.
- Both partners are a healthy weight, with a good waist-to-hip ratio (see page 51).
- Both partners avoid smoking, alcohol and caffeine.

Working out your probable fertile time means keeping a record of your periods for some months, in some cases up to a year, to establish the normal length of your cycle.

Cervical mucus

If your periods are irregular, you may be able to establish when you ovulate by studying your cervical mucus (produced by glands in the cervix's lining). Just before ovulation, it is transparent, thinner and more profuse, and takes on an jelly-like consistency, so that a drop will stretch between your fingers without breaking. After ovulation less, more milky coloured, mucus is produced.

THE MENSTRUAL CYCLE

At the start of the cycle, an egg develops in a follicle in the ovary. At ovulation, the egg is released, and the follicle then turns into a corpus luteum. This secretes hormones that cause the lining of the uterus to thicken. If fertilization does not occur, the corpus luteum decays and the thickened lining is shed with the unfertilized egg.

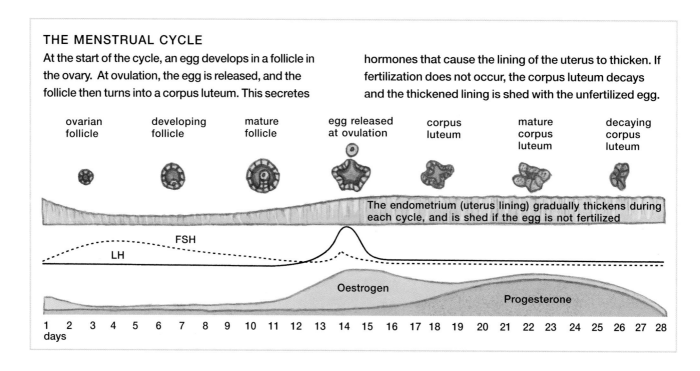

| ovarian follicle | developing follicle | mature follicle | egg released at ovulation | corpus luteum | mature corpus luteum | decaying corpus luteum |

The endometrium (uterus lining) gradually thickens during each cycle, and is shed if the egg is not fertilized

FSH
LH
Oestrogen
Progesterone

1 2 3 4 5 6 7 8 9 10 11 12 13 14 15 16 17 18 19 20 21 22 23 24 25 26 27 28 days

Remember that the consistency of cervical mucus may change for other reasons – for example, if you have an infection. For greater accuracy, it is best to combine this method with the body temperature method.

To test your mucus, insert your finger into your vagina, then gently withdraw it. If the mucus is clear, moist and stretchy, you are probably close to ovulation. Making love within the next 24-36 hours could give a good chance of conception.

Making love around the time of ovulation will maximize your chances of becoming pregnant. All methods for establishing ovulation are approximate, so you should continue to make love at other times.

Body temperature

You can measure changes in your basal body temperature to determine when you are at your most fertile. Basal body temperature (BBT) is your temperature immediately on waking in the morning, before you have got up or eaten or drunk anything. BBT drops just before ovulation and then rises again some 12-24 hours later, once ovulation has occurred. If you record the changes in your BBT each day for several months on a special chart, a pattern is likely to emerge. You can use this to help you predict the time of ovulation.

Remember that your temperature can rise and fall for other reasons. For example, if you are ill or if you take your temperature later in the day, your reading is likely to be inaccurate. Doing both the temperature and cervical-mucus methods at the same time tends to give more accurate results than either method done alone.

Ovulation kits

You can also establish the day of ovulation by using an over-the-counter ovulation prediction device. These kits work by measuring the amount of the LH hormone being produced, which helps to establish when ovulation is about to occur. All you need to do is a urine test. If plenty of LH hormone is being produced, a chemical will change colour. This means you are likely to be ovulating. However, like all the methods, ovulation kits are not foolproof. They can produce a false positive result. They are also expensive.

BODY TEMPERATURE CHART

In the temperature method, a basal thermometer is used to detect minute changes in a woman's body temperature during the ovulatory cycle; regular thermometers are not sensitive enough.

Most basal thermometers are supplied with a chart like this one. Make several copies so that you can keep a record of temperature changes over a few months. You may need help from an expert in order to interpret the results and pinpoint your fertile period.

Preconceptual care

Ideally, both you and your partner should start to prepare for conception a few months before you try for a baby. Nobody can guarantee you a healthy baby but if you and your partner are fit and healthy at the point of conception, you are giving your pregnancy the best start possible.

Your diet, weight and fitness can all impact on your fertility and on the pregnancy. Maintaining a regular fitness programme, eating a healthy diet and reducing stress can all aid your chances of conception, and will also help the woman's body to cope better with pregnancy. The months before conception are also a good time to give up smoking, reduce or give up alcohol, and attend to any other health issues.

The majority of women do not need any supplements other than folic acid either before conception or during their pregnancy. However, it is important that you start taking folic acid, which substantially reduces the risk of spina bifida, for a couple of months before you start trying for a baby – the current recommended dose is 400 micrograms every day.

DENTAL CHECK

Before conceiving, have a full dental check-up. Try to get any treatment done straight away so that you can avoid having X-rays or anaesthetics during pregnancy. Pregnant women are also advised not to have any amalgam (silver) fillings put in or removed during pregnancy since they may leak tiny doses of mercury, which is toxic.

MEDICAL CHECK-UP

Tell your doctor that you want to conceive. Ask about any supplements or medication you are taking – both over-the-counter and prescribed drugs could affect the health of your baby. Your doctor will also be able to provide advice on your diet, health and lifestyle, and advise you on losing or gaining weight, if necessary.

If you have diabetes, epilepsy or any other chronic condition that requires you to take long-term medication, your doctor may recommend changing the drugs or reducing the dosage before conception. He or she may also suggest genetic counselling if you or your partner have a family history of genetic disorders.

SEXUAL HEALTH CHECKS

Some sexually transmitted infections can affect your fertility as well as your general health. As they do not necessarily cause symptoms, you may be unaware that you have been infected. For this reason, all women

Getting plenty of rest and relaxation is an essential element of preconceptual health care. You should also make sure that you have all the vital health checks.

wanting to conceive are advised to have a 'well-woman' screening test. This checks for signs of:
- Bacterial infections such as chlamydia, gonorrhoea and syphilis, which can be cured with antibiotic treatment.
- Viral infections such as warts, herpes, hepatitis, and HIV, which can usually be treated to improve symptoms.

Untreated chlamydia, in particular, is a major cause of female infertility and ectopic pregnancies. It may cause pain on intercourse but is often without other symptoms, so many women only visit their doctor when they have problems conceiving. Up to a third of people are thought to be infected with chlamydia at some point in their lives.

SEXUALLY TRANSMITTED INFECTIONS
Symptoms may include any of these:
- Pain in the lower abdomen.
- Pain during or after sex.
- Bleeding after sex.
- Spotting or bleeding between periods.
- The sudden onset of much heavier periods after starting a new sexual relationship.
- Pain when passing urine.
- Increased or foul-smelling vaginal discharge.
- Rash, spots, lumps, itching or ulcers around the genital area.

RUBELLA

Before you try to get pregnant, you should have a test to ensure that you are immune to rubella (German measles). Rubella is a viral disease that can cause severe abnormalities in babies if their mothers catch it during pregnancy. Have the test even if you are sure that you had rubella as a child – rubella is frequently misdiagnosed, and it is not clear how long immunity achieved in this way lasts. If you are not immune, you can be vaccinated and then retested to make sure that the vaccine has worked. You should not attempt to conceive for at least one month after the vaccination.

CUTTING DOWN ON ALCOHOL

Some doctors recommend that women give up alcohol before trying to conceive as well as during pregnancy, while others say that an occasional drink will do no harm. All experts agree that regular, heavy drinking or binge drinking can have an adverse effect on fertility and also carries high risks for the baby.

Up to two glasses of wine a week may do no harm during pregnancy, so this could be a good limit if you are trying to conceive. Spirits contain much more alcohol than wine or beer and should be avoided completely during conception and pregnancy.

Men should drink no more than two pints of beer or half a bottle of wine daily when trying to conceive. Heavy drinkers may produce weak, inferior sperm, which are unable to negotiate the journey to meet the woman's egg. They may also produce babies with serious defects.

Alcohol crosses the placenta, so a baby is exposed to alcohol when the mother drinks. An occasional drink may do no harm, but babies born to mothers who are heavy

Yoga is an effective and enjoyable route to deep relaxation, and at the same time it increases your stamina, strength and suppleness.

drinkers may be affected by fetal alcohol syndrome. This can cause severe defects such as growth deficiency, facial abnormalities, problems with co-ordination and movement, and mental impairment. In addition, the babies may be born addicted to alcohol – and may suffer withdrawal symptoms and fail to thrive.

If you have had one child with a severe abnormality and are now trying for another baby, you and your partner should stop drinking for three months before attempting to conceive. You should continue to abstain from alcohol until you are sure that you are pregnant. The woman should continue to abstain throughout her pregnancy.

GIVE UP SMOKING

If you smoke, you should give up before trying to conceive. As well as affecting your general health, smoking reduces your fertility. If you smoke while pregnant, you have a higher risk of miscarriage and stillbirth; you also face an increased risk of having a premature or low-birthweight baby. Your partner should also give up to avoid the risk of passive smoking to both mother and baby. See your doctor if you want help with giving up smoking.

For optimum fertility and a healthy baby, it is best to give up alcohol entirely. At the very least, you should cut down to no more than two glasses of wine a week.

Time with your partner

Before you welcome a new baby into your life, it is important to devote special time and energy to your relationship with your partner. The time before conception – as well as the months of pregnancy itself – can be a marvellous opportunity to strengthen the bonds between you, and to work through unresolved emotional issues.

It can be very easy for partners to become focused on the baby that they want, and to forget that they are life partners as well as potential parents. Couples who enjoy each other's company, and respect each other's strengths and aims, tend to make happy and committed parents.

A loving relationship and good communication can help you to face possible delays in conception as well as the challenges that pregnancy can bring. In the weeks and months to come, you may have to undergo a number of tests and checks. Some may raise difficult questions – for example, how you would react if there was something wrong with the baby. The time that you invested in each other before conception will help you cope together, as loving partners.

WORKING TOGETHER

The months before conception may be a good time to complete projects that you wish to carry out in the house or garden. Working together for the future can deepen the relationship and can also help you to prepare both practically and mentally for the likely changes to your lifestyle when you have a family.

Practical projects are also better done before the pregnancy is advanced, and certainly before you have a new baby to care for. Any unresolved long-term problems – such as clearing up financial affairs – would also best be dealt with now rather than later, when you will have less time and energy to devote to them.

ENJOY ONE ANOTHER

How you celebrate and enjoy your relationship with your partner will depend on what you both like doing. You may like to cook delicious food together, go for long walks in the fresh air, swim or exercise, have friends in for dinners and barbecues, or enjoy other shared interests.

Making love is, of course, a wonderful way to express your affection. For many couples, this is the first time that they are able to enjoy sex without having to worry about contraception, which can heighten the pleasure as well as the sense of connection between you.

SHARING MASSAGE

Gentle massage is a great way of deepening the closeness between you and your partner. It is also highly beneficial for pregnant women or those wishing to conceive. Anyone can give a pleasurable massage, and the basic techniques are not difficult to learn. You may like to enrol in a short course to learn from an expert. As well as being extremely relaxing, massage is helpful during pregnancy since it can alleviate common complaints such as backache, insomnia and even morning sickness.

Pregnancy can be an emotional time, with many ups and downs. A close and loving relationship will help you to face any difficulties together.

Giving a relaxing massage

The key to good massage is focus and feedback. Concentrate on what your hands are doing and enjoy the pleasure that you can give. Use the following basic techniques, alternating them in whichever way feels right to you. Ask your partner whether or not the touch feels good – or if they would prefer a lighter or firmer pressure. Then let your intuition guide you. Do not massage over a joint or the spine. Avoid using fast, rhythmic movements on a woman who is pregnant or trying to conceive.

1 Start with slow, rhythmic, stroking movements, using the whole hand. Try applying light pressure with your fingertips, or use your thumbs or knuckles for deeper pressure. If you want to use oil, stroke it evenly over the area that you are massaging.

2 Gently grasp handfuls of flesh or muscle, particularly where you can feel that a muscle is hard or contracted. Use your thumbs and fingers to knead and roll the area, rather like dough. Keep checking that the touch feels good for your partner, and alternate with strokes.

3 Work specific areas by making a series of small circular movements with one or several fingers, the pads of the thumbs, or the heel of the hands. This helps to stimulate the circulation. Alternate with stroking movements, and remember to ask for feedback.

Aromatic massage

Adding a few drops of aromatherapy oil to your massage oil can heighten the pleasure and well-being that receiving a massage can bring. The main, immediate effect of aromatherapy is relaxation, which is very beneficial in conception and pregnancy – neroli or rosewood are excellent soothing oils. You can also use oils in a vaporizer, to create either an uplifting or soothing atmosphere in a room.

Aromatherapy oils can have a powerful effect and not all of them are suitable for women intending to conceive. See pages 230-231 for advice on using aromatherapy oils safely, and a list of oils to avoid in pregnancy.

When not to massage

There are some circumstances in which you should not have a massage. For example:

- If you have an infection.
- If you have a high temperature.
- If you have severe back pain, especially if the pain shoots down the arms or legs.
- If you have a skin infection.

Massage is one of the easiest ways to de-stress and release the tensions of the day. It's also a great way to pamper your partner and enjoy time together.

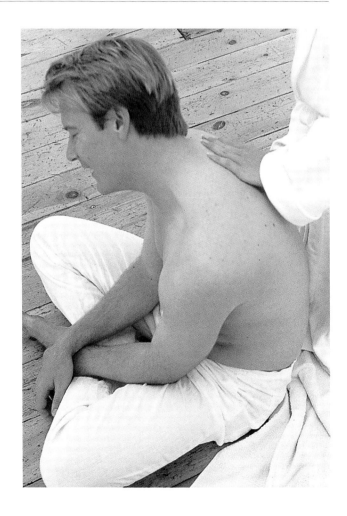

Avoiding hazards

We know that some environmental substances, in particular toxins and radiation, may hinder conception and endanger pregnancy. The research currently available is not clear-cut, and it is by no means the case that all women exposed to a potential hazard will necessarily develop a problem. However, it seems sensible to reduce your exposure to hazards wherever you can, as a safeguard for yourself and your child. If you are trying to conceive or are pregnant, here are some of the things you should avoid.

X-RAYS

Having an X-ray exposes you to a tiny dose of radiation. The dose given is too small to cause problems to you, but it can sometimes have an adverse effect on the developing fetus. Always tell your doctor and your dentist if you are trying to conceive or know that you are pregnant. Wherever possible have any medical or dental investigations carried out before you attempt to conceive to avoid exposing the fetus to any risk.

If you had an X-ray before realizing that you were pregnant, talk to your doctor about the potential effects. In most cases, there is unlikely to be a problem.

OTHER SOURCES OF RADIATION

Computers, VDUs and televisions are sometimes cited as a hazard because they give out small amounts of radiation. However, the general advice is that the radiation you are exposed to in this way is not in sufficient quantity or strength to have an effect on fertility or pregnancy.

The research concerning the effect of mobile phones on the brain and the nervous system is not yet clear, but it would be wise to reduce your use to a minimum. Avoid chatting for long periods and use a hands-free model whenever possible. Do not chat with the mobile held next to your head while in an enclosed area such as a car.

CATS AND KITTENS

The faeces of kittens and young cats may carry the parasite toxoplasmosis. If this is passed to a pregnant woman, it can harm a developing fetus and cause a variety of abnormalities. The faeces is infectious only when kittens or young cats first acquire toxoplasmosis – which is usually while hunting during the first year of life. They then develop antibodies to the infection and excrete the parasite, in which case they are no longer infectious. To protect yourself, avoid contact with kittens and young cats wherever possible. Always wear gloves if you have to

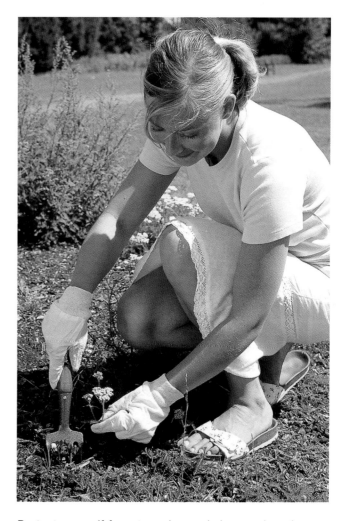

Protect yourself from toxoplasmosis by wearing gloves while gardening, and washing your hands afterwards. Check that your tetanus immunization is up to date.

TOXOPLASMOSIS

This is a form of infection that causes few symptoms – those affected may think they have a mild case of flu. So if you know that you been exposed to kitten faeces, see your doctor for an immunity test straight away. This can detect antibodies to toxoplasmosis in the blood, and will help to establish whether or not you are immune. Unfortunately, the test can sometimes provide borderline results.

If toxoplasmosis is caught during pregnancy, it can cause a miscarriage. It may also cause damage to the unborn baby, including to the brain. If you have already been infected and are immune, toxoplasmosis will not affect future pregnancies.

> **" Complete any renovations before you try for a baby. Chemicals in some decorating products are harmful. "**

empty a cat-litter tray, and disinfect it with boiling water for five minutes every day. There may also be toxoplasmosis in the soil so wear gloves for gardening. Wash your hands thoroughly after contact with soil.

APPLIANCES

It is worth getting appliances such as microwave ovens or gas heaters checked to make sure that they are working properly and are not leaking radiation or carbon monoxide into your home.

CHEMICAL PRODUCTS

Certain room deodorizers, furniture polish, oven cleaners, weedkillers and other products may contain poisonous substances. Always read labels carefully, and seek out household cleaning and garden products that are non-toxic and environment-friendly.

Take special care if you are exposed to chemicals at work – for example, if you are a hairdresser or a gardener. Talk to your doctor or midwife about whether or not any substances you come into contact with could be harmful to your pregnancy.

LIVESTOCK

Do not touch pregnant livestock if you are trying to conceive or may already be pregnant. They may carry bacteria that can cause miscarriage.

LONG-HAUL FLIGHTS

Sitting in one position for a long period – as you do when flying – increases your risk of deep vein thrombosis (DVT). In DVT a blood clot forms in the leg or pelvis. This clot can then become detached and travel to the lungs, a condition that can be life-threatening. It is now known that women are at greater risk of developing DVT when they are pregnant.

To help prevent DVT, get up from your seat every hour or so and move around. At regular intervals in between, flex your wrists and ankles and stretch your neck to left, to right and downwards in order to keep freshly oxygenated blood flowing around the body. Drink plenty of water before, during and after the flight – dehydration has been shown to increase the risk of DVT – and make sure that you do not drink any alcohol.

Home renovations are best done before you start trying for a baby. Choose products that are environment-friendly, to reduce your exposure to toxic substances.

IS YOUR HOME SAFE?

Take time before trying to conceive to make sure your home is a safe place to be. This is a good time to get done any jobs that could expose you to risk in pregnancy – for example, stripping old, lead-based paint from walls. Try to complete any renovations before you try for a baby – chemicals in some home-decorating products, such as paint thinners, strippers and glues are potentially harmful. Wherever possible, choose paints and other products that are child- and environment-friendly.

Many women find it difficult to bend down even early on in their pregnancies, so it is a good idea to complete any jobs that will require you to do so before conceiving. You should also fix any obvious hazards such as loose carpeting on the stairs.

Common Qs and As

Q: How will having a baby change our lives?

A: Almost every aspect of your lifestyle will change to a greater or lesser extent when you have a child to look after. You will have to consider the child as well as yourself in every decision that you make, whether short or long term. For example, whenever you go out of the house, you will have to take a bag with extra clothing, spare nappies and other equipment with you. You may need to wait until the baby has fed, slept or been changed. You will be unable to go to some places, such as the cinema and theatre, with the baby – for those you will need to hire a babysitter or arrange for a friend or relative to look after the baby for you. In general, spontaneous outings will be much more difficult to achieve.

Although you will have less disposable cash and less free time, you will probably find that you will enjoy spending money on the baby and relish the time that you have with him or her. Parenthood often brings with it a very profound change in attitudes and priorities. You may find that your feelings about your career change and that you want to prioritize family life over your work. It may be that you start to feel that you have less in common with certain friends and that you actively seek out other parents to spend time with, or become closer to your family. Whatever the changes in store, many parents say that the joy of having a baby and bringing up a child profoundly outweighs the sacrifices they make.

Q: Once I have a baby, will I ever have time for myself again?

A: You will, but it will take more organization than before, and you will need the help of others to make sure you get it. It is a good idea to persuade your partner or a member of your family or a close friend to look after the baby for a few hours each week to make sure that you get your valuable 'me' time.

Q: My partner is very keen to have a baby and believes that it is a part of any normal human relationship to have children together. I am not so sure... and I don't know what to do.

A: You could say that it is part of most human partnerships to have a baby, but not all. There is nothing abnormal in not having children of your own. If you have doubts about having a child, give yourself and your partner more time to think things over. You may come to realize that your doubts simply reflect a certain anxiety on your part about how you will adapt to parenthood. You may also realize that there are other things you want to do with your life before you have children. Over time, you may discover that you are prepared to welcome this new challenge.

Q: My sister-in-law tells me that having children is nothing but drudgery. She says that if she had known what it is like, she would have thought twice about having her children at all. What do you think?

A: It may be that you caught your sister-in-law at a bad time. Perhaps she was feeling tired after work and knew she was behind with all the washing and housework. It may be that she thought back to her single life, before children, and wished for the luxury of time to herself. If you talked to her again, you might discover that she is happy and proud of her children and would not be without them. On the other hand, it may be that she really does yearn for the apparent freedom and luxury of a child-free life. It is important to remember that whatever someone else feels is no indication of how you would feel in a similar situation.

Q: My mother and my mother-in-law keep telling us that it is best to have children as young as possible. We would like to wait for a few years. Is this safe?

A : The ideal time to conceive is in your twenties. However, many women are having babies in their early thirties without problems. It is only after the age of 35 that a woman's fertility decreases significantly. Should any problem present itself, it could take time to be resolved and, at over 35, time starts to be against you. That said, many women have healthy babies in their late thirties and even their forties.

You should remember that mothers and mothers-in-law are often eager for grandchildren, and this may colour their judgement as to what's best for their daughters and daughters-in-law. You must be your own judge; only when you and your partner feel the time is right should you go ahead.

Q: I am concerned that my partner is talking about giving up her job after she has our baby. I don't think this will be helpful for her sanity or for our finances. What can I say to her?

A : It may be that a compromise solution in which she works part-time is the best option for you both. You may find it helpful to sit down together and work out three different budgets: one based on her returning to work, one on her working part-time and the other on her staying at home.

Your partner will need to work out how much money she will need from you if she is to stay at home full-time. This will help her to appreciate the impact this has on your joint finances. Be sure to include everything in your budget, and allow for extras such as holidays. When you have completed the budget, add at least 10 per cent as a contingency figure.

Q: I have recently got married to a man who has been married before and has two children by his first wife. I do not have any children and would love to start a family. My husband is reluctant to have a baby on the grounds that it could upset his children. I feel that this goes against my nature and is unfair. How can I persuade him?

A : This is an extremely complex issue, made more tricky because it affects a number of people who are bound up together in a potentially sensitive situation. First, it must be said that if you really want to have a child but do not act on that desire, you could regret it for the rest of your life. So it is important that you make it absolutely clear to your husband how important having a child is to you.

Fathers who no longer live with their children, through divorce, often suffer considerable guilt and anxiety as a result. Once they become calm and settled within their new marriage, they are often much more likely to consider positively the idea of having another child. It will help if you tell him that you understand these issues and also that you are in no way trying to cancel out his former marriage by creating another family. Take positive steps to show him that there will always be time and space in your lives for his first two children.

Ask your husband if he would like to encourage some kind of open dialogue with his children, if they are old enough to appreciate the issues. You may also find it beneficial to have one or two counselling sessions, attended by both you and your husband.

Healthy eating

> " What you eat will affect the growth and development of every part of your baby. "

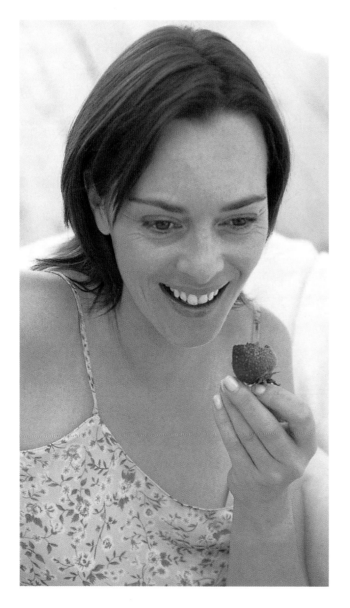

From the very first moment of conception, your baby will benefit from your healthy eating habits, as well as those of your partner. What you eat will affect the growth and development of every part of your baby: his or her bones, muscles, joints, teeth, senses and brain. Many people also believe that certain foods can even boost fertility.

Eating healthily and well is not nearly as complicated as some magazines and books lead us to believe. As you will see in the following chapter, good nutrition depends on a very simple formula indeed: eating a wide range of healthy foods and avoiding junk food.

Certain foods and toxins should be completely avoided before and during pregnancy and these are described in detail in the following pages. As far as supplements are concerned, there are very few – other than folic acid – that the woman who is pregnant or hoping to conceive needs to take.

If you get hungry between meals, try to snack on fruit rather than the many tempting – but usually unhealthy – alternatives that are all too readily available.

Food hygiene and how you prepare food is an important concept for pregnant women and is, in any case, something that all of us need to be fully aware of. Some food bugs may adversely affect the baby's healthy development and in some cases prove fatal to the unborn baby.

We have so much information available to us these days about the effects of food and how it is produced that all of us can take what we need for optimum health, growth and development and avoid harmful foods. Use this chapter as your guide to what and how much to eat and drink, what your weight should be, and how you can treat yourself to a cleansing detox day.

Top: A healthy diet is a well-balanced one, with a good proportion of fruit and vegetables. Make sure that you eat five portions of fruit and vegetables each day.

Drinking plenty of water cannot be over-emphasized. Even those of us who think we drink a great deal are probably not consuming enough.

Sensible eating

Healthy eating is a major cornerstone of preconceptual care. If you are trying for a baby, both partners should eat a healthy diet that provides a good supply of all the vital nutrients. This helps to boost your immune system, aids cell-repair and renewal, and keeps the reproductive organs in good working order.

Do not restrict your food intake in order to lose weight before conception or during pregnancy. Dieting can adversely affect fertility because you may not be taking in enough nutrients to keep the body functioning properly and producing the necessary hormones. If you do want to lose weight, it is generally better to increase your physical activity rather than restricting the amount that you eat. At the same time, do not overeat. Being overweight and eating a poor diet have both been shown to have an adverse effect on fertility.

You should also ensure that you keep to healthy eating habits, which you can then go on to share with your children. Make time for meals, do not rush your food, and

Make time to prepare and enjoy healthy meals made from fresh ingredients. Sitting at the dining table to eat will get you in the habit of taking good, regular meals.

stop eating when you have had enough. Make sure that you do not miss meals. Eat little and often – having four or five small meals a day is much easier on the digestion than eating a couple of larger ones.

EATING IN PREGNANCY

To a degree, your baby's health depends on what you eat and drink just before and during pregnancy. Because of this, mothers-to-be were traditionally advised to 'eat for two'. Experts no longer regard this as sensible advice, but that is not to say that the opposite is true. Some women eat too little during pregnancy to keep their weight down. Undereating can lead to problems such as more difficult labours and underweight babies and an insufficient supply of nutrients and energy to support the pregnancy.

In general, women who gain a reasonable amount of weight tend to have easier pregnancies and labours, and a lower risk of miscarriage and neonatal death (death around the time of delivery). Heavier babies are often healthier than those with a low birthweight, and are usually better able to resist common childhood illnesses. However, pregnant women who gain an excessive amount are at greater risk of developing diabetes, as are their babies.

Pregnancy can have a huge effect on your eating habits.

Remember to eat at least five helpings of fresh fruit and vegetables every day.

ARE YOU A HEALTHY WEIGHT?

Here we provide two ways for you to check whether you are a healthy weight. One quick method is by using the chart on the right. Simply find the point where your height and weight meet and then check the key below. The other method (using the body mass index) is explained below.

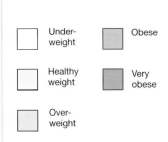

	Under-weight		Obese
	Healthy weight		Very obese
	Over-weight		

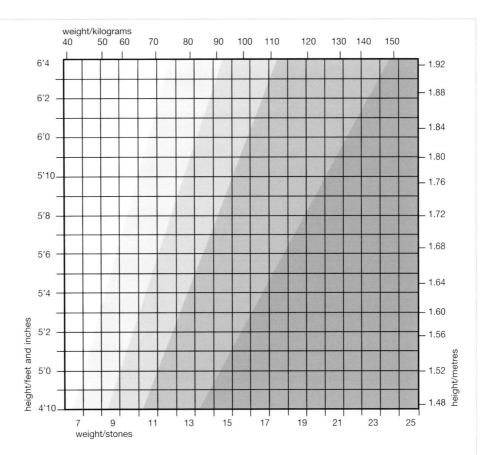

Body Mass Index (BMI)

Healthcare professionals often use a calculation called the body mass index to work out whether a person is a healthy weight for his or her height. You can do this just as easily for yourself.

BMI = your weight in kilograms divided by (your height in metres) squared. (To convert weight from pounds to kilograms multiply by 0.4536; to convert height from feet to metres multiply by 0.3048.)

For example, Sue weighs 65 kg and is 1.64 metres tall, so her BMI is: $65 \div (1.64)^2 = 24.17$

A BMI of over 40 will adversely affect your fertility and is also a serious health risk. The ideal is a BMI of 20-25. Over 30 and you need to lose weight. If your BMI is under 20, concentrate on gaining weight through eating protein and carbohydrate, and having a full cooked breakfast and a generous lunch and dinner.

Some women go off foods they once loved, while others keep eating the same dish or develop highly eccentric tastes. All of this is normal, so long as you have a balanced diet, and eat enough to maintain your energy levels.

WHY WOMEN GAIN WEIGHT IN PREGNANCY

Women lay down fat early in pregnancy as preparation for milk production and breastfeeding. This fat remains after the baby is born, but should gradually disappear, providing that you are following a healthy diet and exercising regularly. Other weight gain comes from the placenta, the fluids surrounding the baby and the baby itself, which accounts for more than half of the total weight gain. During pregnancy, women produce more blood, and this also increases their overall weight. The extra blood is needed to support a healthy pregnancy.

Everyone is different and so there are no strict rules about how much weight pregnant women should put on. Most women tend to gain around 9-13.5kg (20-30lb)

during pregnancy. However, someone who is already overweight may not need to put on as much weight during her pregnancy as a woman who is underweight. That said, the overweight woman should not try to diet once she knows that she is pregnant. Your weight will be monitored through your pregnancy as part of your antenatal checks and advice will be given on whether your weight gain is healthy.

RATE OF WEIGHT GAIN

The following is a rough guide to the rate of weight gain through a normal pregnancy:

0–12 weeks	10 per cent
13–20 weeks	25 per cent
21–28 weeks	45 per cent
29–36 weeks	20 per cent
37–40 weeks	0 per cent

A balanced diet

Eating healthily is a vital part of preconceptual care for men and women, helps women cope better with the demands of pregnancy, and gives a growing baby a healthier diet, too. General guidelines for healthy eating are:

- Eat a balanced diet, including food from each of the main food groups every day.
- Eat five helpings of fruit and vegetables every day.
- Minimize your intake of animal fats and sugars.
- Drink at least eight glasses of water every day.
- Have regular meals.
- Choose natural unprocessed foods wherever possible.
- The only supplement that all women need to take is folic acid.

GROUP 1: BREADS AND OTHER CEREALS

These foods are excellent sources of carbohydrate, which gives us energy, and fibre, which helps to keep the digestive tract healthy. They also provide us with B vitamins, some calcium and iron. Eat whole grains wherever possible – for example, wholewheat breakfast cereals without added sugar, wholemeal bread and wholewheat pasta. Choose brown or wild rice, which have undergone less processing than white varieties.

GROUP 2: FRUIT AND VEGETABLES

Eat five helpings of fruit and vegetables each day. A helping can be a glass of juice, a piece of fruit such as an apple or banana, a small salad or a portion of vegetables. Fruits and vegetables contain a wide range of vitamins and minerals, have almost no fat and are a good source of fibre. Eat them raw or lightly cooked to gain their full nutrient value.

GROUP 3: MEAT, FISH AND ALTERNATIVES

Beef, lamb, pork and bacon are good sources of protein, which the body needs for vital functions such as cell-repair. They also provide minerals such as iron and zinc, and B

vitamins. Opt for lean cuts and trim off visible fat. Grill, roast or microwave meat, so that some of the fat drains off. Add more vegetables than meat to stews and casseroles to gives you a healthier dietary balance.

Fish and poultry also provide protein. Oily fish such as mackerel, salmon and sardines are rich in nutritious fish oils, so try to eat two portions a week. However, avoid eating more than one fresh tuna steak or two medium-sized cans of tuna a week, due to the mercury content (excess mercury can harm a fetus' nervous system). Grill, steam, microwave or bake fish rather than deep frying it.

Nuts, peas, lentils, soya and pulses also contain protein but, unlike meat or fish, they do not contain all the essential amino acids needed for growth. To maximize their nutritional value, serve them with plant foods and whole grains such as wholemeal bread. Some people class pulses as a distinct food group, but nutritionally speaking, they cannot be considered as good for you as meat or fish.

GROUP 4: MILK AND OTHER DAIRY PRODUCTS

Dairy produce such as eggs, cheese, milk and milk products provide calcium, which builds teeth and bones, and some protein. Pregnant women need lots of calcium to build their baby's skeleton. Low-fat dairy products are generally better for you. If you worry about weight gain, reduce your butter intake and avoid cream. Natural yogurt is a healthy option. Women who wish to conceive or who are pregnant should avoid raw or lightly cooked eggs and soft cheeses such Brie and Camembert, because of the risk of food poisoning.

GROUP 5: FAT AND SUGAR

We need some fat in our diet. There are two main types of fat: saturated, which is solid at room temperature, and unsaturated, most of which remain liquid. Saturated fats, such as butter and lard, can increase blood cholesterol and

Try this test to check how healthy a brown loaf is: take the bread between your hands and squeeze gently. If it gives easily, it probably doesn't provide much fibre. As a general rule, the denser the bread, the more fibre it contains – so the healthier it is for you.

ORGANIC FOOD

Many people believe that organic produce tastes better and is more nutritious for you than conventionally grown food. Buying organic means that you are reducing your exposure to chemicals in the foods that you eat: organic fruit and vegetables are produced without the use of chemical fertilizers and pesticides, while animals used for organic meat are not given routine antibiotics or growth hormones.

THE MAIN FOOD GROUPS

This shows the proportions of the five main food groups that parents-to-be should aim to eat.

1 BREADS AND CEREALS
33 per cent

2 FRUIT AND VEGETABLES
33 per cent

3 PROTEIN FOODS
12 per cent

4 DAIRY FOODS
15 per cent

5 FATS AND SUGAR
7 per cent

with it the risk of heart disease. The two forms of unsaturated fat – monounsaturated and polyunsaturated – are better for you and may decrease cholesterol levels. Monounsaturated fats include olive oil and avocado, while polyunsaturated fats include most vegetable oils, fish oil and nuts. As a general rule, pick low-fat dairy products and use olive oil in place of butter.

Sugary foods provide a short-term energy boost, but little nutritional value. Eat sparingly, if at all.

WHY WE NEED FIBRE

Fibre is an indigestible substance that we get from nuts, cereals, fruit and vegetables. It is not broken down or digested in the body, but is vital for speeding up the passage of waste products through the bowel and removing toxins. Constipation is common during pregnancy, when bowel movements slow down, but plenty of fibre-rich food and water will help to prevent this.

DRINK WATER

Make sure that you are drinking enough water to maintain and repair all the body's systems, including the reproductive system. To avoid dehydration, which can lead to irritability, headache, tension, swollen ankles and a bloated stomach, you need to drink at least eight glasses of water every day – more if you are also drinking tea and coffee. This may seem like a lot, but after a few days your body will become accustomed to it.

Can foods boost fertility?

Whether or not certain foods can boost fertility is a matter of great debate. Some natural health practitioners strongly believe that they can. However, many doctors and other health experts profoundly disagree. Leading fertility specialists maintain that no food in the world can actually make you more likely to conceive.

To a certain extent, this is a matter of interpretation. If your diet lacks certain important nutrients, this could lead to fertility problems. A deficiency of zinc, for example, has been linked to low sperm counts. In such cases, eating zinc-rich food – such as eggs and whole grains – may help to improve the man's fertility. In general, however, most health professionals agree that following a healthy balanced diet, drawing on all the main food groups every day, is the best route to optimum fertility for both partners. Remember, too, that this must be combined with regular, sustained exercise.

Foods that are rich in zinc, which is important for male fertility, include sardines, turkey, eggs, brown rice and cheeses such as Parmesan and Cheddar.

FERTILITY FOODS FOR MEN

Prospective fathers should eat a healthy, nutritionally balanced diet that includes foods rich in vitamins A, B, C and E, and essential fatty acids (which are found in oily fish and polyunsaturated fat). Men also need to eat foods that contain the minerals zinc and selenium.

Zinc and vitamin C play particularly important roles in the question of male fertility. Zinc is needed for the production of sperm and the male hormones: several prominent research studies have found that the male sex glands and sperm contain high concentrations of zinc.

HERBAL TEAS FOR FERTILITY
Herbalists recommend the following teas, singly or in combination, three times daily:
- cinnamon
- cramp bark
- ginger
- ginseng
- lemon balm
- lady's mantle
- motherwort
- vervain
- winter cherry

Men can play their part by sticking to five portions of fruit and vegetables a day. A glass of orange juice counts as one portion.

> 66 Drawing on all the main food groups every day is the best route to optimum fertility. 99

To enhance your preconceptual health, make sure you drink enough – but of the right kinds of drinks such as fruit juices, smoothies, herbal teas and lots of water.

Vitamin C is thought to reduce the tendency of sperm to clump together in the woman's body – a common cause of infertility. Modern diets are often low in zinc, and stress, smoking, pollution and alcohol deplete the body's levels further. Zinc-rich foods include oysters and shrimps, as well as other shellfish, sardines, turkey, duck and lean meats. Parmesan and Cheddar cheese are good sources of zinc, as are eggs, wholegrains, brown rice and nuts.

Citrus fruits, strawberries, kiwi fruit and peppers are excellent sources of vitamin C and should be included as part of your five servings of fruit and vegetables a day. Citrus fruits also provide selenium, another nutrient that is needed for fertility. One of the best sources of vitamin A is liver (not to be eaten by pregnant women or those trying to conceive), also found in egg yolks, dairy products, carrots, red peppers and leafy vegetables. You can get B vitamins from meat, green vegetables and wholegrains. Vitamin E is found in nuts and most vegetable oils.

FERTILITY FOODS FOR WOMEN

Any woman who is wanting to conceive should ensure that they follow a balanced, healthy diet. This diet should include foods rich in fatty acids, vitamin C, zinc, iron and folic acid – all easy to obtain from everyday foods. Iron-rich foods include meat, fish, eggs, dark green leafy

The best way to up your intake of vitamin C is to eat as much fruit as possible. Take melon, for example, for breakfast with muesli or as an after-dinner dessert.

vegetables and dried fruit. Good supplies of folic acid are found in green leafy vegetables, and also in nuts and pulses (see also pages 40-41).

If you have been taking the contraceptive pill, it may be helpful to increase your intake of foods containing the mineral manganese (good sources include oats, rye bread and peas) and also vitamin B6 (green vegetables and wholegrain cereals). These foods help to break down oestrogen, an excess of which may be associated with infertility. Eating zinc-rich foods might also be helpful (although shellfish should be avoided).

KEEP IT FRESH AND RAW

Another vital aspect of healthy eating is choosing fresh, unprocessed foods. There is still much research to be done on the effects of an over-refined, chemical-laden diet on fertility and pregnancy, but fresh produce, with fruits and vegetables raw or lightly cooked, is as beneficial to the prospective parent as it is to all of us.

Do I need supplements?

You need more of certain nutrients before conception and during pregnancy. For example, your iron requirement almost doubles while your baby is growing. Many experts believe that pregnant women and those trying for a baby can obtain all the minerals and vitamins they need from a healthy, balanced diet.

The only exception that applies to all women is folic acid. This is needed before conception and during early pregnancy in an amount that is difficult to derive from our food. You should not need to take other supplements, as long as you eat regular, healthy meals.

Some women may be advised to start taking supplements such as iron or calcium as the pregnancy progresses. However, this is only if they cannot obtain sufficient supplies from their diet; supplements are not needed as a matter of course.

FOLIC ACID

An essential B vitamin, folic acid (folate) cannot be produced by the body, so it must be obtained through diet or supplements. Women hoping to conceive and in the early stages of pregnancy need 400 micrograms (mcg) of folic acid every day, to help the baby's spine and brain to develop properly. To ensure that you are getting enough, take a 400mcg supplement before conception and for the first 12 weeks of pregnancy. You should also eat plenty of folate-rich foods such as Brussels sprouts, wholemeal bread and orange juice.

What folic acid does

Folic acid protects the neural tube – which will go on to form the spine and spinal cord – and helps it to close properly. This helps ensure normal brain and spinal cord development. Folic acid can help protect an unborn baby

FOLIC ACID AND THE NEURAL TUBE

Women hoping to conceive need 400mcg of folic acid a day, to ensure the healthy development of the baby's spine and spinal cord.

cross section of
neural tube at 4 weeks

from developing spina bifida (an abnormal development of the spinal cord) and anencephaly (absence of most of the brain). Infants born with anencephaly die shortly after birth, and babies with spina bifida are born with partial or total paralysis.

The neural tube should close between the 25th and 30th day after conception, when women may not realize they are pregnant. This is why all sexually active women of childbearing age should take folic acid each day.

MINERALS AND PREGNANCY

It is important that you obtain a sufficient amount of all vitamins and minerals before and during pregnancy. However, some minerals have particularly important roles to play in the health of both mother and baby, so you should pay particular attention to ensuring that you are getting enough. Eating foods that are rich sources of these minerals is the most natural way of upping your intake, but some women may need to take supplements.

Calcium

You should make sure that you are getting enough calcium before you conceive because once you are pregnant the baby will deplete the reserves of calcium in your bones and teeth. Calcium is essential for the healthy development of your baby's teeth and bones, which begin to form from around weeks four to six.

Your body absorbs calcium more efficiently during pregnancy, and your baby is unlikely to go short. The baby will take what calcium it needs, but this may not leave you enough for your own requirements.

FOODS HIGH IN FOLIC ACID

• spinach and other leafy vegetables	• asparagus	• strawberries
	• Brussels sprouts	• bananas
	• orange juice	• grapefruit
• broccoli	• tomato juice	• wholemeal bread
• green peas	• oranges	

Folate levels decrease over time and with cooking, so do not store fruit or vegetables for long periods before eating. Cook vegetables lightly by steaming, microwaving or stir-frying.

CALCIUM-RICH FOODS

• milk	• sesame seeds	• bread
• yogurt	• pulses	• canned fish
• cheese	• leafy green	with bones
• nuts	vegetables	(eg pilchards)

Make sure that you eat and drink plenty of calcium-rich foods before conceiving and throughout your pregnancy. You will need the equivalent of 600ml (1 pint) milk a day. A small pot of yogurt or 25g (1oz) hard cheese contain as much calcium as about 200ml (⅓ pint) milk.

Vegans and women who never drink milk, either because they are allergic to it or because they simply don't like it, may need calcium supplements. If you are eating well, 600 milligrams (mg) should be enough, but 1200mg may be advised in some cases.

Vitamin D helps the body to absorb vitamin C properly. This vitamin is found in milk, butter and eggs. More importantly, however, the body can manufacture its own vitamin D if it is exposed to the sun. You should therefore take a short walk outdoors each day to expose your face, hands and arms to daylight.

Iron

During pregnancy, your body manufactures extra blood, and your requirement for iron increases at the same time. You will probably need almost twice as much iron as you did before you became pregnant.

Iron is needed for the formation of haemoglobin, the oxygen-carrying pigment in red blood cells. If you don't have enough haemoglobin in your blood, insufficient oxygen may be transported to your organs and your baby. This will also result in your becoming very tired.

Make sure that you are eating plenty of iron-rich foods before conception, particularly red meat and dark poultry meat. Vitamin C helps the body to absorb iron from other, plant-based sources more efficiently, so it is a good idea to have a glass of orange juice or a tomato salad with meals. Another simple way of increasing iron intake is to use iron pans when cooking.

Pregnant women used to be given iron tablets as a matter of course. This should not be necessary so long as you eat a good diet with sufficient iron-rich foods (although

Take a short walk every day so that you receive exposure to sunlight. This enables the body to manufacture vitamin D, which in turn aids the absorption of vitamin C.

Supplements such as iron come in a number of different forms. Chelated supplements are said to be more rapidly absorbed by the body.

it may be necessary if you are expecting two or more babies). If you are worried about iron intake, or feel tired for no apparent reason, see a doctor. A simple blood test will determine if you are deficient (anaemic). It can be hard to get enough iron if you do not eat red meat, so vegetarians and vegans are often advised to take iron supplements.

Zinc

You need zinc to help the baby develop – there is evidence to suggest that an inadequate intake is linked to low birthweight. Make sure you are eating enough zinc-rich foods before conceiving; the body's levels of zinc can fall by as much as 30 per cent during pregnancy.

IRON-RICH FOODS

• red meat; dark	• nuts	• prunes
poultry meat	• dark green	• dark
• wholegrains	and leafy	molasses
• egg yolks	vegetables	• brewer's
• pulses	• dried fruit	yeast

ZINC-RICH FOODS

• oily fish	• molasses	• peas
• onions	• pumpkin	• beans
• oysters	seeds	• wheatgerm
• meat	• walnuts and	• brewer's
• eggs	other nuts	yeast

Foods to avoid and food safety

During pregnancy and the months before you conceive (both men and women), avoid taking in toxic substances if possible. You cannot combat environmental health hazards such as emissions from industrial sites, but you can make sure that you do not spend time in smoky atmospheres and that you avoid foods that may be harmful, are highly processed or lack nutritional value.

WHAT TO AVOID

The following substances may cause harm to you or your baby and should ideally be avoided completely.

- **Soft, blue-veined and unpasteurized cheese** such as Brie and goat's cheese, due to the risk of listeriosis.
- **Raw or lightly cooked eggs and poultry**, as hens may be infected by salmonella and other bacteria. Eggs and chicken must always be well cooked to prevent infection.
- **Raw beef** including steak tartare, rare beef and undercooked beefburgers, regardless of where the meat comes from, because of the risk of BSE.
- **Certain fish**, because they contain mercury, which can harm the developing nervous system in an unborn child. Avoid shark, swordfish and marlin and eat no more than one tuna steak or two medium cans of tuna each week.
- **Shellfish and raw fish**, which carry a higher-than-average risk of food poisoning.
- **Liver**, liver pâté and liver sausage. They are high in vitamin A, which can cause damage to the fetus.

OESTROGEN AND FERTILITY PROBLEMS

The female hormone oestrogen, used in some contraceptive pills, plays a vital role in reproduction. Research suggests that some women who take an oestrogen-containing pill for several years may suffer reduced fertility for a few weeks or months when they stop. Oestrogens are also found in non-organic dairy produce and meat, fish from polluted waters, pesticides, plastic containers and clearfilm.

Increased exposure to synthetic oestrogens may be one reason for the rise in fertility problems. In men, too much oestrogen can lower sperm count, while an excess in women is thought to be associated with conditions such as endometriosis and ovarian cysts, both of which adversely affect fertility.

- **Unpasteurized milk**, which may harbour highly harmful bacteria, including salmonella and listeria (see also section on preventing food poisoning).

Minimize your intake of the following foods and drinks:

- **Alcohol**, which may impede the uptake of B-vitamins, zinc and iron, lower hormone levels, inhibit ovulation and the ability of sperm to move, and harm a fetus.
- **Tea and coffee**, whose caffeine content may harm female fertility. A lot of tea can impede iron uptake.
- **Sugary foods** such as cookies, cakes and other sweet snacks and drinks, which contain few nutrients.

BANISHING CAFFEINE

If you want to conceive, it is a good idea to cut out or cut down on caffeine, tea and chocolate. Researchers have found that they can have an adverse effect on female fertility.

One study found that taking in more than 300mg of caffeine a day lowered a woman's chance of conceiving by as much as 27 per cent. Even modest consumption appears to hinder conception: women who drink only one to two cups daily lowered their chances of conceiving by about 10 per cent.

Another study found that an intake of more than 300mg of caffeine a day may be associated with miscarriage. In addition, pregnant women who drank eight or more

cups of coffee a day were found to have double the risk of stillbirth as women who did not drink coffee.

It is helpful if you have some way of measuring 300mg of caffeine. This 300mg limit is roughly equivalent to the following items:

- Four cups or three mugs of instant coffee.
- Three cups of brewed coffee.
- Six cups of tea.
- Eight cans of regular cola drinks.
- Four cans of energy drinks.
- Two 200g (7oz) bars of chocolate.

There are all kinds of non-caffeine hot drinks available today that form good alternatives to tea and coffee, from herbal tea to barley-based drinks.

- **Fried foods and junk food**, which are high in unhealthy fats and should be avoided where possible.
- **Salt**, from adding salt to food or eating salty snacks such as crisps (US potato chips). Excess salt increases the risk of high blood pressure, which can be harmful.
- **Convenience foods and takeaway meals**, as these have poor nutrient value. Eat fresh, natural foods.

PREVENTING FOOD POISONING

Poor food hygiene is responsible for thousands of cases of food poisoning every year. Most people suffer a bout of diarrhoea or sickness and have no long-term effects. However, pregnant women need to take great care to avoid food poisoning, since there is a real threat to the unborn baby. Infants and children are also at risk.

Food poisoning is usually the result of eating food that has been contaminated by bacteria. These precautions will help prevent bacteria from spreading and multiplying:
- Wash your hands with hot water and an antibacterial soap before and after handling food, especially poultry, raw meat, fish, seafood, salads, vegetables and eggs.
- Wash your hands with hot water and antibacterial soap after handling cats, dogs and other domestic pets.
- Disinfect kitchen surfaces with an antibacterial solution, to kill potentially harmful bacteria.
- Use plastic, not wooden, chopping boards, and disinfect them after each use. Use separate boards for cooked and raw foods.
- Fridges should be kept at under 5°C (41°F). Use a fridge thermometer to be sure the temperature is right.
- Store raw foods separately from ready-to-eat and cooked foods (place raw meat and fish on the bottom shelf of the fridge). Always abide by use-by dates.
- Regularly clean taps, telephones and any gadgets in the kitchen, using an antibacterial solution.

Avoiding listeriosis

Listeriosis is caused by the bacterium *Listeria monocytogenes*. If caught during pregnancy, it can result in miscarriage, stillbirth or severe illness in the baby.

High levels of listeria have been found in some foods, so it is advisable to avoid these. They include:
- Unpasteurized milk.
- Pâté made from meat, fish or vegetables.
- Mould-ripened and blue-veined cheeses.
- Soft-whip ice cream from ice-cream machines.
- Pre-cooked poultry and cook-chill meals unless thoroughly reheated.
- Prepared salads, unless washed thoroughly.

Avoiding Campylobacter pylori

The bacterium *Campylobacter pylori* is the chief cause of food poisoning in both the UK and the USA – it accounts for more than 2.5 million cases of food poisoning in the USA every year. The bacterium is found in raw meat, poultry, wild birds and unpasteurized milk. This is one reason why pregnant women need to avoid raw and lightly cooked eggs and undercooked chicken.

Avoiding salmonella

Salmonella is a bacterium commonly found in hens. Be sure to cook poultry and eggs thoroughly when you are trying for a baby and during pregnancy. Do not eat foods containing raw egg, such as fresh mayonnaise.

Avoiding toxoplasmosis

Toxoplasmosis is an infection caused by a parasite that can cause miscarriage or damage to the unborn baby. It may be present in soil, so fresh fruit, vegetables and lettuce are all potential sources of infection. They should be thoroughly washed under running water.

Be sure to wash your hands with antibacterial soap both before and after handling foods.

Always disinfect kitchen surfaces and chopping boards after preparing food on them.

Use an antibacterial solution to wipe over taps, telephones and kitchen surfaces regularly.

A healthy day

You want to be as healthy and fit as possible before conceiving a baby. This cleansing programme offers a gentle way to eliminate toxins from the body without putting it under any stress. Undertaking a preconceptual detox with your partner can also be a pleasurable way to relax and spend some time together.

Some people associate detoxing with total fasting. However, it is very important that you do not take any extreme measures before conception and during pregnancy. Fasting is not good for the body, and should be avoided, in particular, by anyone wishing to conceive.

This programme emphasizes exercise, rest and relaxation together with healthy eating. Feel free to adapt it according to your individual needs. No special equipment is used, but you will need a soft-bristled brush for the skin, and essential oils of your choice.

A day of detoxing

Set aside a whole day – or even a weekend – for your detox. Choose a time when you know that you won't be interrupted, so you can focus totally on yourselves.

1 As soon as you wake up, drink a glass of hot water with a slice of lemon in it. Lemon possesses cleansing properties so will aid the detox process. (Drinking hot water with lemon when you wake up is a good habit to acquire.) Then eat a piece of fruit or a slice of wholemeal bread – don't add any butter or spread. This will get your digestive system moving.

2 Do some gentle stretching, yoga or warm-up exercises. Then, do 30 minutes of brisk exercise. This could take the form of running, fast walking or any other exercise that makes you slightly breathless (you should still be able to keep up a conversation). Brisk exercise speeds up your circulatory system, bringing oxygen and nutrients to all areas of the body and helping to eliminate toxins. Afterwards, drink a large of glass of water, and some juiced or liquidized fruit or vegetables.

3 Next, dry-brush your whole body in order to remove dead skin cells – either brush your own body or do this for your partner. Brush upwards, using long strokes on the arms and legs. Spend at least five minutes doing this, then take a warm shower. Use a body scrub to help slough off more dead skin cells in the water.

4 After the shower, deep-cleanse your face. Pour some boiling water in a large bowl, add a few drops of essential oil (chamomile, lavender or lemongrass are good oils to choose), then place a towel over your head. Let the steam soak into your skin for a few moments, then remove the towel and pat your face dry. Splash your face with cold water a few times to tighten up the pores again.

5 You and your partner may like to give one another a massage at this point. Massage helps to boost the circulation, which speeds up the elimination process. Enjoy a full body massage, or concentrate on the legs and feet, where toxins tend to collect. A foot massage is easy to do if you are on your own and improving the circulation here will have a knock-on effect for the whole system.

The most important aspect of detoxing is to drink water – and lots of it. Heighten the effect by adding a slice of lemon to each glass.

Wholemeal bread without butter is a wake-up call for the body's digestive system. Drink at least one glass of water, with lemon, beforehand.

Exercise and fresh air are not only an essential part of detoxification, but are important elements of a healthy and enjoyable lifestyle.

Use a soft-bristled brush to energize your skin and remove dead cells. You and your partner can do this for each other if you like.

Give yourself a mini face treatment. Add a drop or two of essential oil to a bowl of boiling water, then allow the steam to cleanse your skin.

6 Spend some time relaxing after your massage; give yourself 30 minutes or an hour of total rest. Then do some gentle yoga or stretching to re-energize yourself. Stretching helps to mobilize the joints; it also increases the flow of blood, and brings nutrients and oxygen to different areas of the body.

7 Have a small lunch of fruit, vegetables and cereals. Stay sitting upright for at least 15 minutes after eating, to help your digestion. Then, go out for a short walk.

8 Do some meditation at this point, or simply sit quietly and focus on your breathing. Breathing deeply helps to get more oxygen to the muscles and organs. Wait two hours after eating, then do another session of exercise.

9 Have a salt rub. Waste products are excreted through the skin and massage, exfoliation and salt rubs all help keep the pores clean and healthy. You can use any type of salt mixed with a little olive oil. Rub into the skin with a circular motion, moving away from the heart. This aids the circulation and elimination systems.

10 Have a long aromatic bath, with your partner or by yourself. Dilute a couple of drops of aromatherapy oil in a carrier and add to the water. Afterwards, moisturize your skin. Combine this with another massage if you like.

11 Spend the rest of the evening quietly, perhaps incorporating some more yoga or stretching. Go to bed early to be sure that you get plenty of rest.

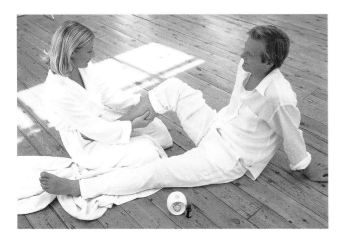

Take it in turns to give each other a relaxing massage. Try a leg and foot treatment, then a back massage.

ESSENTIAL ELEMENTS OF A HEALTHY DAY
Throughout the day:
- Drink only water. You should have at least 2 litres (3½ pints) and preferably more. Have a large bottle for each of you on hand so that you can keep topping up. This will also help you to monitor how much you have drunk.
- Eat lightly every two or three hours. Choose fibre-rich foods: fresh fruits, raw or lightly steamed vegetables, and whole-grain cereals.
- Remember that this is your time to relax – do not read, watch television or answer the telephone, and try not talk about anything contentious.

Common Qs and As

Q: I have found all sorts of weird foods and food remedies for boosting fertility on the Internet. Do they work?

A: Most fertility specialists and gynaecologists would recommend that you eat a wide variety of healthy foods every day with plenty of vegetables and plenty of water. There is no need to single out any one particular food. Refer to pages 32-35 to ensure that you are not missing out on any nutrients.

Q: I have heard that detoxing is a necessary part of preconceptual care. Why?

A: Many people feel healthier, more active and invigorated after a detoxing for a short period, say a weekend. One of the great strengths of detoxing is the focus upon drinking plenty of water and exercising, both of which are very good for us. However, a healthy lifestyle that you can maintain every day is likely to be much more helpful than the occasional short detox.

Q: I was anorexic when I was younger. Could this make a difference to my chances of conceiving now?

A: Provided that your periods have returned to a normal pattern, your previous anorexia shouldn't affect your chances of conceiving. However, in view of your medical history, you may be wise to consider a combined multivitamin and multimineral supplement. Check this with your family doctor, and make sure that any supplement you do take is suitable for pregnant women.

If your periods have not returned to normal, you should consult your family doctor without delay. If necessary, ask your doctor for a referral to a consultant gynaecologist.

Q: I have a very fast-paced job and tend to eat on the wing. Could this adversely affect my chances of conceiving?

A: Eating in this way may not affect your chances of getting pregnant, but it will certainly not help either. Eating snacks hurriedly is not a good or healthy dietary habit, and it makes it hard for you to ensure that you are getting all the nutrients you need. If you have any other underlying medical problem, poor nutrition will tend to exacerbate the problem.

You may like to consider starting to pace yourself now for life with a baby, by eating regularly and well. Snacking as you go will become increasingly difficult and impractical once you have a child to consider.

Remember, too, that stress can affect your fertility and your ability to cope with pregnancy, so you might want to consider slowing down your lifestyle as part of your preconceptual care.

Q: I don't usually want to eat much in the morning, as early-morning eating makes me feel a bit queasy. Now I am trying for a second baby, I want to make sure that I get into eating habits that give me enough nutrients. How can I try to achieve this?

A: First and foremost, ask yourself if there are any foods that seldom make you feel queasy in the morning. You do not have to eat standard 'breakfast' fare. If you find the only thing you can eat is chicken tandoori, so be it. Secondly, make sure you have plenty of fluids, especially water, and try drinking juices or smoothies, for their extra nutritional value. Thirdly, make sure that your other meals include plenty of protein foods such as meat and fish, as well as wholegrain bread and pasta, and fruits and vegetables. These foods will help to keep you going.

Q: I have noticed that most of my friends manage to control their weight gain quite well with their first baby. Once it comes to the second baby, though, some of them have blown up by three stone (nearly 20kg) or more. How can I stop this happening to me?

A: The best thing you can do is to exercise regularly for the duration of the pregnancy and afterwards as well – swimming two or three times a week is ideal. Mothers who are at home with the first baby may find it difficult to take time out to exercise. If this is the case with you, try walking for a good 30 minutes a day with your first baby in a pushchair. Avoid high-calorie foods such as chocolate, biscuits, pastries, cakes, sugary foods, salty foods, fried foods, crisps, peanuts and alcohol.

Q: I shall be going abroad soon for a long vacation. I am worried about what we eat and how it is prepared since we are trying for a baby. Are there any precautions I should take?

A: You should always take care with what you eat and follow good hygiene practices when travelling in a developing country. In particular:
- Do not eat snacks from street stalls.
- Do not eat any salads or peeled fruit or fruit salad.
- Do not eat shellfish, pâté, raw steak, undercooked poultry, raw or lightly cooked eggs, or soft blue-veined cheeses.
- Do not drink local water or have any ice in your drinks. All water should be bought bottled or thoroughly boiled before use.
- Clean your teeth with bottled water.

Check to see if there are any inoculations you need for your country of destination – and how far in advance you need to have them. Ask your doctor how these could impinge upon pregnancy first.

Q: There seems to be a new health scare almost every week about some food or other that pregnant women must not eat. I am becoming increasingly worried about my diet. How can I be sure that what I eat is safe?

A: This is a good question, but nobody can give you a cast-iron assurance that your diet is absolutely safe. The reason for this is that medical research, scientific research and research into nutrition is going on all the time. Scientists do make new discoveries, which they then publish. Newspapers can then seize upon this information and make the most of it – sometimes inflating it into scare stories. This can have the effect of making us think that none of the food we eat is really safe.

It is impossible to live without exposing yourself to any risk at all. The best you can do is to be pragmatic and to take precautions where you can. It has been well-established, for example, that some foods are unsafe or carry a higher risk in pregnancy, so it is sensible to avoid them. These include raw eggs, liver, soft cheeses and some fish and meat. We also know that a diet including whole cereals, fresh fruit and vegetables, most fish, well-cooked chicken and other foods will give you a good range of nutrients, which helps your baby to develop. Making sure that you are following a balanced, healthy diet is therefore very important.

You should also take care to observe the rules of food hygiene. It can be a good idea to avoid eating out or getting takeaways unless you can be sure that good standards of hygiene are practised in the restaurant. Other than that, the best thing to do if you read any stories in the media that worry you is to have a talk with your midwife or doctor. They will help you to decide what, if any, changes to your diet you need to make.

Top fertility factors

66 There is seldom any need to worry if pregnancy doesn't happen right away. *99*

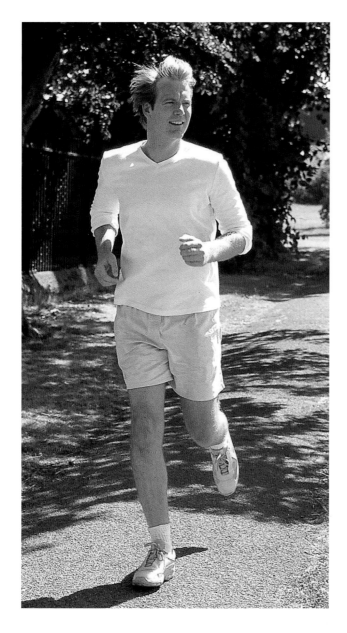

Some women become pregnant while barely thinking about it – it just happens. Others plan the pregnancy and find that they are pregnant within a few months. The remaining few may take well over a year to conceive and some of those may encounter a delay that is even longer than that.

There is seldom any need to worry if pregnancy does not happen straight away – this is very common, and many couples take the best part of a year to conceive. In fact, infertility is officially defined as over a year of regular, unprotected sexual intercourse without conception.

There are many ways in which you can boost your fertility level, as you will see throughout this chapter. De-stressing through complementary therapies is especially beneficial, both before conception and during pregnancy. In addition, you can prepare to eliminate the common causes of infertility before you even attempt to become pregnant. For example,

Keeping in good physical shape – and this includes your partner as well as yourself – is a key aspect of preparing the body properly for conception.

giving up smoking and cutting alcohol down to a very small intake are vital steps towards a healthy conception and pregnancy.

Your weight is another important consideration: extreme thinness and obesity adversely affect fertility levels in both women and men. As with everyone, attention to diet is the key issue here, combined with regular exercise.

There are also much rarer causes of infertility, such as inherited diseases. In these cases, specialist genetic counselling may provide the way forward, and is readily available.

Top: Listening to soothing music is a really easy way to relax and unwind – it is thought that stress is a common cause of decreased fertility.

Simply using candles to create soft light and a calm atmosphere is another way to alleviate the build-up of stress that can creep up on all of us.

Getting pregnant

The best way of achieving a healthy pregnancy is to have sex as frequently as possible during the woman's fertile period, and for both partners to look at all the aspects of their lifestyle with a view to achieving optimum health and vitality.

HOW OFTEN SHOULD YOU HAVE SEX?

It used to be thought that a man would produce weaker sperm if he had sex very frequently. However, doctors now know that this is a myth, and so there is nothing to gain by you and your partner abstaining from sex with a view to producing more vigorous sperm. In fact, it is now well established that the more often you make love, the better the chance you have of getting pregnant.

Statistically, the chances of becoming pregnant in any one act of intercourse are low. However, you can increase your chances of conception by making love every day during the woman's fertile period. It is important to remember that many experts and researchers in the field of infertility are sceptical about the effectiveness of the various methods for calculating the fertile period. So, even if you think that you know when your fertile period is, you should still continue to have regular, unprotected sex at other times.

HOW LONG WILL IT TAKE TO CONCEIVE?

One important study into conception found that couples having sex once a month between the woman's periods took an average of 43 months in which to conceive. With couples having sex three times a month, the average time for conception was 15 months. If the couple made love ten times a month, the average delay was reduced

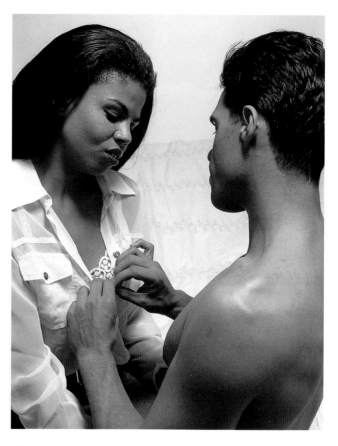

Give yourselves plenty of time to enjoy happy, relaxed lovemaking. The more often that you have sex, the more likely you are to conceive.

to five months. In couples who had sex 15 times or more each month, conception took an average of just three and a half months.

About one in six couples experience some delay or difficulty in becoming pregnant. You should not worry if it takes time for you to conceive, provided that the delay has not continued for more than a year. However, you should ensure that you are making love at least every other day during the woman's fertile period. Eighteen out of every twenty couples who are trying for a baby manage to achieve a pregnancy within a year. Another one in twenty conceive within two years. Others may succeed after trying for more than two years.

Nobody knows why conception can sometimes take a long time, or sometimes fail to happen at all. Many couples who have been trying for a year or two to become pregnant are perfectly healthy and have no obvious fertility problems. Ultimately, you may have to accept that conceiving a baby involves an element of chance – and it sometimes takes time.

THE PILL AND YOUR FERTILITY

Some women experience a delay in conception if they have been taking the Pill before they start trying for a baby. The majority of women find that their periods return to normal within three months of stopping the contraceptive pill, but a few may find it takes longer. If you are planning to conceive in the near future, some experts recommend that you stop the Pill and use alternative methods of contraception for three months before you try to get pregnant.

> " There is nothing to gain by abstaining from sex with a view to producing more vigorous sperm. "

EMOTIONAL FACTORS

It is often impossible to know why a woman does not conceive, but it is certain that emotional factors and stress as well as medical problems can play a part. Events such as moving house, starting a new job or suffering a bereavement in the family can all cause stress. This can reduce your desire to make love, and can also have a temporary effect on your fertility.

Sometimes the very fact that couples are trying for a baby can cause anxiety and so delay the wished-for conception. This is what lies behind the stories everyone has heard of couples who stop trying, and then quickly find that they conceive.

WHEN TO SEEK HELP

Medically, infertility is defined as the inability to conceive after more than a year of regular, unprotected sexual intercourse. You and your partner should see a doctor together if you have not conceived within a year of starting to try – or earlier if you think there may be a medical reason for the delayed conception.

It is a good idea to take a record of the start and finish dates of each period from the time that you started to attempt conception. This will help your GP and any specialist to understand your normal cycle.

Feeling overwhelmed by your work can hinder your chances of conception – you may be too busy to make love at the right time, and stress can affect fertility.

Aside from medical problems, the causes for a delay in conception may include:

- Your age.
- Being overweight.
- Being underweight.
- Having a sexually transmitted disease.
- Drinking alcohol.
- Having a high caffeine intake.
- Smoking.
- Having intercourse at the wrong time – for example, being too busy to have sex during the fertile period.

Your doctor may give you individual advice on how to maximize your chance of conception, for example by helping to pinpoint the woman's fertile period or by advising you to, say, lose weight.

If appropriate, you may also be referred to a specialist for further investigations into the causes (see next chapter). Doctors do not usually refer couples for further treatment until after they have been trying to conceive for a year or more, unless there is a good medical reason to do so.

Don't be surprised if you do not conceive straight away. Many couples take more than a year to become pregnant, even when they are making love regularly.

Risk factors

Nobody knows why some women have difficulty conceiving, develop problems in pregnancy or give birth to babies with certain disorders or defects. But research has established a number of risk factors for pregnancy; these are listed opposite. Being affected by one or more of these risk factors does not mean that you cannot or should not become pregnant. However, it can mean that you may need closer monitoring and more detailed or frequent antenatal care than other women.

ASSESSING THE RISK

The many different risk factors may look daunting, so it is important to remember that over 97 per cent of pregnancies result in a healthy baby. If the medical staff involved in your care know of any risk factors, they can offer you appropriate tests and be fully prepared for any complications that may arise.

In some cases, women and their partners may benefit from genetic counselling before trying to conceive. Genetic counselling gives an individual assessment of your chances of having a baby affected by a congenital (developmental) disorder. This is usually offered to prospective parents who have a medical history that could affect a pregnancy. It may also be offered to women over 35 in order to evaluate the risk factor of age, and to women who have had three or more successive miscarriages.

HIGH BLOOD PRESSURE AND DIABETES

Established diabetes or high blood pressure can put the mother at a higher-than-average risk during pregnancy. These conditions can also develop during pregnancy, and this is one of the reasons that pregnant women need to attend regular antenatal checks before the birth.

High blood pressure

During pregnancy, high blood pressure is risky because it may lead to pre-eclampsia. This condition is one of the most common causes of miscarriage or stillbirth, so it needs to be carefully monitored by medical staff. Pre-eclampsia also poses a risk to the mother since it can lead to eclampsia, a serious condition that causes convulsions and can be fatal.

Symptoms include high blood pressure, swelling (in the face, ankles, wrists and sometimes all over the body) and the appearance of protein in the urine. This is one reason why urine is tested as part of a woman's antenatal care. Pre-eclampsia often develops at 30-34 weeks' pregnancy but it can start earlier or later.

Diabetes

There is no reason why women with diabetes should not bear a child, but they need careful supervision to ensure that their blood sugar and insulin levels are kept under control. Because of this, diabetic women are likely to attend antenatal clinics more frequently than usual. They usually have repeated blood and urine tests, so any problem can be promptly identified and treated.

Women with diabetes have a greater than average risk of such complications as stillbirth, pre-eclampsia, urinary infection and excessively large babies. For these reasons, pregnant women with diabetes are encouraged to attend hospital antenatal care and to have a hospital delivery so that specialist medical staff are on hand to assist.

Pregnancy diabetes is a form of the disease that occurs only in pregnancy and clears up soon after the birth. It carries the same risks as established diabetes.

RUBELLA AND RHESUS INCOMPATIBILITY

Both rubella and rhesus incompatibility can cause serious birth defects. These problems are more common than genetic and chromosomal disorders. However, you can be screened before conception so that both hazards can be avoided. Pregnant women are screened for rubella and rhesus incompatibility as part of their antenatal care.

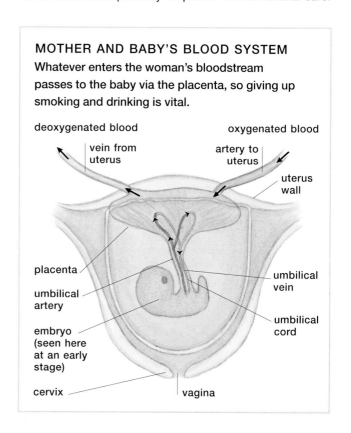

MOTHER AND BABY'S BLOOD SYSTEM
Whatever enters the woman's bloodstream passes to the baby via the placenta, so giving up smoking and drinking is vital.

deoxygenated blood   oxygenated blood

vein from uterus   artery to uterus

uterus wall

placenta

umbilical vein

umbilical artery

umbilical cord

embryo (seen here at an early stage)

cervix   vagina

Your blood pressure will be taken regularly once you are pregnant, because high blood pressure can lead to problems in the pregnancy.

Rubella

Also known as German measles, rubella is a highly infectious viral disease. If a pregnant woman contracts rubella, the virus can attack the baby's nervous system and heart, causing deformities, miscarriage or stillbirth.

Rubella can exist in a very mild form and it is easy to mistake for a cold. Ideally, women should be checked for immunity to rubella before they attempt to become pregnant. If you are not immune, you can be vaccinated and then be checked again to make sure that the vaccine has worked. You should have the rubella immunity test, even if you think that you had rubella as a child. The disease is often misdiagnosed, and the duration of immunity acquired through illness is unknown.

Rhesus incompatibility

The rhesus factor is a substance found in blood: most people have it, and so are described as rhesus positive, but about one in six people do not have rhesus factor in their blood, and are rhesus negative.

Problems can arise when a rhesus-negative woman carries a rhesus-positive baby. In this case, some of the fetal blood cells can pass from the baby's body into yours. This provokes your body to make antibodies to fight the alien cells and destroy them. This reaction does not usually harm either you or the baby. The problem arises with a subsequent pregnancy if the baby is again rhesus positive. The woman's body now contains antibodies to fight and destroy rhesus-positive cells. These antibodies may pass into the circulation of the second baby and attack its blood cells, leading to severe anaemia, heart failure, jaundice or mental impairment. In an extreme case a baby would need a transfusion in the uterus, but women can be monitored for this situation and there are now injections available that help to prevent serious problems from arising.

FACTORS THAT MAY AFFECT YOUR PREGNANCY

The risk factors associated with conception and pregnancy include:

Age
- Being under 18.
- Being 36 or over.

Reproductive medical history
- Previous problem affecting the uterus, such as fibroids.
- Previous Caesarean or myomectomy (removal of fibroids from the uterus).
- Having an IUD in place at conception.
- Three or more miscarriages that occurred before existing pregnancy.
- Four or more previous deliveries.
- In a previous pregnancy, early labour, cervical stitch, late miscarriage, late termination, two or more terminations, stillbirth or neonatal death.
- Previous small or large baby.
- Congenital fetal abnormality in previous baby.
- Developing rhesus antibodies in previous pregnancy.
- Developing problems such as high blood pressure, proteinuria, pre-eclampsia in a previous pregnancy.
- Severe bleeding after giving birth to previous baby or manual removal of placenta.
- Very short labour (less than 2 hours) or long labour (over 12 hours) in previous pregnancy.
- Postnatal depression after birth of previous baby.

Other medical factors
- High blood pressure (140/90 or more, taken after you have been lying down for five minutes).
- Diabetes.
- Hepatitis B, HIV or AIDS.
- Family history of or congenital fetal abnormality.
- Having a heart murmur.
- Pelvic or abdominal abnormalities.
- Being underweight or overweight.
- Being less than 1.5m (5ft) tall.

Lifestyle factors
- Smoking.
- Drinking more than ten units of alcohol a week.
- Illegal drugs taken by either parent.
- Having had a high number of sexual partners or a partner who is bisexual.

Race
- If you are of Afro-Caribbean origin, a test for sickle-cell anaemia is suggested.
- If you or your family is of Mediterranean or Asian origin, a test for thalassaemia is suggested.

What is the best age?

The best time biologically for a woman to have a child is when she is aged between 20 and 25. However, biological fertility is not the only thing that women have to consider when deciding when to try for a baby. Many women do not meet the person they wish to have children with until much later in life, or they may feel unable to cope with the demands of a new baby when they are younger. Women may also wish to concentrate on other aspects of life, such as building a career or ensuring they are financially stable, before they have a family.

Women's fertility decreases with age, particularly after they reach 35. Statistically speaking, both mother and baby also face increased risks as the years go by. However, it is important to remember that statistics give an indication only of the likelihood of a problem occurring in particular circumstances; they cannot predict what will happen to individual women. In other words, women over the age of 35 will not necessarily experience difficulty in conceiving a healthy pregnancy, nor are women guaranteed a problem-free pregnancy if they have children in their twenties. Many women have experienced the successful delivery of a healthy baby when in their late thirties and early forties.

PROBLEMS WITH CONCEPTION

Older women may take longer to conceive for several reasons. Most important is the fact that age can affect the general fertility of both partners. In addition, older couples may make love less frequently, and conception depends on regular and frequent sexual intercourse. At the same time, the menstrual cycle is more likely to become irregular as the woman ages, which may make it more difficult to pinpoint the fertile period.

One problem for women over 35 is that any delay or difficulty with conception may take time to resolve. If, for example, a 36-year-old woman tries to conceive, it will probably be a year before she realizes that there is a problem. She will therefore be 37 by the time that she seeks help. Fertility tests, too, can take time, so she may be 38 by the time a problem is identified. During all this

> **Many women have experienced the safe and successful delivery of a healthy baby when in their late thirties and early forties.**

AGE AND THE LIKELIHOOD OF A DOWN'S BABY

The risk of a woman bearing a baby with Down's syndrome rises sharply as she ages.

Age	Risk factor
20	1 in 2000
25	1 in 1205
30	1 in 885
35	1 in 365
37	1 in 225
39	1 in 140
40	1 in 109
42	1 in 70
45	1 in 32
49	1 in 12

time, the woman's fertility will have continued to decrease. Women who decide to undergo artificial insemination or assisted conception also discover that these procedures are time-consuming. In an ideal world, any fertility treatments and assisted conception should be embarked upon earlier rather than later in the woman's childbearing years.

AGE-RELATED PROBLEMS IN PREGNANCY

One of the most common concerns felt by older mothers is that the baby will have Down's syndrome, a genetic error that causes both physical and mental impairment. The impairment can be such that the child can never lead an independent life. As people with Down's syndrome may live to over the age of 50, this can place an exceptional burden upon the parents.

The possibility of having a Down's syndrome baby is not the only consideration for older mothers. Other risk factors that are linked to age include the increased possibility of:

- High blood pressure, which can lead to pre-eclampsia.
- Diabetes developing in pregnancy.
- Miscarriage and genetic defects – the likelihood of miscarriage rises with age in the same way as the incidence of Down's syndrome, but it is not known why this is so.
- Babies of low birthweight.

Women over the age of 35 are also more likely to develop other general medical ailments that may have an impact on a developing baby. Some disorders may need treating with medication that may be inappropriate during pregnancy. The mother-to-be may also feel very tired and suffer severe fatigue during labour. Pregnancy can also exacerbate any underlying medical condition, such as back pain or anaemia, because of the burden that it exerts upon the mother's body.

AN INDIVIDUAL PERSPECTIVE

All of this may seem highly alarming to the woman over 35 who is pregnant or who hopes to become so. However, you should be aware that all the risks discussed here are based on statistics – your individual risk may actually be much lower. After all, a large number of women over 35 do have extremely successful and trouble-free pregnancies. In general, it may be that the older mother takes a little longer to conceive and that there are more potential health risks both to her and the

While there are additional risks for older mothers-to-be, age brings with it an increased maturity and confidence that will be helpful during pregnancy and parenthood.

baby, but the important thing to remember is that with good antenatal care risks can be identified promptly, monitored and treated.

When it comes to younger mothers-to-be, women under 20 may be physically healthy, but this is not usually the best time to have a baby. The woman's body may not be fully developed, she may not have completed her education and she and the father may not be emotionally mature enough to cope with the demands of bringing up a child. Young mothers also tend to be less aware of the risks of smoking and drinking in pregnancy, and they may be less likely to attend antenatal care.

Your weight

Research shows that women who are underweight or overweight may have difficulty conceiving, and there is also some evidence to show that men's weight can affect their fertility.

THE EFFECT OF BEING UNDERWEIGHT

Being excessively thin may be the result of restricting food intake or of exercising too much. Both can upset the hormonal balance in the body with the result that your fertility is affected. Women need a certain amount of body fat in order to produce the hormones that control ovulation. This is why women who are very thin may stop ovulating and having periods altogether. Men who are very thin may suffer reduced sperm count or function.

The best way to achieve a healthy weight if you are too thin is to add plenty of complex carbohydrates such as wholewheat pasta and bread to a healthy, balanced diet. Do not increase your intake of high-fat foods.

THE EFFECT OF BEING OVERWEIGHT

Excess weight in men can affect their ability to produce sperm, while overweight women may experience difficulty conceiving. Pregnant women who are overweight are at greater risk of suffering birth complications. Also, if you are overweight, it will probably take you longer to recover from the labour and delivery and you will be prone to fatigue both during pregnancy and during the first few months of motherhood.

All of the health risks associated with being overweight can have an adverse impact on conception, on the course

Being a healthy weight helps you to maintain good posture, which in turn reduces fatigue and aids the elimination of toxins from the body.

of the pregnancy and on the delivery itself – the most notable health risks in trying to become pregnant and maintaining a pregnancy are high blood pressure, diabetes and kidney disease.

LOOK TO THE FUTURE

Prospective parents may want to consider the long-term risks of being overweight, both for their own health and for the future well-being of their children. People who are overweight are more likely to die prematurely – and the risks rise with every extra stone that they carry.

If, for example, you weigh 85kg (about 13 stone) instead of the 65kg (10 stone) that would be ideal for your

Being overweight reduces the chance of conceiving. If you weigh more than is ideal, cut out fatty, sugary foods.

height and build, your risk of dying within a given period increases by 60 per cent – statistically speaking, you are likely to die five years before your time.

All parents want to see their children through to a happy, independent adulthood. By looking after yourself, you will maximize the time you have with your children (and grandchildren) and the time they have with you.

CHECKING YOUR WEIGHT

The body mass index (BMI) provides a quick method of assessing whether you are a healthy weight for your height. Being under- or overweight may be harmful to your health and undermine your chances of conceiving. Check the box on page 29 to find out your BMI.

Your waist-to-hip ratio, which shows how much fat is stored in the abdomen, is another guide that you can use to assess your general health. To check your waist to hip ratio, divide your waist circumference by your hip circumference. The ratio should be less than 1 for men and less than 0.8 for women. For example, a man with a 80cm (32in) waist and 92cm (36in) hips would have a ratio of 0.88, which is fine. If his waist was 104cm (41in) and he had a hip measurement of 102cm (40in), the ratio would be 1.02, signifying he was overweight.

Both the BMI and the waist-to-hip ratio should be used as a rough guide only to your health and weight. If you are worried about your weight, it is a good idea to see your doctor for individual advice.

KEEP HEALTHY AND CONTROL YOUR WEIGHT

Diet and exercise should be the twin pillars of any weight-control programme that you may undertake. Natural therapies can help to strengthen and support your physical and emotional well-being, as well as aid weight control. If you want to lose weight, do so slowly and steadily – avoid any rapid weight-loss programmes, food supplements, diet pills or any diet that is based on a particular food group, such as all-protein meals. Ideally, you should reduce your weight to its optimum level and maintain it for several months before conception. You should not be dieting when you are trying to conceive or are pregnant.

- Eat healthily every day, and cut out sugar, salt, alcohol, cakes, biscuits, sweets, chocolate and peanuts. Your doctor may refer you to a dietician if you feel you need help with developing a healthy eating plan.

- Consider acupuncture to stimulate your energy levels, bolster your immune system and boost your lymphatic drainage system, which helps to eliminate toxins. A course of six or twelve sessions with a qualified acupuncturist may be the booster you need to set you on course for a controlled weight loss.

- Try the Alexander technique, a system of posture and balance that improves energy levels, strengthens all the muscles of your body, increases suppleness and helps you to move properly. All these factors may assist your weight control.

- Use essential oils (aromatherapy) to enhance your energy levels. Some oils help to eliminate toxins and some help you to relax and thus improve your posture and movement. Always check that the ones that appeal to you are safe to use during conception and pregnancy before buying.

- Visit a chiropractor or osteopath, who can help to correct poor postural habits and so strengthen muscles. Manipulation of the skeletal and muscular system can also help to remove energy blocks – thus assisting the efficient functioning of the body's processes.

- Take regular exercise at least every other day, but don't exhaust yourself. Walking and swimming are good ways to start exercising. Dance therapy is a fun method you may like to try.

- Consult a herbalist for herbs that help to stimulate the lymphatic draining system and the elimination of toxins. Check that any you use are safe during conception and pregnancy.

- Try a massage or shiatsu. Both techniques can greatly improve the lymphatic drainage system. Toxins are eliminated and your vitality increases, which helps to speed up your metabolism and reduce hunger.

- Practise yoga for increased suppleness so that the muscles start to work at their optimum and your digestive system functions more efficiently.

- Consider homeopathy, focusing on those remedies that help cleanse the system and relieve fatigue. Check that your choices are safe to use in pregnancy.

Fertility hazards

Smoking and drinking are two of the biggest risk factors for conception and pregnancy, but they are under your control. It is essential that you and your partner do not smoke at all if you are trying for a baby or if you are pregnant, and you should not drink more than a small amount before conception.

You should also try to avoid other harmful substances wherever possible. For example, avoid doing anything that brings you into contact with toxic substances and do not take any medication or supplements without discussing this with your doctor. In addition, you should be aware of any signs of poor health that you experience, and see your doctor promptly if you think that you are ill.

SMOKING AND INFERTILITY

It has been shown that smoking by either partner directly affects the chances of conceiving. Both partners should give up smoking some months (ideally at least four months) before attempting to conceive. This gives some time for your bodies to recover from the effects of smoking and also allows you to cope with any withdrawal symptoms that you may experience.

Smoking in the first few months of pregnancy is likely to have a more harmful effect on a baby's health than any other aspect of your lifestyle. Carbon monoxide and other poisonous chemicals will cross the placenta from your bloodstream directly into the baby's. This may affect development, and may make the baby more vulnerable to infection and disease.

Women who smoke during pregnancy are more likely to miscarry or to have a stillbirth. If they carry the baby to term, the baby is likely to be underweight (this is usually referred to as low birthweight) and he or she is more likely to suffer with infections of the respiratory tract, such as bronchitis and colds, in childhood. The child's ability to concentrate and learn may also be affected as may be his or her capacity for memory.

If you are already pregnant and still smoking, don't be tempted to think that it is too late to stop. It is not. You can minimize the damage to your baby by giving up now. Nicotine is a drug, which, like many others, is addictive, and it is undeniably difficult to stop smoking. Your doctor or midwife will offer you advice on good ways to quit. While you are doing so, it may be helpful to remember two things. First, if you give it up now, you will never have to go through the withdrawal symptoms again. Second, you are now doing your best to make sure that you give birth to a healthy child.

The occasional drink may do no harm, but both men and women should give up smoking before conception. Smokers and heavy drinkers may produce weak sperm that are unable to complete the journey to fertilize the woman's egg.

BREATHING IN TOXINS: WHAT SMOKING DOES

Tobacco smoke contains dozens of carcinogens. It also contains carbon monoxide, which is a poisonous gas that lowers the amount of oxygen carried around the body by the blood. Tobacco smoke also contains nicotine, which makes the heart beat faster and work harder than it should. Nicotine adversely affects blood-clotting factors, and so may play a part in heart attacks. In addition, tobacco smoke contains radioactive compounds, which are known to cause cancer. It contains hydrogen cyanide, which kills cilia, the tiny hairs that move together in waves to help keep the lungs clean and working efficiently. All of these toxins are entering your baby's bloodstream via the placenta each time you smoke.

DRINKING ALCOHOL

Fertility experts have different views on whether women trying to conceive should abstain completely from alcohol or merely cut down to a sensible level. The occasional glass of wine or beer is unlikely to cause harm, but most doctors advise women to keep drinking down at least to a minimum if they want to conceive. Two glasses of wine or beer a week is probably a good limit to observe, and spirits should be avoided completely. The man should drink a maximum of two pints of beer or half a bottle of wine a day, and preferably less than that.

If you are experiencing any difficulty in conceiving – that is, if you have been having regular, unprotected intercourse for a year or more but have not achieved a

Strive for a healthy lifestyle, good general fitness and relaxation. A happy, well-balanced relationship is vitally important if you are going to create a new life.

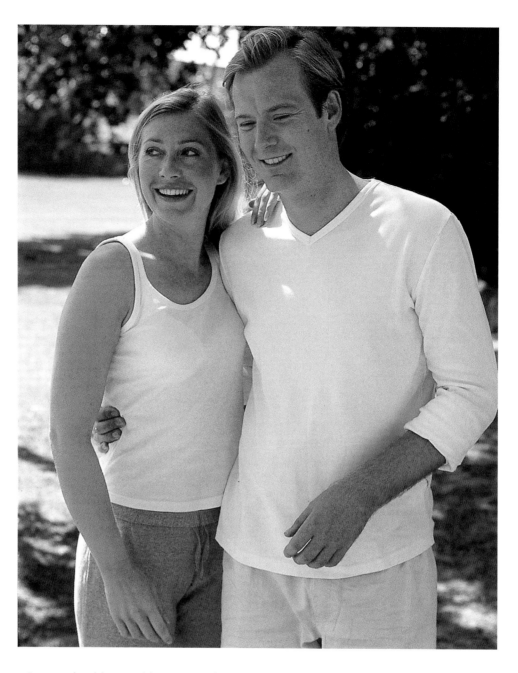

pregnancy – then both partners should consider abstaining from alcohol completely. Heavy drinking can affect both your chances of conception and the pregnancy itself. Men who are heavy drinkers may produce weak sperm and can also produce babies with serious defects. Women who drink excessively around the time of conception and during pregnancy can give birth to severely damaged babies. If you do drink heavily and wish to try for a baby, it is a good idea to see your doctor for advice. He or she may advise you to give up alcohol for several months before attempting to conceive.

YOUR GENERAL HEALTH

Ideally, both partners should be in good physical health before conceiving a child. This will give you the best chance of achieving a healthy pregnancy. A good level of health and fitness will also help the woman's body to cope with the demands of pregnancy and labour. It is

worth seeing your doctor for a check-up, so you can sort out any health problems before conception. This will also help to reduce your risk of having to take medication during pregnancy. Look at the list of symptoms below, and let your doctor know if any apply to you:

- Aches, pains and inflammations.
- Allergy.
- Apathy, feeling overtired, having less zest for life.
- Asthma or shortness of breath.
- Bloating.
- Constipation or other bowel problems, such as diarrhoea.
- Cough, persistent.
- Dark circles under eyes.
- Dental abscess.
- Fluid retention (swollen ankles, legs or fingers).
- Regular indigestion.
- Swelling and pain in the joints.

The role of the genes

Everyone resembles their parents. You only have to look at a family photo album to see how obviously and how often human characteristics are passed on from one generation to the next.

The mechanism by which these resemblances pass down the generations is the gene. Every human being has around 70,000 genes, and each gene contains a piece of information about one detail of a person's inherited make-up. For an embryo in the uterus, the data contained in the genes function as instructions: they tell the growing organism how to organize the multiplying cells into a human baby (as opposed to a frog or a rose); and they make that baby an individual, with a unique set of identifying characteristics inherited from its parents.

These genes are responsible for all that we are at the moment of our birth. They determine physical details such as our build, hair colour and facial features. Genes also govern, for good and ill, our natural propensities. A bookish nature, a gift for football, playing the violin or painting – all these talents can be learned, but they tend to be inborn. That is, somewhere in those 70,000 genes there is one for intelligence, athleticism, musicality or artistry that comes to a child as a birthday gift from its father or mother.

WHERE GENES ARE

There is a complete set of genes within every cell of a human body. Each drop of blood, every hair – every tear, even – contains millions of copies of the total blueprint for each individual. This is why blood tests can tell doctors so much about a person's genetic make-up: all the information about who you are is there to be decoded.

Genes are stored in long strings of DNA, and DNA forms part of the 46 pairs of chromosomes in the core of every cell. Every person inherits 23 chromosomes from their father (via the specialized sex cells in sperm) and 23 from their mother (via the sex cells in ova). The mix is random, and unique from the very moment of conception. Each child in a family gets a different set of 46, and so a different collection of genes. This is why brothers and sisters are not clones of each other.

WHAT CAN GO WRONG

Copies of chromosomes are laid down within sex cells, ready to be passed on to the next generation. But sometimes the copying process can go wrong and a gene mutates. This can have no effect at all, or it may result in an abnormality that manifests itself as a disease in the next generation. If that disease is not fatal, and the person

THE SPIRAL OF LIFE
Genes are stored in the double helix of DNA. There is a complete set of genes in every human cell.

double helix shape resembles a twisted ladder

sides of ladder are sugars and phosphates

rungs of ladder are chemicals called 'bases'

INHERITED DISORDERS
Some of the most common inherited disorders include the following:
- Congenital heart defects.
- Diabetes, type 1.
- Cleft lip and palate.
- Colour blindness.
- Thalassaemia (blood disorder).
- Fragile-X syndrome (the leading cause of mental impairment).
- Sickle-cell anaemia.
- Cystic fibrosis.
- Muscular dystrophy.
- Haemophilia (blood-clotting disorder).
- Polycystic kidney disease.
- Haemochromatosis (iron storage disease).
- Achondroplasia (disorder of bone growth).
- Huntington's disease/Chorea (brain disorder).
- Albinism (lack of the pigment melanin).
- Marfan's syndrome (disorder affecting the heart, eyes and skeleton).
- Tay-Sachs disease (disorder affecting the brain).

affected grows up and has children, then the mutated gene can be passed on with all the others, perpetuating the illness in subsequent generations. So, a hereditary illness represents a tiny flaw in the genetic make-up of a person who may have lived generations ago. That person passed the flaw on by chance, in the natural way, and now it has become a fixture of the genetic make-up of some of his or her descendants.

However, there is another kind of disorder affecting the genetic process. Sometimes something goes wrong not with an individual gene, but with the entire chromosome. Some chromosomal disorders inevitably result in miscarriage, because some vital piece of genetic information has been lost. There are some chromosomal disorders which are not fatal or life-threatening, but do result in illness or some other medical disorder for the child. The best-known example is Down's syndrome, which results when an embryo inherits an extra chromosome from the parents, and so has 47 instead of the usual 46.

It is important to understand that chromosomal disorders are not hereditary. A hereditary disorder is one where all the genetic information has been passed on correctly to the embryo, but it just so happens that one of the characteristics that has been passed on is flawed or damaged from a health point of view. A chromosomal disorder, on the other hand, is one where the process has gone awry at the moment of conception. It is a genetic accident, not an inherited condition.

These disorders are rare: about one in every 100 births includes such a single gene disorder. Chromosomal abnormality occurs in about one in every 150 births.

WHAT IS GENETIC COUNSELLING?

Genetic counselling is a consultation with a doctor at which the possible effects of any genetic disorder, as well as your individual risk of passing a particular disorder on to your children, will be explained to you. You may also want to talk about the effect an inherited disorder may have on your child's quality of life; and how that disorder could be treated afterwards.

You may be offered genetic counselling if there is any condition within your own personal medical history, or the medical history of your partner or either of your families, that could suggest a risk. Genetic counselling may also be offered to older women, particularly those over 40, whose babies are statistically more prone to chromosomal disorders. Couples who are first cousins may be offered counselling, because they share a greater proportion of the same genes (inherited from their mutual grandparents) so there is more chance of any hereditary disorder being passed on.

Sometimes, entire communities are at greater risk of specific disorders. These are groups that, historically,

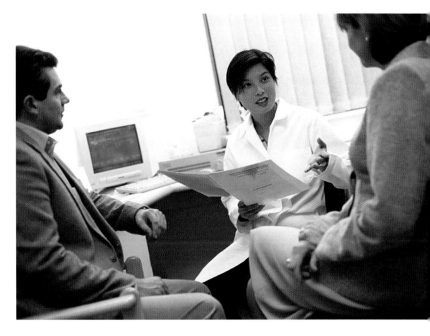

A genetic counsellor will help you and your partner to interpret scans and test results, in the context of your two families' histories. You will be given probabilities rather than forecasts; genetics cannot predict the future.

tend to intermarry for strong cultural or religious reasons, with the result that all the families in the group are genetically related to each other.

The genetic consequence of this is that the gene pool is smaller, and this has the effect of increasing the chance that any disorder that may exist will become more widely distributed than usual within the community. This increased risk will persist even after the cultural circumstances that created it have changed. So, for example, Ashkenazi Jews are more at risk than other people of Tay-Sachs disease. People of Mediterranean or Asian origin are statistically more likely to inherit thalassaemia.

GENETICS AND PROBABILITY

On its own, the fact that there is an inherited disorder in your family does not mean that you are a carrier of the disease, nor that you will inevitably pass it on to the next generation. Remember, only half your genes come from each parent, so there is only a 50:50 chance of any single gene being passed from a parent to you, or from you to your child. Moreover, the mere presence of a gene in your genetic make-up does not of itself mean that you will display that characteristic: not all genes are active in every person or every generation.

In the case of some hereditary diseases, you can be tested to determine whether or not you or your partner is a carrier. This is done by means of a blood test. You cannot be given a simple yes or no answer to the question 'Will my child develop a hereditary disease?'. All that can be determined is a statistical probability, and this can be used to advise you.

Relaxation and fertility

Stress and anxiety can delay conception, so it is important that you incorporate plenty of rest and relaxation into your life when you are trying to conceive. Exercise, too, is an essential part of your preconceptual and pregnancy care. Moderate physical activity not only contributes to general good health, but it also relieves stress and tension, thus helping to keep your hormones and menstrual cycle functioning normally.

EXERCISE

Incorporate three or four exercise sessions of about 30 minutes into every week. Walking in the fresh air and swimming are good options for women who are pregnant or hoping to become so, because they can be done for long periods without causing excessive tiredness. Whichever activity you choose, avoid exhausting yourself. Make sure that you combine your fitness programme with a healthy diet and drinking plenty of water.

SLEEP

How much sleep we need varies depending on our age, health and particular constitution. Most adults need about eight to ten hours a night in order to feel fully rested. Good-quality regular sleep is an absolute must for good health. As we sleep, our blood pressure decreases. The

> " Exercise can relieve stress and tension, thus helping to keep your hormones and menstrual cycle functioning normally. "

body's repair systems work more quickly and efficiently, so sleep is the time when damage is repaired. In addition, the body's natural elimination systems (the liver, the kidneys and the circulation) can carry out their work without having to process more toxins from the air we breathe or food we eat.

To help ensure a good night's rest, try the following:
- Establish a good sleep routine. Go to bed and get up at roughly the same time each day, even if you have had a bad night.
- Eat your last meal of the day at least three hours before bedtime. You can have a small snack before bed if necessary.
- Avoid stimulants in the evening, such as tea, coffee, alcohol and nicotine. Having a milky drink before bed can help you to get to sleep.
- Make sure the bedroom is well ventilated – open the window a little at night.
- Clear any daytime clutter, such as a computer, TV, newspapers or work papers, from the bedroom. If you can't clear them away, cover them up with a throw.
- Make sure that your bed gives you good support without being too hard.
- Avoid having stimulating discussions or arguments before bedtime – put them off until the next day.
- If you can't sleep, get up and go into another room. Try again in a few minutes or when you feel sleepy.

ACHIEVING PEACE OF MIND

Relaxation and peace of mind are important elements of your preconceptual care. Some psychologists say that there are three basic elements of happiness: having a good relationship, having something to do and having something to look forward to. Those are three important goals to work towards, but, whatever your circumstances, you can develop a relaxed attitude.

One step to peace of mind is to look at your present problems, worries, and dilemmas. If you feel anxious

Relaxation is an important aspect of improving your fertility. An aromatherapy bath, with candles, can be a wonderful way to release the strains of the day.

about any area of your life, sit down and write a list of the issues that worry you. Put them into categories: practical, financial, emotional, family and so on.

Now consider how you may be able to deal with those worries. Nagging long-term problems can be both destructive and extremely fatiguing: it is much better to deal with them if you are able to, or at least try and adopt a more relaxed attitude towards them. If you feel overwhelmed by a particular problem, it may be worth getting some additional help from either a complementary therapist or a counsellor.

Assess your priorities and take steps to deal with them in order of importance. List problems, too, so that you can seek help if necessary to resolve them.

MONITOR YOUR STRESS RATING

Everybody has some stress in their life. However, it is possible to put a figure on your stress levels, as shown in this test devised by Holmes and Rahe in 1967.

Tick those events you have experienced in the last year, then add up your total. This will give an indication of the source and degree of stress in your life.

EVENT	SCORE	EVENT	SCORE
☐ Death of spouse	100	☐ Change in residence	20
☐ Divorce	73	☐ Change in school	20
☐ Marital separation	65	☐ Change in recreational habits	19
☐ Prison term	63	☐ Change in church activities	19
☐ Death of a close family member	63	☐ Change in social activities	18
☐ Personal injury or illness	53	☐ Taking out a small mortgage/loan	17
☐ Marriage	50	☐ Change in sleeping habits	16
☐ Loss of job	47	☐ More or fewer family gatherings	15
☐ Marital reconciliation	45	☐ Change in eating habits	15
☐ Retirement	45	☐ Holiday	13
☐ Change in family member's health	44	☐ Christmas	12
☐ Pregnancy	40	☐ Minor violation of the law	11
☐ Sex difficulties	39		
☐ Addition to family	39	**TOTAL SCORE**	
☐ Business readjustment	39		
☐ Change in financial state	38		
☐ Death of a close friend	37		
☐ Change to different type of work	36		
☐ More or fewer marital arguments	35		
☐ Taking out a large mortgage or loan	31		
☐ Foreclosure on mortgage or loan	30		
☐ Change in work responsibilities	29		
☐ Son or daughter leaving home	29		
☐ Trouble with in-laws	29		
☐ Outstanding personal achievement	28		
☐ Spouse begins or stops work	26		
☐ Starting or finishing school	26		
☐ Change in living conditions	25		
☐ Change of personal habits	24		
☐ Trouble with boss	23		
☐ Change in work hours or conditions	20		

Assess your stress rating by adding up the figures for each life event that you have experienced. If your total comes to less than 150, your rating is normal. If your rating comes to 150–299, you are experiencing more stressful events than the average person. A high level of stress can undermine your chances of getting pregnant, and you may be at risk of developing a stress-related condition. A score of 300 or more is very high, and your risk of becoming ill is much greater than normal.

If you have a high stress rating – or if you are feeling anxious, stressed or overwhelmed – make sure that you dedicate time each day to de-stressing and relaxing. There are many ways to do this – what is important is to find one that works for you. For example, you may need to do more exercise, take up yoga or meditation, or simply incorporate some 'me-time' into your day.

Preconception yoga stretches

Many doctors recommend yoga exercises such as these as an effective way to relax, which may help those trying to conceive. These exercises also increase blood flow (and so the supply of oxygen and nutrients and removal of accumulated waste products, which may cause imbalances), flexibility and strength in areas vital to conception, pregnancy and birth – the pelvic region, hips, abdomen and spine. Many yoga instructors believe that this approach encourages energy to flow freely around the body in a way that makes it more open to conception.

Pelvic movements with focused awareness

These relaxing movements encourage increased awareness, blood flow and flexibility in the pelvic area.

Feel that you are opening up to new healing energy and letting go of any tension there.

1 Lie down, with a large book and three cushions beside you. Place one cushion under your head and tuck in your chin to lengthen the neck. Bend your knees and plant the feet hip-width apart on the floor. Place the book on your lower abdomen, so it is evenly balanced on the hip and pubic bones. Place your arms alongside your body, with palms facing down to support you. As you breathe in, press on your hands and arch your lower back so that the navel and hip bones rise and your pelvis (and the book) tips towards your feet.

2 As you breathe out, gently pull in the navel towards the spine and press on your hands to lift the sitting bone (coccyx) just off the floor. With this movement, the pelvis (and the book) is now tipped backwards, towards your head. Keep your waist against the floor and move the lower spine only. Repeat these two movements several times. As you do so, bring real awareness of thought to your body. This will help you to do the movements in a focused way. Breathe naturally as you work; do not hold your breath.

3 Now place your hands, in a relaxed pose, on top of the book. Breathe deeply, bringing your awareness to the pelvic region. Feel the movements of the book over the pelvic area as you breathe in and out slowly for several minutes.

4 Remove the book and bring the soles of your feet together so that your knees fall outward. Support them with the remaining two cushions. Place your hands, palms up, beside you in a gesture of openness and complete surrender. Relax for several minutes.

Improving flexibility and muscle tone in the lower body

These three simple exercises improve flexibility in the spine and hips and strengthen the abdominal muscles. Work gently at first; your strength and flexibility will improve with practice. Relax afterwards and feel the effect of the exercises on your muscles and breath. Keep your coccyx on the floor throughout.

1 Lie on your back with a cushion under your head and your arms, palms down, alongside the body. Bend your right leg, keeping the left leg stretched with the ankle flexed. Make large cycling circles with your right leg until you feel tired. Then rest for a few moments with both legs stretched out – be aware of the muscles in the right side of the lower abdomen. Repeat the same number of circles with your left leg, and then rest again.

2 With your left knee bent and your left foot planted firmly on the floor, take hold of your right knee and move the right leg in circles from the hip. This releases any tightness in the groin and hip joint. Keep breathing naturally and work very gently, especially if the area feels stiff. It doesn't matter if the movements are very small, since your flexibility will gradually improve. Rest, then repeat the movements on the other side.

3 Now work with both knees and the breath. Breathe in as you take the knees out to the sides. Breathe out as you pull your knees close to your chest to stretch your lower back. Again, work very gently and build up your ability slowly – in yoga the point is always to work with the body, not to force it into uncomfortable positions. Repeat several times, then rest.

Lying twist

This powerful but simple twisting exercise opens up and relaxes both the shoulders and the hips. This in turn helps to make the entire spine more flexible, creating space between the vertebrae.

Lie down, raise your arms, bend them at the elbows, and place them on the floor above or beside your head. This position opens and lifts the chest. Bend your knees and place your feet together on the floor. Breathe in. As you breathe out, lower both knees to the right, ensuring that you keep them together. The aim is to place your right knee on the floor without letting your left elbow leave the floor, but only take it as far as feels comfortable. As you breathe in, raise your knees to the centre, still keeping them pressed together. As you breathe out, lower them to the left and raise them again as you breathe in. Repeat several times, then relax for several minutes.

Common Qs and As

Q: I had a pregnancy terminated when I was 17 – I am now 29 and married and wish to have my first baby. But I am worried that I may not be able to conceive because of the termination.

A: There is probably no reason for you to worry: many women have had a termination – even several terminations – and then gone on to have a healthy baby later on. The best advice is to go ahead and start trying, although you may wish to visit your family doctor to discuss your particular medical history.

Q: I have had thrush and a number of other infections in the past and wonder if this will affect my chances of becoming pregnant.

A: Many women suffer from regular thrush, and there is no reason why this should stop you from conceiving. However, a sexual health check is recommended for all women before attempting to conceive. Explain your circumstances to your family doctor and make sure that you have the full range of checks – especially the one for chlamydia, which often has no symptoms but frequently causes infertility.

Q: I have had two miscarriages early on in my pregnancies. I am now trying to conceive for the third time. Is it likely to happen again?

A: Miscarriage is very distressing, and it is not surprising that you are anxious about conceiving again. However, you may find it reassuring to know that having two successive miscarriages is quite common – you have only a slightly higher than normal risk of having another one. Doctors do not consider that you have a problem until you have had three successive miscarriages.

Get plenty of support before and after conception. If using natural therapies, choose a practitioner who is experienced in treating pregnant women.

Q: How do you know if you have one of the risk factors for pregnancy?

A: Most risk factors cause unusual symptoms. If you notice anything worrying, you should see your family doctor so that any problem can be identified and treated.

Some conditions, however, cause few or no distinctive symptoms. These include fibroids and ovarian cancer. If you are aware of any conditions that have affected members of your family, you should tell your doctor. He or she may recommend a specialist check-up before you try to become pregnant.

Q: We are always so busy, we are often too tired to make love, but I desperately want to have a baby.

A: So, something has to give. Take a look at your daily routine and your weekly schedule – both your own and your partner's – and decide what you can edge out in order to make more time for you and your partner. Beware leaving it too late: if you should encounter problems in conceiving, you may need additional months (or more) for these to be resolved.

You might find it helpful to make a list of all the things you have to do. Put them in order of priority to you. Now see whether you can leave any undone – if so, delete them. Think whether any can be delegated to other people – and do so. Then set yourself a reasonable timescale in which to achieve the rest.

Q: We want to start a family but I am terrified when I read about all the things that can go wrong.

A: Remind yourself that 97 per cent of all pregnancies result in the safe and successful delivery of a normal and healthy baby. With today's antenatal care (which represents preventative health care at its best), problems can be detected and resolved. You really have no reason to be terrified. Starting a family is one of life's great adventures.

Q: We want to start a family but I am scared of the pain of birth.

A: There are now a wide range of pain relief options for labour and delivery. You will be able to tell those responsible for your care that you want maximum pain relief and make sure that that statement is entered on your hospital birth plan. You may also want to consider a water birth, which is thought to reduce the pain. At this stage, it is a good idea for you to confide in your partner and perhaps an additional friend or relative as well.

You may wish to discuss with them who you would like to be with you for the labour and delivery. You could, for example, have your partner as well as your mother or sister or good friend. You may wish to have an acupuncturist or hypnotist with you as well as – or instead of – your partner or relative. It would also be a good idea for your partner to accompany you to antenatal checks and, of course, to the antenatal (parent craft) classes as well.

On the issue of fearing the pain and discomfort of childbirth, there is another reason for you to act now and not delay conceiving. This is because, the younger you are when you give birth, the easier it is likely to be for you. As you get older, your energy levels will be lower and your muscles and joints will be weaker and less flexible.

Q: I have read that Pilates and yoga are particularly helpful in conception and pregnancy. Why is this?

A: Pilates is a system of conditioning exercise that focuses on low impact and relaxing routines. In essence it consists of a series of controlled movements performed within the frame of your body so that no movement will pull you from the centre of your body. Yoga also teaches you to focus, balance and 'centre' both your mind and body. Relaxing Pilates and yoga routines are especially helpful because relief from stress is of vital importance during pregnancy, and when trying to conceive.

If you want to practise Pilates or yoga when you are pregnant, it is important that you start before you conceive, and build up your strength, flexibility and body awareness. Experts say that you should not start Pilates, yoga or any other new form of exercise in the first three months of pregnancy. However, if you already have an established routine, you can usually continue provided that you modify certain positions – a trained yoga or Pilates teacher must advise you on how to do this.

Pilates and yoga also increase the circulation to your growing baby rather than diverting blood from it like other exercises. They develop your overall muscle strength and also increase your flexibility. This helps to prevent lower back pain during pregnancy and also improves your balance. Because Pilates and yoga help you to relax and teach you to breathe deeply and evenly, delivery may prove easier. These forms of exercise can also strengthen the abdominal muscles, making it easier for you to recover from childbirth and regain your pre-pregnancy fitness.

Women who are overweight may find Pilates and yoga particularly useful means of starting to exercise. Having improved their muscle strength and flexibility, they can then progress more easily to regular walking and swimming regimes.

Delayed conception

❝ Professional help often resolves the problem, leading to a successful pregnancy. **❞**

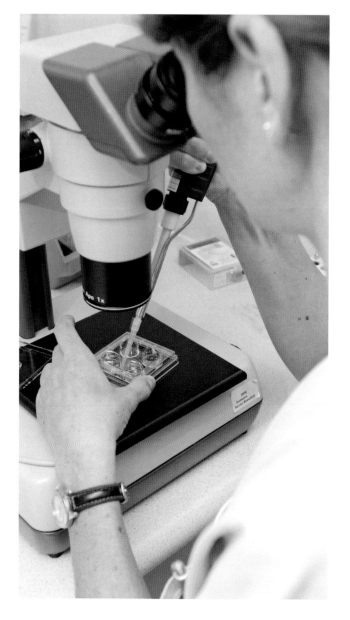

If you and your partner experience a delay in conceiving, remember first and foremost that this is nothing unusual. For especially long delays, professional help often resolves the problem, leading to a successful pregnancy.

Many people immediately think of IVF (in-vitro fertilization) as the solution to infertility, but this is very much a last-resort solution with a fairly low success rate. Infertility can be caused by all kinds of different problems, outlined in the following pages, and some of these can be resolved relatively simply.

The first step is for both partners to consult the family doctor and ask for a referral to a specialist. In the meantime, the chances of becoming pregnant will be enhanced by both partners doing everything they can to improve their general health and fitness. This means of course giving up smoking, cutting out alcohol, eating healthily, and exercising regularly. Relaxation is also a prime consideration. It can be

All kinds of tests and investigations can be undertaken to understand infertility, so do not worry needlessly without seeking medical advice.

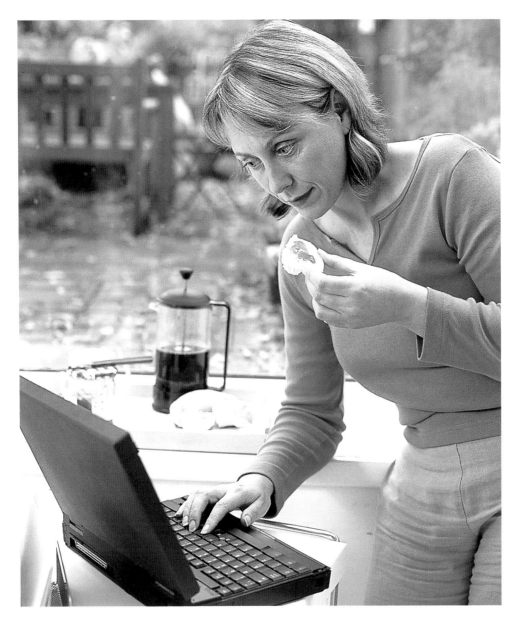

Many people believe that a stressful modern lifestyle, trying to juggle too many tasks and not taking time out for ourselves, contributes to infertility problems.

Meditation is the perfect way to relax and cope with the anxieties that may accompany infertility problems. The simplest form of meditation is simply to focus on gazing at an object such as a flower or crystal.

difficult to maintain a happy, balanced attitude to life while trying to deal with your feelings about delayed conception. However, do whatever you can to relax and have fun with your partner by focusing on those things that you normally enjoy together. Choose activities that you enjoy out of the home to try and take the focus off lovemaking.

About one-third of infertility problems are caused by the woman's reproductive system, one-third by the man's and one-third may be unexplained. Once the problem is found, relatively simple surgery may be the answer. Even unexplained infertility often gives way to unexplained fertility after a period of time. There are lots of good reasons to feel hopeful.

Problems with conceiving

Many couples naturally start to worry if conception does not happen within the first two or three months of trying for a baby. However, delayed conception is extremely common and there is very often no need for a couple to feel anxious.

The months of trying to get pregnant can be an extremely stressful time for both partners. It is all too easy to allow your thoughts to be dominated completely by your desire to have a baby, and to become increasingly worried when conception does not occur. Unfortunately, anxiety can become part of the problem and delay conception still further.

SEEKING MEDICAL HELP
You should see your family doctor if you have been having regular, unprotected sex for a year or longer but have not conceived. Your doctor may check that you are making love at the correct time, and will also ask about your general health and lifestyle – in particular whether you smoke or drink. He or she may also carry out some preliminary tests to rule out some of the obvious causes of infertility.

If these tests do not provide answers, ask to be referred to a consultant gynaecologist. It is very important that both partners attend all these consultations – because the problem may be with either partner or, sometimes, with both of you. In one-third of cases, failure or delay in conceiving arises from the woman's reproductive system; in another third there is a problem with the man's reproductive system; in the remaining third the problem lies with both partners or its cause simply cannot be identified. A gynaecologist will take a detailed medical history and will also check lifestyle factors that could be the reason for

WORKING TOGETHER
Trying for a baby can involve many moments of both expectation and disappointment. It is difficult to cope with a specific problem with conception, but also hard to bear a failure to conceive where the cause simply cannot be identified. It is extremely important that you both find ways to relax as much as you can and to enjoy your relationship fully, so that trying for a baby does not become a negative and unhappy experience.

> **Delayed conception is extremely common and there is very often no need for a couple to feel anxious.**

delayed conception. Various checks may be done on your blood and on the man's blood and semen. The reproductive organs of both partners are likely to be checked for damage, blockages and other problems.

These investigations may be invasive and time-consuming. However, they and any subsequent treatment can be very fruitful: up to 40 per cent of couples who seek specialist help achieve a pregnancy within two years. The major causes of infertility, together with their treatments, are discussed on the pages that follow.

MISCARRIAGE
In some cases, the woman may actually have conceived, but she may have had a miscarriage without realizing it. A high proportion of miscarriages occur within the first two months of pregnancy, often before the woman knows that she is pregnant. The loss of a baby through early miscarriage is much more common than many people believe, and may account for many cases of what is thought to be delayed conception. It could be that as many as over a half of all early pregnancies end in miscarriage.

The warning signs for an impending miscarriage include vaginal bleeding, abdominal cramps and backache similar to those of a period. Excessive vomiting can also be a symptom. Once a miscarriage starts, there is little that can be done to halt it. However, it is important that you seek medical advice immediately because there is a risk of infection and complications.

INVESTIGATING MISCARRIAGE
Having a miscarriage can be a very traumatic experience. For some women it is just as distressing as a bereavement, even when it occurs in the early stages of pregnancy. It may be of some comfort to know that miscarriage, particularly in the early months, is very common. It does not mean that there is anything inherently wrong with you, or that you are likely to miscarry next time you become pregnant. The vast majority of women go on to have successful pregnancies after experiencing a miscarriage. For this reason, having one or even two early miscarriages is not usually seen as a reason for medical investigation.

Tests are usually done if a woman experiences repeated miscarriages: this is defined as three or more successive miscarriages with no successful pregnancy occurring in between. After suffering three miscarriages, you should seek specialist help and advice. A late miscarriage – one that occurs after 14 weeks – should also be investigated.

Your family doctor will be able to refer you to a consultant gynaecologist if you have had recurrent miscarriages. In some cases, couples may then be referred to a genetic counsellor. Genetic counselling may help to determine the level or risk of future pregnancies, and to discuss the best way forwards.

WHY MISCARRIAGE HAPPENS

Doctors do not know why so many pregnancies end unsuccessfully, and determining the cause of a miscarriage can be very difficult or even impossible. Some of the known causes of early miscarriage include:

- A major abnormality in the baby. About three in every five early miscarriages are thought to be connected to fetal abnormality.
- The mother contracting rubella, listeriosis or chlamydia during the pregnancy.

It can be very distressing for both partners when pregnancy does not happen straight away, especially if you have delayed having a baby. It is essential to be totally supportive of each other.

- The failure of the fertilized egg to implant successfully in the lining of the uterus.
- The mother having a low level of progesterone, which is needed to sustain the pregnancy.

Later miscarriage (after 14 weeks) can be the result of:
- An abnormality in the uterus, such as a large fibroid.
- A weak (incompetent) cervix. This is a condition in which the cervix dilates instead of remaining tightly closed during pregnancy.
- Certain antenatal tests; amniocentesis, for example, carries a 1 in 200 risk of miscarriage.
- The mother having diabetes, epilepsy, asthma, kidney disease or high blood pressure.

Miscarriages are more common in very young women or women over 35. Many people think that minor injuries or distress can cause a miscarriage, but there is no medical evidence to support this.

WOMEN'S REPRODUCTIVE PROBLEMS

The conditions listed below include the most common reasons for female infertility. However, that is not to say that all women affected by them necessarily become infertile – some women with small fibroids, say, may have successful pregnancies without treatment. Treatment is an option in the case of most disorders.

Polycystic ovaries

This is a common condition in which many small cysts form in the ovaries. Polycystic ovary syndrome affects about one in ten women. Some of these women will encounter a variety of hormone-related problems, including infertility.

Women with polycystic ovaries may have no symptoms – with the result that they only know that they have the condition when fertility tests are done. However, symptoms can include:

- Obesity.
- Excessive hair growth on the face or body.
- Acne.
- Infrequent or no menstrual periods.
- Male-pattern baldness (the form of hair loss that is most commonly found in males – namely, losing hair first from the temples and then from the crown, with the bald area on the crown gradually widening).

Drug treatment is sometimes used to induce ovulation in women with polycystic ovaries. Otherwise, the cysts may be treated by being cauterized with a needle. This procedure is done by laparoscopy, in which a fibre-optic tube is inserted into the pelvic area through a small incision made just below the navel. This enables doctors to examine the woman's reproductive organs, take samples and carry out some minor surgery. A general anaesthetic is given.

Endometriosis

One in ten of all women referred for fertility testing turns out to be affected by endometriosis, making it a major cause of infertility. In this condition, cells similar to those of the lining of the uterus (the endometrium) become established outside it. They can grow anywhere in the pelvic area – for example, on the ovaries, in the Fallopian tubes, bladder, uterus, bowel, peritoneum or on the pelvic wall.

These stray endometrial cells respond to natural changes in hormone levels in the same way as those inside the uterus. That is, they increase during part of the month and break down when the lining is being shed (the period). However, because these cells are trapped inside the pelvic area, they cannot leave the body. Instead, they become inflamed and cause adhesions, which can cause one internal organ to become stuck to another. They may also form swellings which fill with dark blood – chocolate cysts.

ENDOMETRIOSIS

If you suffer with severe back ache, abdominal pain or strong cramps during menstruation, ask your doctor to refer you for a specialist check for endometriosis. In this condition, cells like those of the uterus lining grow elsewhere in the pelvis, in the areas shown below.

Possible endometriosis sites include: abdominal wall, intestines, Fallopian tubes, ovaries, appendix, uterus, peritoneum (lining of abdomen), cervix, rectum, bladder and vulva.

Many women who are affected by endometriosis think that they merely have painful periods, with the result that the condition often goes undetected for a long time – until fertility testing starts, in fact. The symptoms of endometriosis can include severe backache, abdominal pain and cramps during periods, and pain at ovulation, during bowel movements and during sex. The woman may sometimes also experience nausea and dizziness. Endometriosis is diagnosed by close examination of the pelvis, using a laparoscope.

The condition is usually treated by hormone therapy or by surgery. The procedure known as thermal coagulator treatment uses helium gas ionized by an electric current to dry out the endometrial cells. This procedure has had good results, and its other advantage is that it can be performed quickly.

Pelvic inflammatory disease (PID)

Infection can often cause inflammation in the uterus, Fallopian tubes and ovaries – a condition known as pelvic inflammatory disease. This is a common cause of infertility and other pregnancy-related complications. It is estimated that women who have suffered with PID have a seven-fold risk of ectopic pregnancy.

The bacteria that cause gonorrhoea and chlamydia are thought to be the main causes of PID, although bacteria that normally exist harmlessly in the bowel or gut may also be the culprit. The bacteria enter the body through the vagina and then work up through the cervix into the pelvic cavity. The infection may occur as a consequence of sexually transmitted chlamydia, childbirth, miscarriage, termination or the fitting of an IUD.

In some cases, PID causes no symptoms other than the woman's inability to become pregnant. It is therefore often not detected until fertility testing starts. The condition is also sometimes misdiagnosed as either endometriosis or appendicitis because it can cause similar symptoms. Where symptoms occur, they can include abdominal pain, exhaustion, high temperatures and very heavy, painful periods. The pain has been described as a dull ache across the lower abdomen. In some cases, it may be so intense that the woman is unable to move. The scar tissue caused by PID can increase the risk of recurrent infection and it can cause pain during sex.

PID is diagnosed by means of an internal examination and a laparoscopy. It is usually treated with antibiotics. In severe cases, the woman may need to be admitted to hospital so that antibiotics can be given to her intravenously (directly into the veins).

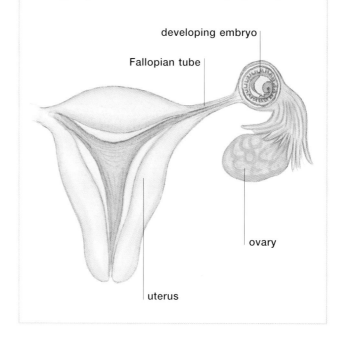

ECTOPIC PREGNANCY

Sometimes a pregnancy can start to develop in the Fallopian tubes rather than in the uterus. An ectopic pregnancy is normally accompanied by severe abdominal pain, and the woman will need emergency treatment to remove the pregnancy.

developing embryo

Fallopian tube

ovary

uterus

Ectopic pregnancy

An ectopic pregnancy is one that starts to develop in one of the Fallopian tubes or, more rarely, in another site in the abdominal cavity rather than in the uterus. It can cause permanent damage to the tube, leading to infertility. Doctors do not know why an ectopic pregnancy occurs. However, it is more common if the Fallopian tube has already been damaged by infection, surgery or by a previous ectopic pregnancy.

An ectopic pregnancy can be extremely serious, even life-threatening, and so the woman must get immediate medical treatment. The symptoms can include intense pain in the abdominal area and vaginal bleeding. Ectopic pregnancies are sometimes initially diagnosed as appendicitis or miscarriage.

An ectopic pregnancy cannot develop normally. Once an ectopic pregnancy is confirmed, surgery is needed to remove it. Sometimes, part of the Fallopian tube and part of the ovary may have to be removed as well, although doctors will avoid this whenever possible. Women who have suffered one ectopic pregnancy are at a higher risk of experiencing another one. However, many women who have had an ectopic pregnancy go on to have a perfectly healthy pregnancy.

Many women suffer menstrual cramps. However, severe abdominal pain should always be investigated. It may be a sign of one of several serious conditions.

Polyps and fibroids

Different forms of benign (non-cancerous) tumours or growths, polyps and fibroids can cause infertility in women. Doctors do not know why these grow.

Polyps have a stalk by which they attach themselves to the membrane lining the cervix or uterus. They may cause no symptoms, or the woman may experience a watery discharge streaked with blood between her periods and after intercourse.

Fibroids are bundles of muscle fibres that develop in the muscular wall of the uterus. They can vary in size from a small marble to a large ball. Fibroids are very common – one in five women over the age of 30 develops them. Like polyps, they may cause no symptoms. Where symptoms do occur, they may include long-lasting periods and heavy menstrual bleeding, including flooding and passing clots. The woman may also develop anaemia because of the excessive blood loss, which can then lead to feelings of exhaustion, breathlessness and depression. Other symptoms include severe cramps, incontinence, constipation and cystitis.

Polyps and fibroids are diagnosed by internal examination, ultrasound scan or laparoscopy. The woman may also be given a hysteroscopy, in which a viewing instrument is passed up the vagina into the uterus, or she may be offered a hysterosalpingogram, in which a dye is injected through the cervix so that X-rays of the reproductive organs can be taken. Polyps and fibroids are usually removed surgically. Drug treatment may be recommended to shrink large fibroids before surgery.

Early menopause

The menopause usually starts in the woman's late forties but some women may stop having periods in their thirties or even in their twenties. Women affected may at first think that they are pregnant. However, as well as the periods stopping, other symptoms can include hot flushes, night sweats, insomnia, vaginal drying, painful intercourse, loss of libido, genito-urinary infections, thinning of the skin, splitting of the nails, aches and pains, and incontinence. Women may also experience mood changes, anxiety, irritability, poor memory and poor concentration as well as subsequent loss of confidence.

If a doctor suspects premature menopause, the woman will be referred for a laparoscopy. In this procedure, the ovaries are examined by a laparoscope (a fibre-optic tube); this allows the doctor to see if the woman's ovaries contain follicles with eggs. Women who experience premature menopause may still achieve a pregnancy, but only through assisted conception.

Incompatibility

Failure to conceive may be due to an incompatibility between a man's sperm and a woman's cervical mucus. In these cases, the mucus contains antibodies that destroy the man's sperm before it can reach the egg. A post-coital test may be needed in which a sample of fluid is taken from the woman's cervix six to thirty-six hours after intercourse. This may be treated with drugs or the man's semen may be injected into the woman's uterus to avoid contact with the cervix. Assisted conception may also be an option.

INFERTILITY IN MEN

The reason for male infertility is usually defective sperm or a problem with delivering the sperm to the woman's vagina. It is rare for there to be no sperm at all. Usually the problem is that not enough sperm are being produced or that they are not strong enough to make the journey.

Abnormal sperm production

Sperm may be defective in:
- Quantity – if there are fewer than 20 million sperm per millilitre of ejaculate, the sperm count is said to be low.
- Motility – at least 40 per cent of the sperm should be moving in a healthy sample.
- Normality – the sperm should not be deformed.

If you are having difficulty conceiving, the man's semen will be analysed under a microscope for numbers of

FIBROIDS

These are bundles of muscle that have grown in the muscular wall of the uterus. They can delay or prevent conception, so early treatment is essential for women wishing to have a family.

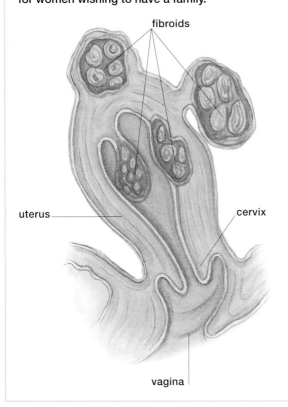

fibroids

uterus

cervix

vagina

sperm, motility, normality, infection and antibodies. The temperature of the testicles may be assessed by thermography. Some experts maintain that temperature is a defining factor in fertility, while many others disagree.

The man will also be screened for a number of diseases such as diabetes and kidney disease, for example, which can affect sperm production. Other male fertility tests include testicular biopsy and testicular X-ray in case of a genetic problem or childhood disease such as mumps, which may have led to problems with the sperm. Often the cause of low sperm count cannot be identified, and so cannot be treated. In some cases, therefore, assisted conception may be recommended.

Sperm delivery problems

There can be problems that stop the sperm from reaching the vagina. The major one is impotence, but another cause may be damage to the man's reproductive tubes, which may be due to a sexually transmitted disease or to some other cause.

Some cases of impotence and erectile problems may be treated by medication such as Viagra. Counselling may be offered if the impotence is thought to have a psychological cause. More often, however, male impotence is associated with a physical problem. Some of these conditions can be quite serious – they include heart disease, narrowing of the arteries, diabetes and high blood pressure – so it is important that men suffering from impotence should see their doctor. If the cause of the impotence is not treatable, artificial insemination may be an option.

Stress and fatigue may adversely affect a man's sperm count and the quality of the sperm he produces, as well as diminishing his desire to make love.

Damage to the tubes that transport sperm – the epididymis or vas deferens – may be remedied by microsurgery. If the man has had a vasectomy, this can be reversed. However, the chances of this reversal procedure being successful are relatively low.

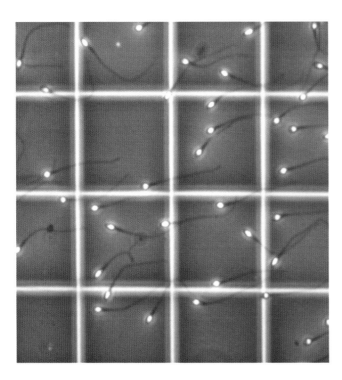

This shows human sperm occurring in a normal quantity – at least 30 million sperm per millilitre ejaculate. The lines on the screen assist counting.

By comparison, this sample shows a low sperm count of under 20 million sperm. A temporary low count may be caused by excess alcohol, smoking, stress or illness.

Fertility treatment

Many couples who have sought professional help with conception go on to have a child naturally. Others may learn that the cause of the infertility cannot be treated or that it cannot be explained. In these cases, assisted conception may be an option. It should be remembered that infertility investigations and treatments can take a great deal of time, and they can also be very intrusive. It is important that both partners take steps to care for themselves and to support each other during what can be a difficult time.

SEEING A SPECIALIST

Various tests need to be done before a decision is made to start fertility treatment. Your family doctor may carry out some preliminary investigations. These tests may uncover a simple problem that the doctor can treat. If not, you should be referred to a specialist for further investigation.

A specialist will want to ensure that the woman is ovulating, the man is producing healthy sperm in sufficient quantities and that the sperm and egg are able to meet. The specialist will investigate the woman's menstrual cycle and ovulatory cycle, the health of her reproductive system and her general health. If the specialist suspects that she is not ovulating, he or she may take blood tests to check her hormone levels at frequent intervals during her menstrual cycle; her ovaries may also be scanned using ultrasound to check when and if ovulation takes place.

The man will be asked to provide two or more samples of semen. These will be analysed under a microscope to check that there is a sufficient quantity of sperm and that they are healthy. If the sperm count is low, the man's testosterone levels may be checked – a lack of this hormone can affect sperm production.

If the woman is ovulating and there is not a problem with the man's sperm, the doctor will carry out further tests to see why sperm and egg are not meeting. A sample of cervical mucus may be collected after the couple have sex and tested to see if there is any obvious incompatibility. The woman's reproductive system may be examined by laparoscopy to detect any blockages or damage, and the man's reproductive organs will also be checked.

Before starting fertility treatment, a specialist will discuss your general health and lifestyle to ensure that these are not factors in any delay in conception. Sometimes you may be given general health advice to carry out before or during treatment, which may include the following guidelines.

Common health advice for men
A specialist may advise:
- Losing weight if overweight.
- Stopping smoking – if you continue to smoke while receiving fertility treatment, it may be less effective.
- Reducing alcohol intake.
- Avoiding caffeine.
- Abstaining from any drugs – cannabis and cocaine, for example, affect sperm quality and quantity.
- Avoiding excessive exercise.
- Having a healthy diet.
- Monitoring the temperature of the testicles – overheating may affect sperm production.
- Reducing stress and getting enough rest.
- Stopping any non-essential medication that may interfere with sperm production.

In general, the man should comply with this advice for about 70 days before the semen analysis takes place. This is the length of time that it takes to produce sperm.

Common health advice for women
A specialist may advise:
- Losing excess weight if overweight.
- Stopping smoking.
- Giving up alcohol for the time being.
- Avoiding caffeine.
- Abstaining from drugs.
- Having a healthy diet.
- Taking regular, moderate exercise.
- Getting enough regular sleep and relaxation.

ROUTINE FERTILITY TREATMENTS
In many cases, the problem is straightforward and treatable. Fertility treatments may include the following:
- Fertility medication to stimulate ovulation.
- Hormone treatment to encourage sperm production.
- Drug treatment with corticosteroids to suppress production of antibodies to the man's sperm.
- Microsurgery – for example, to repair damage to the Fallopian tubes or male reproductive tubes.
- Other surgery – for example, to remove fibroids.

ASSISTED FERTILITY
If the specialist thinks that a couple are unlikely to achieve a pregnancy naturally, he or she may recommend that they start assisted fertility treatment. This treatment may take the form of artificial insemination or one of the other

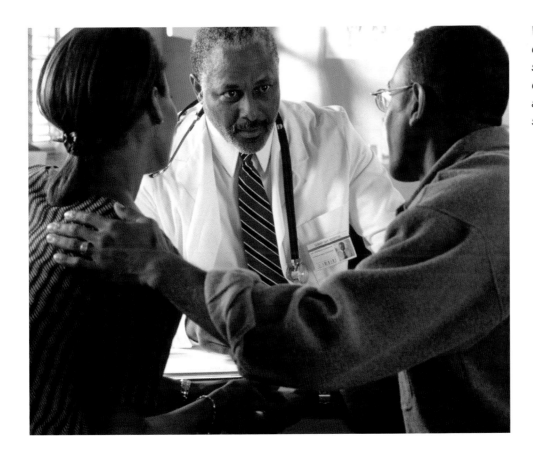

methods listed, depending on the cause of the problem. It is extremely important that a couple understand exactly what is involved in any assisted fertility treatment. They need to appreciate its chances of success, and the financial cost that they will need to bear. They will be offered counselling, which is intended to help them to explore their feelings and to be honest with each other about their anxieties and fears.

ARTIFICIAL INSEMINATION

AI, or artificial insemination, involves introducing the partner's sperm into the woman's cervical channel or directly into the uterus when she is ovulating. This is done in hospital, using a syringe. No anaesthetic is necessary for this procedure. Sometimes the semen may be treated in order to remove defective or poor-quality sperm before they are inserted into the woman's body.

Artificial insemination is a useful method for couples in which the woman's body makes antibodies to her partner's sperm, and also for couples who experience sexual difficulties such as impotence or premature ejaculation, low sperm count or blockages in the male reproductive organs. It is sometimes used for cases of unexplained infertility.

DONOR INSEMINATION

Sometimes a donor's sperm may be used instead of that of a male partner. This is known as donor insemination (DI). The method can be used in cases of impotence or defective sperm, as well as by single and lesbian women who wish to have a child.

> **❝** In many cases, the problem is straightforward and treatable. **❞**

IN-VITRO FERTILIZATION (IVF)

So-called test-tube babies are a result of this procedure, which involves mixing the woman's eggs with sperm outside her body.

Before IVF is carried out, the woman will take fertility drugs to stimulate her ovaries into producing more than one egg. The eggs are then collected. One method of doing this involves inserting a laparoscope through a small cut in the abdomen to draw off the egg-producing follicles. This is done under general anaesthetic. Alternatively, a needle is inserted through the abdomen and is then guided with ultrasound to draw off the follicles. This method requires only a local anaesthetic.

The eggs are mixed with sperm in a laboratory and left to incubate for two days at normal body temperature. Provided that both the eggs and the sperm are healthy, 60 per cent of the eggs may be fertilized. A few of the resulting embryos will then be inserted into the uterus via a syringe. No anaesthetic is needed for this procedure. If there are additional eggs that have been fertilized, they may be frozen for future attempts.

The embryos then need to attach themselves to the lining of the uterus – implantation – for a pregnancy to take place. If all the inserted embryos do implant, doctors may recommend removing all but one to give the pregnancy the best chance of success.

When IVF is used

In-vitro fertilization may be used if the man is producing poor quality sperm, if the woman's body is making antibodies to the sperm, or if she has blocked or scarred Fallopian tubes or irregular ovulation. It is also sometimes recommended for cases of unexplained infertility. IVF can be done using the male partner's or a donor's sperm. Donor eggs can also be used if the woman is not producing her own. In some cases, donor embryos – that is, embryos made from both donor sperm and eggs – may be used.

IVF was successfully used for the first time in 1978, in the UK. It resulted in the birth of the world's first test-tube baby – Louise Brown. Like all assisted conception methods, the success rate of IVF is not high. When two embryos are transferred, there is a one in four (25 per cent) chance of a pregnancy occurring. However, just as pregnancies achieved naturally can end in miscarriage, so too can those that occur as a result of IVF. The percentage of IVF treatments that end in the delivery of a baby is about 15 per cent – in other words, there is a one in seven chance of an IVF treatment resulting in a baby. Most couples who opt for IVF have to go through several treatment cycles.

GAMETE INTRA-FALLOPIAN TRANSFER (GIFT)

GIFT is a variation of IVF that is used when no reason can be found for female infertility, or if the man has a low sperm count. In this procedure, the eggs and sperm are collected as in IVF. Doctors examine the eggs to ensure they are healthy and select up to three for insertion. The eggs are mixed with the sperm, and are then placed immediately in one of the Fallopian tubes, where they are left to fertilize naturally. This procedure is done by laparoscopy, under a general anaesthetic.

GIFT has a success rate of about 25 per cent, which is higher than that of IVF. However, it can be carried out only if the woman's Fallopian tubes are clear.

ZYGOTE INTRA-FALLOPIAN TRANSFER (ZIFT)

This method is very similar to GIFT; the woman's eggs are collected and the eggs mixed with sperm in the same way. However, in this method doctors check that fertilization has taken place before injecting the fused eggs and sperm into the Fallopian tubes.

ZIFT is used when GIFT either hasn't worked or is considered unlikely to work. Again, the woman's Fallopian tubes must be healthy and functioning. The success rate is about 25 per cent. Both GIFT and ZIFT can be done with donor eggs or sperm.

In GIFT, the gynaecologist places selected eggs and sperm in the woman's Fallopian tube, with the aim of fertilization followed by implantation in the uterus.

INTRA-CYTOPLASM SPERM INJECTION (ICSI)

This technique is especially suitable when the man has a low sperm count or produces sperm either of poor quality or low motility. In ICSI, the eggs and sperm are collected in the same way as for IVF. A single sperm is then injected into an egg to ensure that fertilization takes place. The resulting embryo is then placed in the uterus so that implantation can take place. The success rate for each ICSI treatment is about 22 per cent.

DONOR SPERM, EGGS AND EMBRYOS

Sometimes, donated sperm is needed to facilitate a pregnancy. This may be because the male partner may pass on a genetic disease or has a very low sperm count. Donor sperm is also used by lesbian and single women who wish to conceive a child. The donor may be known to the couple. However, more often, the sperm comes from an anonymous donor via a sperm bank.

Another woman's eggs may be used in fertility treatment. The eggs may be fertilized by the male partner's sperm or that of a donor. A few of the resulting embryos are placed in the woman's uterus and she is given hormonal drugs to help maintain the pregnancy. Egg donation is the only assisted conception technique

In ICSI, the woman's egg is placed in a dish and injected with a sperm before being transferred into the uterus in the hope of successful implantation.

viable embryos during IVF or other methods. They may also be produced by fertilizing donated eggs with donated sperm. They are used when neither the woman's eggs nor the man's sperm can be used to achieve a healthy pregnancy.

OTHER OPTIONS

Surrogacy and adoption are two options when assisted conception fails. In surrogacy, another woman is used to carry the fertilized egg and give birth to the baby. In some cases, the surrogate conceives using her own egg and the male partner's sperm, and then hands over the baby at birth. Surrogacy can be fraught with legal difficulties, and it works only if all parties are in full agreement about the arrangement and stick to it. Payment is illegal in some countries, including the UK.

Another alternative is adoption. The legal situation surrounding adoption is much clearer than that of surrogacy. However, there are many more couples wanting to adopt a baby than there are babies available. Often, older couples are not eligible for adopting babies.

available for women who are not producing eggs at all, although surrogacy and adoption may be considered. Egg donation may also be used by women who may pass on a genetic disorder to their children.

Egg donation is a complex procedure, requiring the same drug treatment and monitoring as IVF or GIFT. Egg donors are usually women under the age of 35 who have already had their own children. The donor may be a relative or close friend of the couple, or may be anonymous. The use of the technique is limited because of a shortage of donors.

Donor embryos are also used in fertility treatment. They may come from couples who are themselves undergoing fertility treatment and have produced several

ACCEPTING THE SITUATION

Some couples may decide to go ahead with fertility treatments, but others may choose not to do so. Still more may call a halt to the treatment after undergoing several unsuccessful attempts. Counselling should always be offered to couples who are undergoing fertility investigations and treatments. It may also be beneficial to seek support from a complementary therapist as well.

It is sometimes the case that a couple who accept their infertility suddenly conceive – much to their joy and surprise. Others come to terms with their infertility, finding other ways to have a fulfilling and happy life.

Infertility, which may continue for many years, almost always proves distressing and exhausting. A close friend can be a good source of support. However, be prepared to seek professional counselling via your family doctor if you feel the need to talk through the complex and deeply personal issues involved.

How natural therapies help

Some complementary practitioners believe that therapies may actively assist conception. Most infertility experts and gynaecologists would dispute this. However, there is no doubt that the natural therapies have their part to play in supporting people during the time that they are attempting to conceive.

First and foremost, many complementary therapies, including acupuncture and reflexology, encourage good general health and well-being. They may be useful to those trying to give up smoking and reduce their alcohol consumption, or they may simply help you to feel healthier and more alive, as with the detoxing effects produced by lymphatic massage. Many natural therapies, including massage, aromatherapy, reflexology and yoga, help with relaxation and de-stressing, which can play an important part in conception.

USING THERAPIES FOR EMOTIONAL SUPPORT

Natural therapies, and especially meditation, yoga and relaxation techniques, can be very helpful if you are having difficulty conceiving, allowing you space to express your feelings and come to terms with them. Some people are able to accept the difficulties in becoming pregnant with calm and equanimity, but others are deeply distressed by any delay and need extra support. There is plenty of research and anecdotal evidence to suggest that you are more likely to conceive if you are relaxed, at peace with yourself and able to deal with any negative feelings and anxieties. For example, it is not uncommon for women who have had problems conceiving to get pregnant once

Plants provide a range of gentle remedies that may support conception. For example, certain Bach Flower Remedies aim to promote the kind of relaxed, open state of mind said to increase the chances of falling pregnant.

Reflexology can help to boost immunity and energy levels, creating a state of optimum health that is ideal for conception. Always seek medical advice before receiving reflexology during pregnancy (especially within the first three months) or possible pregnancy.

they are on a referral list for specialist advice – the pressure has been taken off them slightly. Negative feelings can all too easily take over. Women who have difficulty conceiving may rapidly find their lives dominated by thoughts of their ovulatory cycle. The start of each month may bring new hope, and the woman may feel determined to ensure that lovemaking coincides with her fertile period. As the time for menstruation approaches, she may become alternately anxious and hopeful, only to feel bitterly disappointed when she knows that she has not conceived. All this can be exhausting and stressful, and her self-esteem may drop.

Having children is seen as a natural process. Many women, in particular, feel very angry when it does not happen for them. It can be particularly hard to accept if they have spent years using contraception so as not to become pregnant at the wrong time or with the wrong partner. At the same time, a woman may start to feel guilty or inadequate. She may look for reasons in her past – wondering, for example, if the delay is somehow due to a previous termination or a past infection. Doctors can often be reassuring on these points.

At the same time, the man may be unhappy about the way his sex life with his partner is dominated by ovulation charts. He may feel taken for granted, wonder if his partner is more interested in having a child than in a happy relationship, and suppress his own feelings about a longed-for conception so that he is able to support the woman. From a conception standpoint, he too may benefit from supportive natural therapies, to improve his general well-being and keep him de-stressed.

Part of the holistic approach to health means that, as well as specific therapies, partners must learn to open up and speak to each other, in order to receive loving support and reassurance from each other. Friends or relatives can also be very helpful, although it is important to remember that not everyone has sufficient understanding and sensitivity in this situation. It can be an excellent idea to seek help from a professional counsellor, who will help you to explore any complex feelings and emotions you may have.

USING AFFIRMATION AND VISUALIZATION

Controlled breathing, meditation, visualization and affirmation work can all help both partners to get into the best mental and physical state to deal with the pre-conception period. Try the following exercise, adapting it to suit your personal situation:

- Choose a place where you will not be interrupted. Sit comfortably, with your back straight, perhaps sitting on a cushion cross-legged, or seated in a chair.
- Take a few deep breaths. Close your eyes. As you breathe, relax your shoulders and your face muscles. Concentrate on your breathing. You can focus on the air passing in and out of your nostrils or the rise and fall of your chest – whichever is easier for you.
- Bring your attention to the centre of your chest, the heart area. Notice how it feels as your breathe in and out – is there tension or pain here? Just notice the feeling, but don't try to change it. If you find focusing difficult, place your hands on your chest, and feel them rise and fall with your breath.
- As you continue to breathe, wish yourself well. There are several ways you can do this: some people like to imagine a pink light in the heart area that slowly expands and grows to encompass their entire body; others like to repeat affirmative phrases in their head. Try the following phrases: "May I be happy, May I be well, May I be safe, May I be at ease in the world". If you prefer, make up your own affirmation.
- Continue for a few minutes. Now visualize your partner in front of you. Imagine the pink light growing

Feel completely free to include whatever elements you wish in pre-conception meditations or visualizations – only you know what feels calming and positive.

to encompass you both, and spend a few moments enjoying its warm loving embrace. If you are using the affirmation technique, turn your good wishes towards your partner: "May you be happy…" etc. After a few minutes, wish both yourself and your partner well: "May we be happy..." etc.
- Now, slowly let the pink light or the words fade away. Bring your attention back to your breathing. Continue sitting quietly for a minute or two, then get up slowly.

Common Qs and As

Q: After several months of trying to get pregnant, I am now starting to think about nothing else. I wait for my fertile period, both of us have cut down on alcohol to a couple of glasses of wine a week, I make sure that neither of us is tired out before my fertile period... and then within two or three weeks, I get yet another period. I am starting to feel depressed about this and am beginning to believe that we will never have a family. What can we do?

A: First and foremost, try to relax, by any means that appeals to you. Make sure that you get enough exercise, and join a yoga or relaxation class. Make sure that both you and your partner are sleeping well: invest in a better bed if necessary.

Some couples do not become pregnant for two or more years, even though there is nothing wrong with either partner. Most gynaecologists know of hundreds of cases in which conception is delayed and, then, for no obvious reason, the problem resolves and the woman becomes pregnant.

The single most important thing for couples in this situation to remember is that they should never give up hope. What is known as unexplained infertility can just as easily, in time, give way to unexplained fertility. In the meantime, it is important to recognize the effect of repeated monthly disappointments on one's partner and the impact of delayed conception on you in respect of your other relationships and your family, as well as on how you manage at work.

Beware of damaging your relationship with your life partner for the sake of a need that may develop into an obsession with fertility and having children at some time in the future. If you are not pregnant after one year of trying, consult your family doctor with a view to a specialist referral.

Q: We have been trying for a baby now for four months and I am becoming increasingly worried and upset. Should we visit our family doctor, or is it too soon?

A: One in six couples experience delays and difficulties in conception. This is nothing unusual. It may take a year or more for you to become pregnant. See your doctor now if you prefer to do so, but you could probably afford to wait for a few months. It may well be that you find yourself pregnant before you see him or her.

Q: We have been trying for a baby for over one year now. I want to consult our family doctor but my partner is unwilling to do so. What can I do? Do you think this is a sign that he is less committed to the idea of starting a family than I am?

A: The fact that you are not yet pregnant may be worrying him. He may be feeling inadequate and disappointed. Talk to him and try to find out why he is so unwilling. He may fear that the issue lies with him, rather than you. Tell him that male fertility problems account for only one-third of cases – even a low sperm count, if that is what it turns out to be, does not make pregnancy impossible. Explain that there may be a relatively simple problem, such as a cyst or a blocked tube. Once he knows some of the facts, he may be more willing to seek help.

It might be helpful to drop the subject and concentrate on reassuring your partner and showing him that you love him for a month or so. However, you would be wise to see your doctor before too much more time passes. If your partner is still unwilling, make an appointment for yourself.

Q: I am getting very worried that there is a problem with me as my wife and I have been trying to get pregnant for nearly a year now, with no success. I'm concerned that I may be doing something wrong. I eat well and have given up smoking, but I have had a very pressured time at work over the last year and am probably drinking more than I should. I also had some kidney problems a year or so ago.

A: There are many reasons why conception does not happen straight away, but it may well be that your sperm count is low as a combined result of tiredness and alcohol. Alcohol has been shown to contribute to lower sperm counts, and fatigue can also do this, at least partly because it is probably making you less inclined to make love. However, kidney disease is another possible factor, as it can also lower sperm production, so do consult your family doctor about this.

Q: Both of my aunts had fibroids and this affected their ability to get pregnant. How do you know if you have them?

A: The problem with fibroids (non-cancerous growths) is that you don't know they are there. The only symptoms tend to be heavy menstrual bleeding, including flooding, very long-lasting periods, and feelings of exhaustion or depression. If you suffer any of these symptoms, you should see your family doctor without delay for diagnosis and treatment.

Q: My partner and I are discussing the possibility of assisted conception treatment. We are concerned that the success rates are so low, and are not sure whether it is worth going ahead or not.

A: Assisted conception treatments do have a low success rate, and most couples have to undergo several cycles of treatment before conceiving. There are obviously no guarantees of success here.

Some couples decide that assisted conception is not for them, and find other ways of coming to terms with their infertility. Only you can decide whether or not you want to go ahead. You should be offered counselling so that you can explore the issues fully – ask your specialist for a referral.

Q: I am not sure how keen my partner is to start a family, although he has agreed that we should and we have been trying for a while. Almost like clockwork, as soon as my fertile period is about to start, we have a row and do not make love for a few days. Then – once I am no longer fertile – we make it up. I have been thinking that it is simply coincidence, but now I am not sure. How can I stop this happening?

A: Consider whether your anxiety about conceiving is playing a part in this situation. It could be that you feel so tense when approaching your fertile period that a disagreement becomes inevitable. Alternatively, it could be that your partner does have real doubts about having a family.

The only way through this is to talk about the issue. Choose a time when you are both calm, and make sure that you listen to what he has to say. You may find it helpful to seek relationship counselling (via your family doctor or specialist organizations) to explore the issues further.

section two

your natural pregnancy

Understanding exactly what is taking place during each stage of your pregnancy makes it even more thrilling and fascinating than it already is. Knowledge of how your baby is growing, what is happening to your body, and how diet, natural therapies and other treatments can support your pregnancy is all part of the journey of discovery on which you and your partner are now embarked.

The first trimester

❝ Having a baby is one of the most exciting experiences that you will ever have. ❞

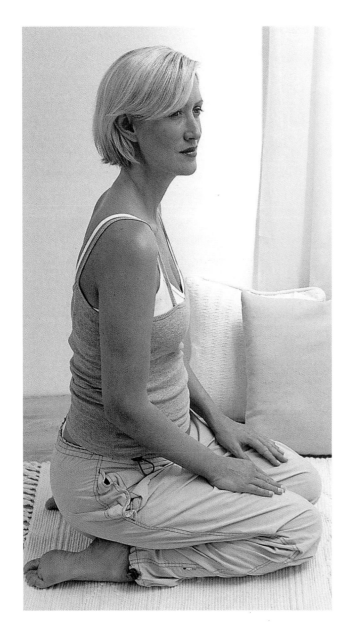

The first term of pregnancy, known as the first trimester, is roughly the first three months. This is an immensely thrilling time for a couple who have decided they want to start a family.

You and your partner will undoubtedly have many questions. Hopefully, this book will answer the majority of them but you should not hesitate to see your family doctor if you have any persistent worries. You will gain understanding, too, from your own experience. As every day passes, you will learn more about your body, your feelings about the pregnancy and the new life that you will soon be introducing into the world.

Pregnant women often experience minor physical disorders such as nausea and backache. There are often simple measures that you can take to relieve any discomfort that you may have, leaving you free to enjoy your pregnancy. In particular, complementary therapies can help to alleviate many

The first 12 or 13 weeks of pregnancy is known as the first trimester. Many women have hardly any visible signs at all, while others do start to 'show'.

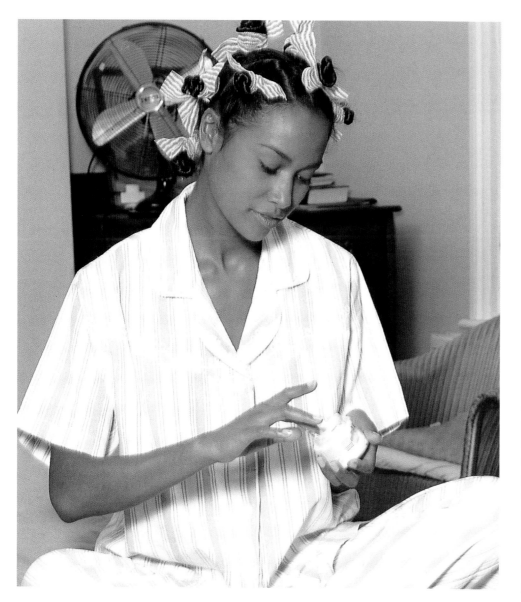

Don't stint on pampering yourself whenever you can, and get plenty of rest and relaxation.

What you eat and drink remains as important as ever in these early formative weeks. Make sure you get your five portions of fruit and vegetables each day. Freshly squeezed fruit and vegetable juices are an especially enjoyable way to include these in your daily diet.

pregnancy-related complaints and also enhance your well-being. The reference section on pages 226–248 will help you to choose the therapy most suitable for you.

Having a baby is one of the most exciting experiences that you will ever have. These few weeks are precious, not least because you and your partner will see your baby's heart beating on ultrasound for the first time. This is living proof of the new life within you.

Don't forget that your body needs at least the first 12 weeks to adjust to this new state. As your hormonal balance shifts and you experience a whole new range of feelings, look after yourself as much as possible – put yourself and your baby first.

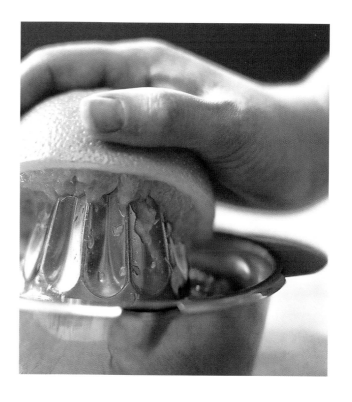

Am I really pregnant?

Some women believe that they sensed the conception of their babies: they did not need to wait for a missed period or other symptoms to know that they were pregnant. This feeling could simply be intuition, or it is possible that these women are able to detect tiny changes inside the body that are associated with the first secretions of the pregnancy hormones. However, most women cannot be sure that they are pregnant until they have had it confirmed by a pregnancy test.

EARLY SIGNS AND SYMPTOMS

The first definite sign of pregnancy is a missed period, known medically as amenorrhoea. Pregnancy is the most likely reason for a missed period, but it is not the only one – stress is another possible explanation. It is therefore best not to assume that you are pregnant just because you have missed your period. The following signs are other early indicators of pregnancy, some of which may occur before you miss a period. However, many women do not notice them until later in the pregnancy:

- Increased tiredness.
- Feeling nauseous, particularly in the mornings.
- Urinating more frequently than usual.
- Tenderness in the breasts.
- Changes in taste, such as a sudden craving for a particular food or a metallic taste in the mouth.

CONFIRMING A PREGNANCY

Most women do their first pregnancy test at home. Pregnancy-testing kits are available from any pharmacy, and they are very accurate. The tests work by measuring the amount of one of the pregnancy hormones, human chorionic gonadotrophin (HCG), in your urine. If enough HCG is present, it triggers a reaction in the test. This is

WHEN YOUR BABY IS DUE

If you know the date of your last period, you can work out your estimated date of delivery using the chart below. The delivery date is normally 40 weeks from the date of your last period but it can be up to two weeks earlier or later. A delivery outside those dates would be considered premature or post-mature.

MONTH	ESTIMATED DATE OF DELIVERY	MONTH
January	1 2 3 4 5 6 7 8 9 10 11 12 13 14 15 16 17 18 19 20 21 22 23 24 25 26 27 28 29 30 31	January
October	8 9 10 11 12 13 14 15 16 17 18 19 20 21 22 23 24 25 26 27 28 29 30 31 1 2 3 4 5 6 7	November
February	1 2 3 4 5 6 7 8 9 10 11 12 13 14 15 16 17 18 19 20 21 22 23 24 25 26 27 28	February
November	8 9 10 11 12 13 14 15 16 17 18 19 20 21 22 23 24 25 26 27 28 29 30 1 2 3 4 5	December
March	1 2 3 4 5 6 7 8 9 10 11 12 13 14 15 16 17 18 19 20 21 22 23 24 25 26 27 28 29 30 31	March
December	6 7 8 9 10 11 12 13 14 15 16 17 18 19 20 21 22 23 24 25 26 27 28 29 30 31 1 2 3 4 5	January
April	1 2 3 4 5 6 7 8 9 10 11 12 13 14 15 16 17 18 19 20 21 22 23 24 25 26 27 28 29 30	April
January	6 7 8 9 10 11 12 13 14 15 16 17 18 19 20 21 22 23 24 25 26 27 28 29 30 31 1 2 3 4	February
May	1 2 3 4 5 6 7 8 9 10 11 12 13 14 15 16 17 18 19 20 21 22 23 24 25 26 27 28 29 30 31	May
February	5 6 7 8 9 10 11 12 13 14 15 16 17 18 19 20 21 22 23 24 25 26 27 28 1 2 3 4 5 6 7	March
June	1 2 3 4 5 6 7 8 9 10 11 12 13 14 15 16 17 18 19 20 21 22 23 24 25 26 27 28 29 30	June
March	8 9 10 11 12 13 14 15 16 17 18 19 20 21 22 23 24 25 26 27 28 29 30 31 1 2 3 4 5 6	April
July	1 2 3 4 5 6 7 8 9 10 11 12 13 14 15 16 17 18 19 20 21 22 23 24 25 26 27 28 29 30 31	July
April	7 8 9 10 11 12 13 14 15 16 17 18 19 20 21 22 23 24 25 26 27 28 29 30 1 2 3 4 5 6 7	May
August	1 2 3 4 5 6 7 8 9 10 11 12 13 14 15 16 17 18 19 20 21 22 23 24 25 26 27 28 29 30 31	August
May	8 9 10 11 12 13 14 15 16 17 18 19 20 21 22 23 24 25 26 27 28 29 30 31 1 2 3 4 5 6 7	June
September	1 2 3 4 5 6 7 8 9 10 11 12 13 14 15 16 17 18 19 20 21 22 23 24 25 26 27 28 29 30	September
June	8 9 10 11 12 13 14 15 16 17 18 19 20 21 22 23 24 25 26 27 28 29 30 1 2 3 4 5 6 7	July
October	1 2 3 4 5 6 7 8 9 10 11 12 13 14 15 16 17 18 19 20 21 22 23 24 25 26 27 28 29 30 31	October
July	8 9 10 11 12 13 14 15 16 17 18 19 20 21 22 23 24 25 26 27 28 29 30 31 1 2 3 4 5 6 7	August
November	1 2 3 4 5 6 7 8 9 10 11 12 13 14 15 16 17 18 19 20 21 22 23 24 25 26 27 28 29 30	November
August	8 9 10 11 12 13 14 15 16 17 18 19 20 21 22 23 24 25 26 27 28 29 30 31 1 2 3 4 5 6	September
December	1 2 3 4 5 6 7 8 9 10 11 12 13 14 15 16 17 18 19 20 21 22 23 24 25 26 27 28 29 30 31	December
September	7 8 9 10 11 12 13 14 15 16 17 18 19 20 21 22 23 24 25 26 27 28 29 30 1 2 3 4 5 6 7	October

Find the first day of your last period on the pink band. The date on the lighter tint below is your estimated date of delivery (EDD).

usually shown as a coloured line in the window of the testing strip. The colour may be quite faint, particularly if you are doing the test early on. However, this still counts as a positive result.

The amount of HCG in a woman's body doubles every two or three days during the first six weeks of pregnancy. If a test is negative but your period still does not start, it is worth repeating the test in another two or three days. If the second result is also negative, you are probably not pregnant. See your family doctor for confirmation if you are still unsure.

For optimum results, it can be helpful to do a pregnancy test early in the morning, when HCG is present in its greatest concentrations. However, most modern tests are very sensitive, and they should give an accurate reading at any time of day. You can do the test on the day that your period is due.

How reliable are pregnancy tests?

Pregnancy tests are extremely reliable – if you get a positive result you are almost certainly pregnant. However sometimes women do the test wrongly or read the result incorrectly. Very occasionally the test fails to work properly or there is not enough HCG to show a positive result. If you are unsure about a result, you can ask your doctor to do a test for you: you will need to provide a urine sample while you are at the surgery.

Finding out that you are not pregnant can be be very disappointing. It is important for you and your partner to take some time to recover from the disappointment and to talk about how you both feel.

A POSITIVE RESULT

If the result of your test is positive, make an appointment to see your doctor two or three weeks later – when you are about eight weeks pregnant. If you are on any medication, see your doctor sooner – the medication may need to be adjusted to ensure that it does not interfere with the healthy development of your baby.

What a doctor will do

Your doctor will confirm the pregnancy by doing another pregnancy test. He or she will check that you are taking folic acid and will also ask you about your general health.

You may be offered an ultrasound scan to date the pregnancy if you are not sure when your last period started. A scan through the abdominal wall will show the baby's heartbeat at seven weeks from the last period, so long as you are not overweight. If you are overweight or if the pregnancy is less than seven weeks, a scan through the vagina may be recommended. A vaginal scan can feel slightly uncomfortable, but it does not increase the risk of miscarriage nor does it cause any harm to the baby.

If you have symptoms such as bleeding or pelvic discomfort, a vaginal scan may be done to check that the pregnancy has not established itself outside the uterus (an ectopic pregnancy). This is important because an ectopic pregnancy can be life-threatening if left untreated.

Early development

By the fourth week of its life, your developing baby is showing the first beginnings of the human form that will develop over the months to come. The sex of your child, the colour of its hair and eyes, its build and potential height, and other genetic characteristics are already decided. The embryo is firmly embedded in the wall of your uterus. Soon, he or she will be floating in a protective sac of warm amniotic fluid.

At this stage, the tiny embryo consists of three layers of tissues, which will develop into different parts of the body. The outer layer of tissue (known as the ectoderm) will grow into the baby's skin and nervous system, as well as its ears and eyes. The middle layer (called the mesoderm) will form the cartilage, bones, connective tissues, muscles and the circulatory system, which includes the heart, the kidneys and the sex organs. The inner layer (the endoderm) will develop into your baby's intestinal tract and digestive system, the lungs and the bladder.

A CRUCIAL TIME

Many vital tissues and organs form between the fourth and eighth week, making this the most important period in the development of the baby. A harmful substance or an infection is more likely to cause a serious problem at

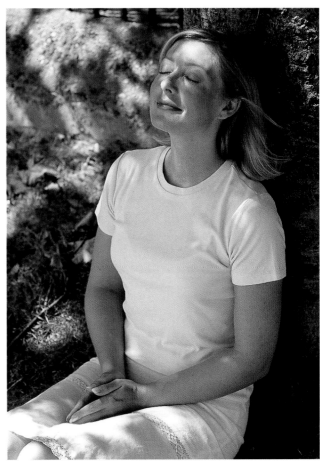

Your baby develops rapidly during the first few weeks of pregnancy, which is why women tend to feel so tired in the first trimester. To help your baby thrive, you need plenty of rest and early nights, as well as fresh air, regular exercise and a healthy diet.

this stage rather than later in the pregnancy, when the baby's organs are in place. This is why it is so important for women to look after their general health when they are trying to conceive – because they could already be carrying a baby and not be aware of it.

Weeks 5-8

Between the fourth and fifth week of its life, the embryo more than doubles in size. By week five, it measures 5-6mm (about ¼in) in length. Despite its tiny size, it has the beginnings of a brain and spinal cord. This develops

As soon as you know that you have conceived, your pregnancy may dominate your thoughts. Confiding in a close friend allows you to share your joy and also to voice any mixed feelings or anxieties.

EARLY DEVELOPMENT OF THE EMBRYO

Your baby's life starts from the moment that the sperm penetrates the egg – conception. At this point the egg is still in the Fallopian tube, but it will make its way to the uterus over the next few days. As it journeys towards the uterus, the fertilized egg is undergoing the first stages of its development.

WEEK 1
FERTILIZATION

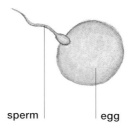

sperm | egg

Conception occurs when a sperm fertilizes the egg in the Fallopian tube. It will take four days for the fertilized egg to make its way to the uterus.

WEEK 2
CELL DIVISION

ball of eight cells   blastocyst

The fertilized egg divides again and again, forming a ball of cells. Eventually, there is a mass of 150 cells, arranged in two sections: the outer cells will develop into the placenta and amniotic sac, while the inner cells become the baby. The blastocyst, as it is now known, attaches itself to the uterus lining.

WEEK 4 +
DEVELOPING EMBRYO

The tiny embryo begins to take shape. Its brain and spinal cord are starting to develop, and its heart is beating. It is attached to the placenta by a tiny stalk, which will develop into the umbilical cord.

WEEK 3
THREE LAYERS

The inner cells are in three layers. The outer layer will become the baby's skin and nerves; the middle one will be the muscles, heart and skeleton; and the inner one develops into other organs.

from the neural tube, which has started to form. At this stage, the baby's heart has already started to beat, although it will not be detectable by ultrasound for another week or two. The heart has only two chambers rather than the four that will develop within another week or so.

The embryo is connected to the developing placenta by a thin stalk, which is the rudimentary beginning of the umbilical cord. Blood vessels are already forming here. From this lifeline, the baby will derive essential nutrients and oxygen, which are needed for its healthy development and growth. At this early stage the placenta is larger than the embryo.

WHAT THE DOCTORS SAY

Medically, your growing baby is known as an embryo until the eighth week of pregnancy, when all the internal organs are formed. It is then known as a fetus until the delivery.

Medical terms can sound baffling. Always ask about unfamiliar terms and abbreviations that you do not understand. Your doctors and midwife should be happy to explain what they mean.

Development from six weeks

The embryo develops rapidly from the sixth to eighth week of pregnancy. It passes through a number of phases that some theorists believe resemble the stages of human evolution – from "tadpole" through a fish-like stage to primitive mammal and finally a tiny human being.

Week 6

During the sixth week, the baby's head forms, rapidly followed by the chest and abdominal cavities. Its rudimentary brain is completed and a spinal column, as well as a spinal cord, is properly formed. The circulation is about to begin functioning. The embryo's heart is now beating steadily, much faster than your own. The stomach is forming, the kidneys are maturing and the liver has grown so much that it almost fills the entire abdominal cavity.

It is also in the sixth week that the baby's face starts to take shape. This is a process that will take several more weeks to complete. Small depressions are appearing where the eyes and ears will be situated. The mouth and jaw are beginning to develop. The embryo is now, incredibly, 10,000 times larger than the fertilized cell from which it originated.

Week 7

The kidneys and lungs start to develop and the head continues to grow, forming a more recognizably human shape. The buds that will form arms and legs are apparent.

Week 8

All the internal organs are now formed, although they will continue to mature. The baby now measures 2.5cm (1in) in length. Doctors will now start referring to it as a fetus.

Weeks 10-11

The baby is moving about a great deal, although you will not yet be able to feel this. The fingers and toes are forming, but are still joined by webs of skin. The facial features are more distinct, and the baby now has eyes.

EARLY DEVELOPMENT, WEEKS 6–13
By week 7, the embryo can be seen on an ultrasound scan. The tiny heart is beating, and the major organs have started to develop. By week 12 or 13, the embryo is a tiny recognizable human with facial features.

6 WEEKS

placenta

eye depression

head and face starting to form

umbilical cord

spine

arm bud starting to appear

7-8 WEEKS

head becoming more clearly defined

arm and leg buds developing into stalks

Weeks 12-13

The external genitals have formed and all facial features are in place. Your baby measures about 7.5cm (3in) in length (roughly the size of an avocado). The muscles are getting stronger, so movements are more vigorous.

SEEING YOUR BABY

Ultrasound enables you to see your baby while it is in the uterus. Most people find this a very moving experience, and it can help to strengthen your feelings of connection with your developing baby.

An ultrasound is invaluable in determining the definite existence of a pregnancy as well as the age of the embryo or fetus. You will be offered an early scan to date the pregnancy if you do not know the day of your last period. Otherwise, most women have their first scan at 10-12 weeks. This scan is used to confirm that the baby is able to develop – in medical terms, whether the fetus is viable. The scan can also identify the existence of a multiple pregnancy, so you will know early on if you are carrying twins, triplets or more.

Another scan is usually carried out at about 18 weeks. This scan is used to identify any developmental and structural abnormalities that may not have been apparent at an earlier stage of the pregnancy.

This is what your baby will look like 12 weeks into your pregnancy – you can see the face at the upper left of the picture. The baby weighs about 45g (1½oz).

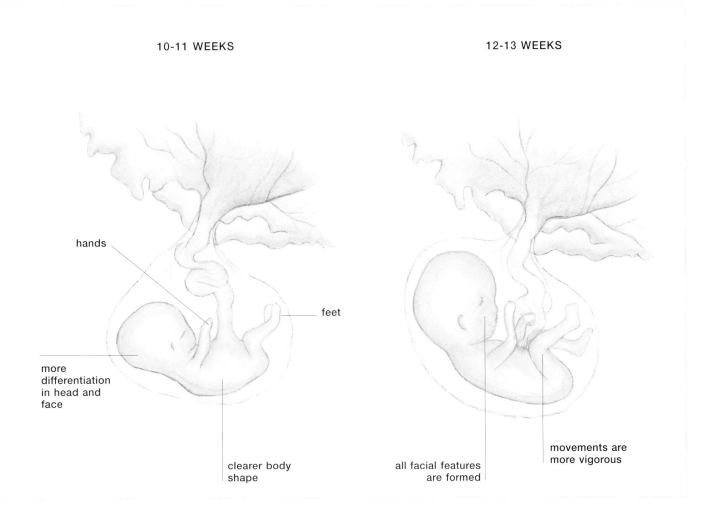

10-11 WEEKS

hands

feet

more differentiation in head and face

clearer body shape

12-13 WEEKS

all facial features are formed

movements are more vigorous

How your body is changing

Your baby grows rapidly during the first three months of pregnancy, and your body changes at the same time. However, most of these developments will go unnoticed by anyone except you and, to a lesser extent, your partner. Many women find it hard to believe that they look much the same as normal, but they do.

Your uterus grows to accommodate the developing baby, but by the end of the first trimester it is still no bigger than an avocado pear. Few people will see any difference in your outward appearance. However, when you are naked, you and your partner may notice that your breasts are fuller, and that your nipples have increased in size and darkened. Some women do fill out a little.

The most noticeable effects of your pregnancy, though, will be in the way you feel rather than in the way that you look. Your breasts may tingle. You may experience a feeling of fullness in your abdomen. You are likely to want to pass water more frequently, and you may feel nauseous some or perhaps all of the time. You will probably feel alternately anxious and excited as you come to terms with the fact that you are pregnant.

FATIGUE

The rapid development rate of the baby in the first weeks of pregnancy is bound to make you feel tired. To help yourself to cope – and to ensure that your baby thrives – you need early nights, regular exercise and a good, healthy diet. Some women feel energized during early

MEETING YOUR NEEDS

Your body will undergo various changes in the first trimester and you will almost certainly need extra sleep. You may also benefit from doing some of the following:

- Take a rest in the afternoon.
- Drink lots of fruit and vegetable juices.
- Go for a short walk every morning before you start work.
- Swim at lunchtime or after work, two or three times a week.
- Avoid doing any everyday tasks that are not vitally important – for example, ironing or dusting. Ask your partner or friends for help when you need it.
- Wear flat, comfortable shoes.
- Go to bed an hour earlier every night – read in bed for a bit if you don't feel sleepy immediately.
- Treat yourself to an aromatherapy massage or acupuncture session (always seek professional advice about such treatments).
- Buy some relaxing herbal bath preparations and pamper yourself.
- Show your partner that you love, respect and desire him.

pregnancy, but most feel very tired in a way that feels new. You may feel an overwhelming desire to nap in the afternoon, or to get to bed much earlier than usual. The best way to deal with this is to give in to it – rest as much as you can.

MORNING SICKNESS

Some women sail through their pregnancies without having any nausea, but most experience at least some morning sickness. There are various theories about why this nausea occurs, and some doctors maintain that it is purely psychological. However, most experts think that it is connected to the increased level of hormones circulating in the blood. Morning sickness most commonly affects women in the morning – hence its

Swimming – say, two or three times a week – is one of the best forms of exercise in pregnancy. It works all your muscles, and increases flexibility and stamina.

> **❝ Your baby grows rapidly during the first three months, and your body changes at the same time. Most of these developments will go unnoticed. ❞**

name – but it can also occur at other times of day. Some women feel nauseous all day for the first few weeks. Morning sickness usually starts during the sixth week and continues until the twelfth or fourteenth. However, it sometimes continues throughout pregnancy.

Eating little and often can be helpful, and it is usually best to eat something to raise your blood sugar levels before you get up in the morning. A dry biscuit or piece of toast is ideal. Many women find drinking ginger tea or sucking on a piece of raw ginger can help. You should also make sure you drink plenty of fluids, particularly if you are vomiting.

Morning sickness may be exacerbated by kitchen smells, tobacco smoke and alcohol, so these should be avoided. It is not uncommon to notice flecks of blood in the vomit. This is because repeated vomiting may cause breakage of tiny blood vessels in the throat or gullet. The blood vessels will heal by themselves so there is no need to be alarmed by this. However, if your sickness is very severe, tell your doctor.

URINATION

One of the earliest signs of pregnancy is an increased frequency in urination. This is known medically as micturition. Some women notice they are passing water more often as early as one week after conception. The increase is due partly to the growing uterus pressing against the nearby bladder, and partly because alterations in hormone levels lead to changes in muscle tone. The increase in frequency of urination is often particularly pronounced in the first nine weeks. After this, the uterus tends to moves upwards, which relieves the pressure on the bladder until much later in the pregnancy.

Some women find that they need to pass water more often throughout their whole pregnancy. It is also quite common to pass a small amount of urine when you laugh or cough. Wearing well-fitting briefs with a light sanitary towel or incontinence pad will help.

TENDER BREASTS

Your breasts may feel heavy and tender, and they often increase in size early on so it is worth investing in a new bra. Your nipples may feel sore and sensitive. They are likely to become harder and may darken in colour. Small white spots may become more pronounced. Breast tenderness is usually relieved after the eighth week.

You will soon start to see subtle changes in your body shape as your baby grows and your uterus increases in size to accommodate him or her.

TASTE

Pregnant women often report experiencing a strange metallic taste in the mouth. You may also develop new preferences for certain foods and drinks, and go off others – particularly coffee, alcohol and fried foods. Try to resist any cravings for sugary or high-fat snacks since these are high in calories but low in nutrients.

Emotional changes

The first few months of pregnancy are a time when you and your partner will be discussing all sorts of practical as well as emotional issues. For example, should you stay in the same home or should you move somewhere bigger or closer to family? If you are staying put, do you need to make changes? Will you want to start decorating a nursery?

You need to consider whether you tell close family and friends straight away, or whether you keep the news to yourselves for a few weeks. Keeping quiet can give you a precious opportunity to enjoy and look forward to this very special journey together. Many couples wait until they are past the twelfth week, and they know that the pregnancy is well established, before sharing the news.

FEELING ANXIOUS

Almost everyone experiences anxiety at some stage of their pregnancy, and most women find that different worries crop up throughout. It is very common to have underlying fears about the health of the baby, particularly before you have gone through any of the antenatal tests. Many women feel anxious about how they will cope with the pregnancy, and how they will deal with the labour and delivery. In addition, couples often doubt their ability to be

Most pregnant women find that they want to sleep more; dreams can be very important now, allowing your mind to adapt to the profound life changes ahead.

good parents and worry about how they will cope with all the practicalities of caring for a child. Concern about the impact that a child will have on your financial situation, sexual relationship, careers and social lives can all surface during pregnancy.

It is important to keep a sense of perspective, and to realize that doubts and worries are perfectly normal. After all, you are embarking on a life-changing event. However, if anxiety starts to dominate your thinking, it can be helpful to confide in a close friend or relative who has had a child, or to talk to your midwife.

You may also experience strange dreams about giving birth or becoming a mother. These dreams reflect the natural anxiety that you feel, and they are also a way of preparing psychologically for the new role ahead of you.

Fluctuating hormone levels may play havoc with your emotions and stability. Get plenty of rest and recognize any volatility for the biological phenomenon that it is.

COMMUNICATING WITH YOUR BABY

Some women find that they do not experience a sense of connection with their baby until later in their pregnancy – and occasionally only after the birth. However, many women feel a bond with the growing baby early on, perhaps as soon as they know they are pregnant. This can be a very special feeling; suddenly the most important thing in the world is the health and well-being of the tiny baby inside you.

Fathers often do not feel a sense of bonding in the first months, when there is little outward sign of the baby's presence. This is understandable, but many women find it hard to accept their partner is not quite so fascinated with the pregnancy as they are. Both partners may need to exercise some tolerance about the different ways that they react to the pregnancy.

It usually helps if the father gets involved right from the start. Ideally he will attend any scans so that he can see the baby on screen. Some men like to talk to the baby through the mother's abdomen. Stroking the mother's

> " Suddenly the most important thing in the world is the health and well-being of the tiny baby inside you. "

belly or playing music to the baby can also help fathers to feel more connected with the life they have created.

Nobody knows how much unborn babies can hear or feel in the uterus, but some research shows that they learn to recognize their parents' voices before they are born. The ears are formed by the seventh week, and it is known that external sounds filter through. Researchers have now found that unborn babies can also distinguish different intonation patterns – so they may be able to recognize the speech sounds you and your partner make.

Communicating with your baby can help you and your partner to bond with your unborn child, long before he or she comes into the world to be part of your family.

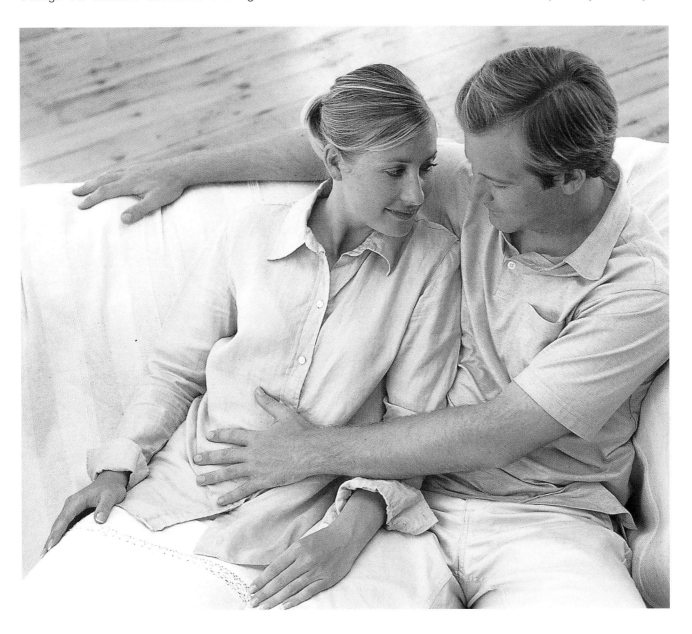

Pregnancy and eating

For the whole of your pregnancy, and longer if you are breastfeeding, your baby is dependent on you for essential nutrients such as protein, calcium, folic acid and water. These nutrients come either from your current diet or from the stores you built up before conception.

Providing for your own and your baby's needs is not complicated. All you need to do is eat a variety of wholesome foods that are fresh (or minimally processed) from the essential food groups. These are listed on pages 30-31. You also need to avoid a few potentially harmful foods, which are listed on pages 36-37.

The amount of food that you need to eat does not increase that much during pregnancy. However, make sure that you are eating enough to receive certain essential nutrients – especially plenty of fruit and vegetables, so that you get a wide range of vitamins. Other important nutrients for pregnancy are protein, calcium and iron.

Drink plenty of fluid, especially water, unsweetened fruit juices and smoothies. Cut out tea, coffee and alcohol completely for optimum health.

If you feel like a snack, take some healthy protein in the form of almonds or other whole nuts. Combine them with some dried fruit for extra nutrients.

PROTEIN

You need 60-100g (2¼-3¾oz) protein per day, and high-protein foods should constitute about 25 per cent of your diet. Good sources of protein include vegetables, lean meat, chicken, fish, eggs, skimmed milk, nuts, cheese, dried peas, beans and grains.

IRON

Pregnancy results in a large increase in the volume of blood in the mother's body. This means that extra iron is needed to make haemoglobin, the oxygen-carrying pigment found in red blood cells. The more haemoglobin that blood contains, the more oxygen it can carry to the various tissues, including the placenta.

The recommended daily amount (RDA) of iron required during pregnancy is 30mg. The need for iron increases

Iron is an important element of your diet, especially when you are pregnant. Broccoli is a good source, and it also contains essential folic acid.

WHEN NAUSEA STRIKES
If you are suffering from morning sickness, try eating little meals at frequent intervals rather than having one or two large meals. This will help to prevent indigestion and heartburn, too.

particularly in the second and third trimester. Good food sources include breads, cereals, dried peas and beans, broccoli and green leafy vegetables.

CALCIUM

Your daily need for calcium is about 1200mg in pregnancy. Good food sources include milk, all other dairy products and green vegetables. Your growing baby needs calcium to build strong bones and teeth. If you do not take in sufficient from your diet, the baby will take calcium from your bones and teeth. You also need vitamin D – produced in the body after exposure to sunlight and also found in some foods – to help your body to process this mineral.

FOLIC ACID

Your folic acid requirement increases considerably in pregnancy, to 400mcg. High intake before conception will also help reduce the risk of neural tube defects in your baby. You can make sure that you receive enough by taking a daily supplement of 400mcg. You should also try to eat at least one dark green vegetable, such as spinach or broccoli, and two to three servings of fruit a day. Sprinkling wheatgerm on your food and not overcooking it will also help maximize your intake – overcooking food destroys any folic acid.

PROTECTING YOUR BABY

The baby will take the nutrients it needs from the mother's bloodstream through the placenta. Researchers are now learning that the developing baby is much more sensitive to the mother's nutritional status than previously thought. Occasional treats do no harm, but it makes sense to follow a healthy diet throughout your pregnancy. Poor intake of one or more essential nutrients during critical periods in an organ's growth can alter the structure, size and functions of that organ. Mothers who eat an excessive amount and who consume a diet high in saturated fat could be putting their unborn babies at greater risk of heart disease, diabetes and high blood pressure later in life.

AVOIDING CONSTIPATION

Pregnant women often suffer from constipation, which contributes to a general sense of lethargy and bloating. It is caused by hormonal changes, which make the muscles of the digestive and gastrointestinal systems less efficient.

Do not take any drugs for constipation. Instead drink eight to ten glasses of water every day and follow a healthy diet: make sure that you are eating five helpings of fruit and vegetables each day and that you include high-fibre wholegrain cereals in your diet. It can also be helpful to avoid bananas, hard-boiled eggs, Brussels sprouts and red meat for a few days.

ESSENTIAL VITAMINS AND MINERALS

Certain vitamins and minerals are vital for a healthy pregnancy. You may need a higher-than-average daily intake of some nutrients, such as vitamin B1. Use the following list to help you to plan your pregnancy diet:

- **Vitamin B1 or thiamine:** about 1.4mg a day – from enriched breads, cereals, grain products, seeds and nuts.
- **Vitamin B2 or riboflavin:** 1.4mg a day – from meat, dairy produce and cereals.
- **Vitamin B3 or niacin:** from fish, meat, nuts, and wholegrains.
- **Vitamin B6 or pyridoxine:** from chicken, fish, soya beans and oats.
- **Vitamin B12 or cobalamin:** from meat, fish, eggs and milk and also from enriched grain products.
- **Vitamin C:** 50mg – from citrus fruit, tomatoes, red and green peppers, broccoli, cauliflower, spinach and strawberries.
- **Vitamin D:** 10mg a day – from milk, eggs, butter and fortified margarine.
- **Vitamin E:** from margarine, vegetable oils, wholegrains and nuts.
- **Magnesium:** 300mg a day – from dairy products, vegetables and meat.
- **Zinc:** 7-15mg a day – from nuts, wholegrains, legumes and eggs.
- **Vitamin A:** 700mcg a day – from fortified milk, eggs, carrots and dark green leafy vegetables.

Plums and other fruits provide you with beneficial vitamins and help to combat constipation. They can also give you a quick boost when you feel tired.

Your lifestyle checklist

Pregnancy is an exciting time, but it can also be stressful, too. Monitoring the different aspects of your lifestyle is an essential element of good antenatal care. By prioritizing your health, you can make the experience of pregnancy much easier. In particular, you need to be:

- Eating well.
- Sleeping well.
- De-stressing and relaxing.
- Exercising regularly.

YOUR EATING HABITS

Have regular meals and give yourself time to eat in a relaxed way. Avoid eating heavy, fatty foods late at night and do not go out on an empty stomach in the morning. Think about what you are eating and drinking and ask yourself if your daily diet is nurturing you and your baby. Are you providing yourself with sufficient nutrients to maintain your energy and well-being?

Try to cut out snacks that are high in sugar or saturated fat. In particular, avoid the following, or have them only as an occasional treat:

- Crisps.
- Cakes and biscuits.
- Coffee and tea.
- Sweetened drinks.
- Red meat (once a week is ample).
- Fried foods.
- Foods containing white sugar.
- White bread.
- Chocolate.
- Convenience foods and ready meals.
- Salt (particularly in snacks).
- Fast food takeaways.
- Sugar and sweets.

SLEEPING

You need to rest as much as possible to combat the fatigue that is typical of the first trimester. This will help to keep you in good shape for the pregnancy and the birth. Consider whether you are getting enough rest. Ask yourself if you are:

- Tired on waking up.
- Using chocolate or other high-calorie snacks to keep you going during the day.
- Sleepy in the middle of the afternoon.
- Exhausted by a day at work.
- Falling asleep in front of the television.
- Unable to sleep when you get to bed.

All these are signs that you need more sleep and more exercise. Try going to bed half an hour earlier for a week. In the second week, continue going to bed earlier than normal and then get up half an hour earlier every morning as well. Have a drink of water or juice and eat a slice or two of toast, then go for a short walk or practise some stretches at home.

ELIMINATING TOXINS WITH JUICES

Whip up your own juices or smoothies. Most of the body is made up of water, so it can quickly become dehydrated. The vitamins and minerals contained in fruit and uncooked vegetables, together with their high liquid content, make them the ideal food for you and your growing baby. At the same time, nutritious raw juices will help to eliminate potentially harmful toxins from your body. Try the following combinations:

- Cranberry, peach and mango.
- Papaya and melon.
- Gooseberry and apple.
- Radish and cucumber.
- Spinach and lemon.
- Carrot, apple and ginger.
- Pineapple and pink grapefruit.
- Strawberry and nectarine.
- Banana and lemon.
- Carrot and beetroot.
- Cucumber and celery.
- Banana and kiwi fruit.
- Red cabbage, apple and lemon.

A juicer is a great investment, letting you prepare fresh, health-boosting drinks whenever you like.

DE-STRESSING

Stress is not good for you or the baby. Many women feel anxious about whether the baby is developing properly, about whether they are doing the right things to maintain the pregnancy, and about how they will cope with having a baby. In addition, you have to cope with all the normal demands of daily life – at a time when you may be feeling unwell or very tired.

If you are feeling unduly stressed or simply don't seem to be able to relax, then it may help to get some extra support from a complementary therapist. Acupuncture, aromatherapy massage, reflexology, shiatsu and homeopathy can all help to relieve anxiety and stress. It is also important to make sure that you have time to do things that you enjoy – whether that is going for a walk or seeing a film. Try to earmark time for yourself each day. Use this for activities that you really enjoy, or just to sit quietly and rest.

EXERCISE

Gentle exercise helps to boost your circulation, which increases the oxygen and nutrients reaching your baby. It also helps to build muscular strength and stamina, which you need to cope with pregnancy and birth. Any form of exercise will help: walking, swimming and cycling are ideal because they are sustained and rhythmic, providing a workout for the heart and lungs. Exercise taken early in the day will set you up and get the circulation going for the rest of the day. Exercising in the evening will help you to unwind and may enhance sleep, so long as it is not too vigorous.

Chest opener

This Pilates-influenced chest stretch is good to practise if you are feeling stressed or tense during the day. It opens up the upper body, soothing tired muscles, making breathing easier and promoting relaxation and a straight spine – very important for the expectant woman. It is especially helpful if you have been sitting at a desk all day.

1 Standing side-on to a wall, stretch your arm out and place your hand against it as shown. If it feels more comfortable, place your hand so that the fingers are pointing towards the ceiling.

2 Now turn away from the wall, keeping your hand on the wall. This gives a gentle stretch to your chest. Do not force anything, and keep your shoulders relaxed as you turn. Repeat on the other side.

Good ways to exercise

The following forms of exercise can be of particular benefit during pregnancy:

- dancing
- swimming
- walking
- t'ai chi
- Pilates
- yoga

If you are not used to exercising, confine yourself to regular walking or swimming in the first three months. Thereafter, it should be fine to try a new form of exercise provided that you have not experienced any bleeding or other problems. Check with your midwife or doctor first, build up your fitness slowly, and do not to overstretch yourself. Seek out a professional instructor who is used to working with pregnant women.

SWIMMING

A few lengths at your local pool can be remarkably energizing. The water will take the weight of your body so that you can move freely. Swimming helps to improve your suppleness as well as your stamina. It also helps to stimulate blood flow around your body, and thus increases the delivery of oxygen to your growing baby.

You may like to consider taking swimming classes to improve your technique, and to ensure that you are not putting unnecessary strain on your body. The Shaw method is based on Alexander technique, and will help you to use your body in the most efficient way possible. Another great form of water exercise is aqua yoga – literally, yoga in water – and many local pools and leisure clubs offer classes in this.

WALKING

Like swimming, walking is a great form of exercise when you are pregnant. A brisk walk really helps to stimulate your respiratory and cardiovascular systems, which need to be in good form when you are carrying a baby and in preparation for the birth itself. Walking is also good for encouraging circulation in the legs – thus helping to prevent varicose veins – and it gets you out into the open air, which usually encourages good sleep and relaxation. Cycling offers many of the same benefits.

DANCE THERAPY

Going to dance classes is usually good fun, and a great way of socializing, making new friends and maintaining fitness at the same time. You will find a number of

Exercising in water

Doing simple exercises and stretches in water is an especially good idea when you are pregnant because the water is so supportive. The two steps shown below use the water's resistance to help tone your upper

arms, which can accumulate fat during pregnancy. This exercise will also open the chest, helping the heart to work faster as your baby grows, and strengthen the upper body in general, aiding your posture.

1 The water should come up to your neck, so stand with your knees slightly bent, if necessary, or kneel if the water is shallow. Now, with both palms touching, stretch your arms right out in front of you.

2 Turn your hands out and open your arms in a wide, circling movement. Take them as far back as possible, then return to the centre. Repeat several times. Inhale as you stretch out and exhale as you return to the centre.

different dance classes on offer at all kinds of places in your local area, and private classes may also be available – a good way to start if you are self-conscious.

One exciting way of keeping fit during pregnancy could be belly dancing. This gentle, rhythmic exercise promotes muscle strength and stamina, so it can help you to manage pregnancy and labour. Belly dancing originated from a combination of symbolic rituals and sexual display. The undulating movements of the pelvis and abdomen, which involve considerable muscular control, are thought by some to be symbolic of conception and birth. These are usually beneficial during a normal pregnancy, but check with your midwife or doctor first. Look out for classes aimed specifically at pregnant women.

PILATES

A gentle form of exercise that improves flexibility, strength and stamina, Pilates places a strong emphasis on posture and alignment. Pilates works on both mind and body, so it can induce deep relaxation and a sense of greater control over your body, which may be helpful during labour.

Exercises can be tailored to individual needs, so Pilates can be practised safely throughout pregnancy as long as you already understand the basic techniques and avoid certain postures. Seek advice from an experienced, qualified teacher, and be sure to tell them that you are pregnant. If you are new to Pilates, do not start in the first three months of pregnancy.

YOGA

Certain types of yoga are widely recommended for pregnancy, particularly the second and third trimesters. Practised regularly, it strengthens muscles, enhances suppleness and improves posture – all of which are helpful during pregnancy and labour. Yoga also involves breathing exercises, which can help with relaxation.

Specific yoga postures, such as squatting, are particularly helpful for pregnant women; others are not suitable and may be harmful. It is therefore best to attend special antenatal yoga classes, or ask your teacher how to adapt the poses. Do not go to general classes if you are new to yoga, particularly in the first trimester.

T'AI CHI

Sometimes described as 'meditation in motion', t'ai chi is a non-combative martial art that involves moving very slowly through a set routine of postures. You repeat the routine over and over again, producing a flowing, synchronized series of movements.

T'ai chi involves controlled, slow movements, which aim to improve the body's flow of energy. It helps mobilize the joints, improve posture and enhance well-being. T'ai chi aids relaxation and enhances body-awareness. It is generally considered safe in pregnancy.

T'ai chi's flowing, meditative movements will help to enhance your awareness of what is happening to your body and mind during pregnancy.

EXERCISING DURING PREGNANCY

You should exercise regularly (ideally for at least 30 minutes, three times a week) in order to work the muscles and circulation, raise energy and endorphin levels and combat stress.

If you have an established exercise routine, it is safe to continue it provided that there are no problems with the pregnancy, but tell any instructors that you are pregnant. However, you may need to reduce the amount or the intensity of any exercise as you must not overexert or exhaust yourself when pregnant (so avoid long periods of aerobic exercise). Do not let yourself become overheated or dehydrated, as this can reduce blood flow and in turn the supply of oxygen to your baby (drink plenty of water as you exercise). If you experience problems with your pregnancy, such as bleeding or abdominal pain, ask your doctor about the advisability of exercising.

In general, it is not a good idea to start a new, unfamiliar form of exercise in the first months of pregnancy. This is because you can easily cause yourself harm if your technique is incorrect.

Keeping your joints mobile

It is important to keep your body open and flexible, in order to enjoy a pregnancy that is as free as possible from aches and pains, and to help pave the way towards a good, comfortable birth.

Releasing the head, neck and shoulders will help to get you into good posture habits, ease stress and minimize certain kinds of tension headache. It will also help to expand the chest, improving breathing and circulation and so making you feel more energetic and helping to bring plenty of nourishing, oxygen-rich blood to your developing baby. The beauty of the neck and shoulder exercises shown below is that they can be done virtually anywhere, any time, as you sit at your desk at work, watch television or sit on the bus, for example.

Loosening the joints

Anyone can do the following easy stretches, which will help to keep your joints mobile and flexible. They make a good short loosening-up routine for the morning, and can help you to warm up for more aerobic exercise, such as brisk walking on the spot or cycling. Work very gently and go only as far as feels comfortable to you.

RELEASING THE HEAD AND NECK

1 Sit comfortably on the floor, cross-legged or with one leg in front of the other. Place one cushion under your buttocks and another under each knee.

2 Slowly turn your head to the right and bring it back to the centre. Now turn it slowly to the left. Repeat several times, breathing normally as you do so.

3 Now slowly drop your head so that your ear is close to your right shoulder. Return it to the centre, then repeat on the left. Repeat several times.

4 Turn your head to the right, drop your chin close to your chest, then move over to the left. Repeat in the opposite direction. Repeat several times.

RELEASING THE SHOULDERS

1 Bring your shoulders upwards and slightly forwards, until they are close to your ears. Keep breathing as you do so.

2 Then move the shoulders back and down, to make a rotating movement. Repeat this several times.

3 Raise your right arm, bending the elbow. Drop your forearm down so that you can place your palm in your upper back.

4 Hold the elbow with the left hand. Relax the shoulders, and hold for a few moments, breathing deeply. Repeat on the left.

Loosening up the spine helps to keep it strong and supple. A flexible spine is the lynchpin of good, upright posture, which can start to suffer with the weight of a growing baby. Correct posture brings these benefits:

- It holds the uterus in the correct position and opens up more space in the abdominal area, so making pregancy more comfortable for both you and your baby and ensuring that the blood supply to the uterus is not constricted.
- It opens up the chest cavity, which becomes more restricted as your baby grows in size, and so improves breathing and circulation, the benefits of which have been covered opposite.

- It makes you feel and look better and minimizes the backache, cramp and sciatica suffered by so many pregnant women.

Loosening up the hips and legs brings vital benefits. The exercise shown below helps to:

- Rest the lower back and legs, which often feel tired and achy during pregnancy.
- Open up your entire pelvic region, exercising and toning the all-important muscles of the pelvic floor area. Well-toned pelvic muscles help to: keep you comfortable when the baby is pressing against the pelvic floor; ease the baby's actual birth; prevent certain post-natal problems.

RELEASING THE SPINE

1 Place your left hand on your right knee, gently turn the upper body and look over your right shoulder.

2 Drop your shoulders, hold for a few moments, then return to the centre. Keep breathing deeply.

3 Repeat on the other side. Be very gentle, and take care not to push your body into a strong twist.

RELEASING THE HIPS AND LEGS

1 Sit next to a wall, so that the side of your body is facing it. Lie down, moving from your side to your back, and slowly swinging your legs up the wall as you do so. Your buttocks should touch the wall. Rest your head on a cushion and breathe.

2 Bend your knees, bringing the soles of your feet together. Place your hands on your knees and press gently towards the wall. Hold for a few moments, or longer if you like, then release. Do not force this: your flexibility will improve with practice.

3 Slide your legs back up the wall. Remain in this posture for a few minutes if you like, breathing deeply and letting any tension drain away. To come up, bend your knees again and then roll on to your side, before getting up slowly.

Yoga for the first trimester

These easy yoga exercises help to improve the posture, which can be adversely affected during pregnancy. Always take care when practising yoga poses, even simple ones like these. Go only as far as feels comfortable, and keep breathing evenly throughout. Lie down and relax for five minutes afterwards.

Grounding

Your hips, legs and feet take your weight, while the pelvis helps support the upper body. These important muscle groups can be strengthened by this grounding exercise, which allows your weight to pass through the legs and feet into the ground. Practised regularly, it will help you cope with the growing weight of your baby.

1 Stand with the feet apart and knees slightly bent. Keep an upright spine, tucking in your chin and tail bone, and keeping the head erect.

2 Bring your hands into a prayer position. Press your palms firmly together with elbows out to the sides. Do not tense the shoulders.

3 Now spread your hands wide, keeping your elbows bent and opening up your chest area. Breathe in deeply as you do this.

4 Left: Stretch your arms out to the sides and lower them to your sides, breathing out. Repeat steps 2 to 4 several times.

5 Right: For a stronger version of this exercise, place one foot on a low chair and bend the other knee. Change legs after a few breaths and repeat with the other foot on the chair.

Standing stretches

By extending up from the hips and through the waist, you create space for the diaphragm, which helps you to take deeper breaths. Gently turn and sway rhythmically as if you are dancing, but do not go into a strong twist.

1 Left: Stand in an upright, relaxed posture with your knees loosely bent. Stretch your arms overhead, first one and then the other. Feel your ribs and waist opening and releasing.

2 Right: Now bring your arms out at shoulder level and swing round from the waist, first to one side and then the other, without changing your leg or arm position. Repeat both movements.

Adapted easy triangle sequence

This sequence works out your abdominal muscles and increases flexibility in the lower spine. This can help to prevent backache and tone up your muscles. However, make sure that you proceed very gently.

1 Stand tall with feet wide and knees bent. Place your hands on your hips. Sway from side to side, tipping your pelvis up to the right as you sway to the right and up to the left as you sway to the left in a rhythmical movement. Keep your spine erect, coccyx tucked under and chest lifted. Repeat several times.

2 Now bend to your right side without tipping forwards – keep your back straight and do not push yourself further than feels comfortable. Place your right hand along your leg and bring your left elbow back to open the left side of the waist and chest as you look up. Keep breathing rhythmically.

3 Without losing the extension in your back, stretch your left arm up and back to open the left side of your body. Keep your abdomen relaxed and do not tense the right shoulder. Breathe deeply. Now come up slowly and repeat the bend on your left side. Do the exercise several times on both sides.

Creating a balanced life

Being pregnant may mean that you have less energy than usual. It is very important to make time for relaxation and exercise, and this may mean that you have to make adjustments to your daily life.

Your list of priorities will probably run something like this:

- My health and my baby's health.
- My partner.
- My family and friends.
- Work commitments and any other must-do activities.
- Socializing.

Bear this list in mind if you are feeling overwhelmed. Decide what you are going to do – and remind yourself that you cannot do everything. Some things may need to be left undone, others may have to be delegated. Make the following your motto: prioritize, delegate, eliminate.

YOUR QUALITY TIME

You are likely to feel tired when you are pregnant and coping with all the demands of everyday life can sometimes be difficult. Make sure that you prioritize time for yourself, or your own needs are likely to be eclipsed by home and work.

Think about what you would most enjoy, and what would help you to relax most. This could be singing, walking, going for acupuncture treatment, joining a pottery class, salsa, swimming or having a facial. Make sure that you incorporate regular 'me time' into your week so that you can do what gives you pleasure. In addition, make sure you spend at least half an hour, and preferably more, relaxing at home every day.

SHORTCUTS AT HOME

Some things have to give when you are pregnant – and household chores are often a good place to compromise. Cut back so that you do the bare minimum. Ask your partner to do more, or consider hiring some extra help. Here are some good ways to reduce the time you spend.

Shopping

Don't fritter away your time by shopping for food every day or two. Keep shopping down to the minimum – if possible, do one big shop per week. Ask your partner or a friend to come with you, or to do the shopping for you. Wherever possible, get your groceries delivered: investigate local vegetable-box schemes and shop via the Internet for non-perishable items that you don't need to select yourself. Buying teabags, toilet paper, washing

View regular pampering as an important part of your pregnancy care. Relaxing moments and treats help to lift your spirits and raise your energy levels.

powder, tins and other essential items in bulk can save you both time and money.

Cooking

If you can get a good lunch during the working day, you may need only a healthy snack and lots of liquid in the evening. When cooking at home, concentrate on quick and easy, nutritious dishes rather than complex meals. Try the following:

- Home-made soups with wholemeal bread.
- Baked potato and cottage cheese.
- Fish risotto.
- Grilled bacon and tomatoes on wholemeal toast.
- Baked potato with baked beans and poached egg.
- Spaghetti with pancetta and tomatoes.
- Poached salmon with salad and new potatoes.
- Poached chicken with tomatoes and red peppers.
- Fish pie (if made in advance) and vegetables.
- Grilled trout with salad and new potatoes.
- Casseroles (beef, lamb, chicken) or other dishes that you can make ahead of time.

If you feel like a dessert, have something healthy such as:
- Fresh fruit and natural yogurt.
- Bananas and crème fraîche.
- Baked apples.

When cooking dishes such as casseroles or pasta sauces, make double the quantity and freeze the rest for another day. That way, you cook less often and will always have a stock of nourishing food in the house.

Housework
- Wash clothes twice a week at most, and preferably only once.
- Change your bedlinen less often than usual. Once every 10–14 days is fine.
- Iron only what you really have to – don't worry about bedlinen, tea towels, hand towels, undersheets, duvet covers, underwear or T-shirts. If you take washing off the line or out of the dryer as soon as it is dry and fold it immediately, you should not have to iron.
- Remember that your home doesn't have to be pristine – a bit of dust won't harm you.

Take regular time out when you are working – an afternoon break with a cup of herbal tea and a cereal bar can help to refresh you for the rest of the day.

GETTING ON TOP OF WORK
Many women find work a struggle, particularly in the early months of pregnancy when they may be feeling exhausted and nauseous. Here are some ways that can help to make it easier.
- Get to work a little early so that you have some quiet time to yourself to get your breath back from the journey, and have a nutritious drink (chamomile tea, for example, or fresh fruit juice).
- If you control your workload, tackle the most demanding jobs early in the day if possible. Remember the first rule of management: 'Don't touch any piece of paper more than once'. Deal with it, file it or bin it straight away. Treat emails in the same way.
- Do not stand for long periods at work – sit down whenever you can. If you work sitting down, stand up and stretch at regular intervals.
- Take at least 45 minutes for your lunch break. Make this a time to eat and rest rather than an opportunity to go shopping. If you feel very tired, see if you can find a place to take a nap.
- Be sure to get some fresh air at lunchtime – just walking once round the block will really help to refresh you – so that you don't start to feel sleepy halfway through the afternoon.
- Counter a mid-afternoon energy dip with a healthy cereal bar and a cup of herbal tea (keep your favourite herbal tea bags at work). If possible, use this time to do any easier jobs, such as making routine phone calls.
- Take your holiday as and when you should. Don't allow your holiday allocation to slip over from one year to the next.
- Take some of your holiday as single days – say, one day every couple of weeks. Use this time to rest, not to rush around trying to catch up at home.
- Take sick days if you need them. Don't struggle into work if you are feeling poorly. Consider telling your manager why you are taking time off.
- If feasible, work from home at least one day a week, in order to give you a break from travelling.
- When you get home from work, try not to jump straight into your next task. Instead, sit down for half an hour and rest, relax with the newspaper or a book, have a bath, or go for a walk.

66 Remind yourself that you cannot do everything. Some things may need to be left undone, others may have to be delegated. 99

Bonding with your partner

It is important to share feelings and activities with your partner during the long weeks and months of pregnancy. Naturally, most of the attention – from your family doctor, hospital staff and midwives, and from family and friends – will be focused on you. You need to make sure that your partner is fully involved with the pregnancy, the birth itself and of course the baby.

Some men are less interested than women in the physical aspects of pregnancy and birth. However, most will not wish to be excluded from enjoying the growing life inside you – your baby has received the gift of life from both its parents, after all. Do not worry if your partner does seem less excited about the pregnancy than you – at the moment, the baby could seem very abstract to him. As time goes on, and the pregnancy becomes more visible, men tend to become more involved.

ENJOYING THE EARLY DAYS OF PREGNANCY

The baby at eight weeks is now the classic curled shape you see in pictures, with the ears starting to form and little hands that are at the moment webbed.

The highlights of early pregnancy will probably include the first pregnancy test, your doctor's confirmation of the test and then the first signs of the changes that your body is now undergoing.

Then comes the ultrasound scan. At 12 weeks you may not be able to discern a human form, but around 20 weeks you will probably be able to see the baby's head, perhaps in profile, and the shape of his or her body. Most men and women find these milestones completely fascinating. You may find that you study the ultrasound photograph and talk about it endlessly – Is it a boy or a girl? How much detail can you see clearly?

To outsiders, these kinds of intimate chats would seem trivial and pointless, but in fact they perform an important function for you as a couple. They allow you to get used to the idea that your life is about to change. They give you a chance to bring your imagination to bear on the transforming effect of having a baby in your life. They are, in other words, mental preparation.

YOUR PARTNER'S WORRIES

Men often have specific worries about childbirth and the early days of fatherhood. Some men, for example, are not sure in the early stages that they want to be present at the birth. It is not that they do not want to support their partner. Usually, any apprehension is centred on the fear of feeling helpless or useless at a time when their partner is in pain or distress.

This kind of anxiety is normal. It takes most men time to get used to the idea of seeing their child born, and most men are glad, after the event, that they were there.

Conversely, neither of you should forget that men are not in any sense obliged to be there, and should not be railroaded into something that they feel uncomfortable about. Although it is now considered normal for a man to attend the birth, it is not so long since this was considered completely out of the question.

Some men even now will find it less distressing to pace the corridors in the hospital than to hold your hand in the delivery room, and you may decide that this is the best

Remember that your life is not solely concerned with pregnancy. Make a point of going out with your friends and enjoying yourselves when you can.

way to do it for both of you. The main thing is that you and your partner should be able to discuss all of his anxieties frankly and openly. The chances are that, in the drama of it all, his reaction will be completely different from anything that you or he have anticipated.

LIFE OUTSIDE PREGNANCY

Things don't stop – for you or for your partner – just because you are having a baby. Continue to share your other interests, and to enjoy time together as a couple. Show your partner you are still interested in him by continuing to talk about his work, his ups and downs, and all the things that you used to chat about before you became pregnant.

Going for a walk or a swim together before or after work will benefit both of you and the baby, too. Make a point of doing things that are just for fun, and don't neglect your friends: you can still go out and enjoy yourselves. In fact, you should grab the chance, because in the first three months or so of parenthood your attention will focus solely on the baby and it may seem to your friends that you have dropped off the social radar.

> ❝ Things don't stop – for you or for your partner – just because you are having a baby. ❞

CARING FOR YOUR PARTNER

Don't stop supporting your partner just because you are pregnant. It is tempting to put your own needs and emotions first, but remember that he may feel ill or depressed some days, and needs you as much as ever.

Think of ways to make your partner feel special: for example, take time to show a real interest in one of his hobbies; go to see the films he wants to see several times in a row and generally give in to him a little more than usual. Encourage him to share his feelings with you and share yours with him. Show him that you care about him all the more now that you are expecting a baby together.

Affection and companionship are the cement that binds a couple together. A good relationship helps us feel secure and strong, and ready for parenthood.

Routine antenatal care

By the eighth or ninth week of your pregnancy, you should have seen your family doctor and registered for antenatal care. If not, then make an appointment as soon as possible. Where you actually receive your antenatal care, and the type of care that you receive, is usually linked with where you ultimately want your baby to be delivered. The first consultation – commonly called the booking-in appointment – is usually held at the maternity unit of your local hospital, where you can discuss your future care. You will be referred here by your family doctor.

It is useful to have an idea of where you would like the baby to be born, and to have discussed this with your partner, before the first antenatal appointment. However, don't worry if you are not sure – there is plenty of time to make a decision and you can, of course, change your mind at a later date.

HOSPITAL-BASED CARE
If you have chosen to have your baby in hospital, then you will probably see hospital staff two or three times during your whole pregnancy. Your family doctor or community midwife will undertake the rest of the care. You will probably be seen at the hospital for a booking-in appointment at around 10 to 12 weeks, then again at about 34 or 36 weeks and once more when your baby is finally due.

If you prefer all the antenatal visits to be carried out at the hospital where you will have your baby, your family doctor can arrange this for you.

FAMILY DOCTOR OR COMMUNITY CARE
You may be able to have all your antenatal care in your family doctor's surgery or at the community midwives' office, particularly if you have decided to have your baby at home and so long as there are no problems with your pregnancy. You should discuss your preferences at the first booking appointment.

DOMINO SCHEME
The word Domino stands for Domiciliary In/Out. This is a scheme in which a community midwife shares your antenatal care with the hospital and your family doctor, sometimes visiting you at home to do the routine antenatal checks. The midwife will look after you at home, take you into hospital, deliver your baby and then arrange for you to return home within 48 hours of the birth.

MIDWIFE DELIVERY
You may choose to have a midwife be responsible for all your antenatal care and the delivery. In this case, you may not see a doctor during your pregnancy, except for the initial referral and unless the midwife becomes concerned about the pregnancy.

Your midwife or doctor should be happy to discuss any fears or questions that you have about your pregnancy.

TESTS

By around 12 weeks, you will have an appointment at your antenatal clinic – probably the first of several. This first visit is intended to ascertain whether or not your pregnancy and delivery are likely to be normal. Routine checks will be done, including your weight, blood pressure, urine and blood. You may be offered an HIV test. The midwife will examine your abdomen to check the size of your uterus.

You can discuss screening procedures during this visit and are likely to be offered a routine ultrasound scan, usually done around weeks 10 to 12, to check the baby is developing normally. There are other diagnostic tests available, such as nuchal fold ultrasound, triple alphafetoprotein (AFP) and amniocentesis. You don't need to decide what tests, if any, you would like to go ahead with straight away: take time to consider the options.

YOUR FIRST ULTRASOUND

You will be asked to drink a pint of water before your appointment so that you have a full bladder for the ultrasound. This causes the uterus to be pushed outwards so that it – and the baby – can be clearly seen.

You lie down for the scan with your abdomen bared. Your skin is covered with a gel, because soundwaves cannot travel through air. The sensor or probe has to make direct airtight contact with your skin. The probe is placed on your abdomen and you will see an almost incomprehensible picture on a screen next to you.

The operator will explain what you can see. You should be able to see the baby moving and you will see its heart beating from the seventh week and hear it from the tenth week. Because the baby is so small, it is not possible to see if it is a boy or girl at this stage.

It is important to drink plenty of water before an ultrasound. A full bladder pushes the uterus outwards so that the baby can be seen clearly.

WHO'S WHO IN THE ANTENATAL TEAM

These are the people who may be involved in your pregnancy care:

- **Consultant obstetrician:** senior hospital specialist in charge of maternity care.

- **Consultant pediatrician:** senior hospital specialist in charge of newborn babies and children.

- **Registrar:** senior doctor who is junior to the consultant and resident in the hospital.

- **Senior house officer:** junior hospital doctor undertaking next level of training and able to call upon the registrar for advice if necessary.

- **Midwife:** nurse specializing in the management of normal pregnancy and labour.

- **Family doctor:** many family doctors undertake much of the antenatal work but few supervise delivery.

- **Health visitor:** about ten days after midwife care finishes, the health visitor takes over. She will advise on the care of your baby and help you deal with any problems.

- **Anaesthetist:** doctor specially trained in giving general and local anaesthesia, including epidurals.

- **Radiologist:** doctor who interprets pictures from imaging techniques, such as X-rays and ultrasounds.

- **Radiographer:** health professional, not a doctor, who performs imaging techniques.

- **Physiotherapist:** health professional who teaches antenatal care and exercises, helps to combat the pain of labour and is skilled in teaching muscle-strengthening exercises and dealing with other ligament and joint problems that occur during or after pregnancy.

- **Social worker:** assists with social problems that may occur during or after pregnancy. Social workers have special counselling skills for women who have emotional or social problems and bridge the gap between the family doctor and the health visitor.

- **Medical students:** may observe antenatal care, labour and delivery as part of their training. Students are required to undertake a certain number of normal deliveries under supervision and to learn certain procedures such as repairing an episiotomy. You have the right to ask for students not to be present.

Tests and specialist care

It is natural to worry about whether your baby is developing normally, but remind yourself that around 97 per cent of pregnancies end in the safe delivery of a healthy baby – and that your antenatal team is there to ensure that any problems are picked up quickly. As well as routine antenatal care, you will be offered diagnostic tests, used to identify serious problems with the baby.

SPECIALIST TESTS

Many women find it reassuring to have diagnostic tests done, but some do not. You are under no obligation to have any of the tests you are offered: you and your partner have the right to decide what is best for you. It is important to remember that no test is 100 per cent accurate, and tests cannot detect all abnormalities.

Chorionic villus sampling

This test is usually carried out at nine to ten weeks (or at any rate not after week 13) and can be used to diagnose Down's syndrome. It can also detect the same chromosome abnormalities as amniocentesis and other genetic disorders such as sickle-cell anaemia and thalassaemia. It is also possible to detect the sex of the

> **“ Around 97 per cent of pregnancies end in the safe delivery of a healthy baby. ”**

fetus and this may be of value if there is a known sex-linked condition in the family.

A narrow plastic tube is passed into the uterus through the cervix and some cells from the developing placenta are drawn off. Some doctors may insert a needle through the abdominal wall rather like amniocentesis, using ultrasound to guide them. The results should be known after ten days. The risk of miscarriage after the test is one in 100, which is higher than with amniocentesis.

Nuchal fold ultrasound

The nuchal fold ultrasound is also known as the nuchal fold or the translucency scan. It is done at about 11-14 weeks, and it is used to predict Down's syndrome cases. The procedure is the same as that for a routine ultrasound, but the operator concentrates on getting a good image of the fetus's neck on the screen and then measures a layer of fluid at the back of the neck. The thicker this layer is, the greater the chance the baby will have Down's syndrome. The chance or risk is expressed as a probability such as a one in 10,000 chance or a one in 100 chance. Depending on the risk identified, you may be advised to have further tests such as amniocentesis.

Doppler ultrasound

This ultrasound is an advanced form of ultrasound imaging and is available only in some specialist hospitals. It can be used to diagnose more accurately the well-being of the baby if previous tests have shown that it is not growing sufficiently well.

The Doppler scanner can identify the veins and arteries through which blood flows and can detect the speed at which the blood is travelling. As this indicates how much oxygen the baby is receiving, it also predicts if a placenta is not functioning well. Colour Doppler is a more sophisticated technique than standard Doppler, and its benefits are still being evaluated.

Later tests

Amniocentesis or the alphafetoprotein test may also be offered as part of your antenatal care. These tests are carried out in the second trimester – see pages 138-141.

WHAT IS DOWN'S SYNDROME?

Normal babies have 23 pairs of chromosomes: 46 in total. In Down's syndrome, there is an extra chromosome – usually in the 21st pair. This causes various physical and mental abnormalities.

pair of chromosomes

extra chromosome

RISK FACTORS

Some women have a higher risk of carrying a baby with abnormalities than others. Doctors have identified certain risk factors, including the mother's age, her or her partner's medical history and the outcome of previous pregnancies. These factors do not mean that you will develop problems in this pregnancy, only that you have a statistically higher risk of doing so than women who are not affected by the same risk factors. Because of this, you may be monitored more closely by the medical team.

TWINS AND MULTIPLE PREGNANCIES

If you are expecting twins or more, you will be more closely monitored throughout your pregnancy. You will probably need more assistance during and after the delivery, so a home birth may not be advisable. Fatigue and nausea may be increased throughout the pregnancy. Twin or multiple pregnancies are usually shorter than the norm: about 37 weeks rather than 40.

INHERITED DISEASES

You should tell the doctor at your first antenatal check if any of the following or any inherited diseases are known in your family or in your partner's family:

- Single gene defects such as Huntington's chorea/disease, cystic fibrosis and sickle-cell anaemia.
- Disorders linked to damage on the X-chromosome such as haemophilia and muscular dystrophy.

During an ultrasound, the operator will explain what you can see on the screen. You will be able to ask any questions that you have and discuss the findings.

- Chromosomal defects such as Down's syndrome.
- Neural tube defects, which include anencephaly and spina bifida.

GENETIC COUNSELLING

You may be offered this to assess the likelihood of certain problems in your pregnancy. It is most often offered to:
- Women over the age of 35, because there is an greater risk of the baby being affected by Down's.
- Parents of a child with a genetic abnormality, a neural tube defect or other form of physical impairment.
- Women who have a tendency to miscarry.
- Couples with known chromosome abnormalities.
- Women who may be carriers of X-linked disorders (such as haemophilia).
- Couples whose family members have a high incidence of a certain disease.
- Couples whose ethnic or racial backgrounds increase the likelihood of a particular problem such as sickle-cell anaemia, thalassaemia or Tay-Sachs disease.

If you believe you need genetic counselling but you have not been offered it, discuss the reasons with your family doctor or consultant.

Checklist of common problems

The first trimester brings its own distinct symptoms. Many first-trimester complaints can be eased by complementary therapies, but always seek advice from a qualified therapist and check any therapies and remedies with your midwife or doctor.

If a complaint persists or troubles you, or you are not sure what it is, consult your family doctor. In any case, mention any problem at your next antenatal check. Do not take any over-the-counter drugs (or prescription drugs left over from pre-pregnancy) unless you have checked that they are safe in pregnancy with the pharmacist, your doctor or a consultant.

Anxiety There are many things that women worry about while pregnant, and anxiety is especially common during the early stages of pregnancy because the whole experience is new and unfamiliar and also because miscarriage is most common during the first trimester. Discuss particular worries or persistent anxiety with your doctor or midwife. You will also find that breathing exercises and meditation will lower general anxiety levels very effectively.

Bleeding Bleeding or spotting is not uncommon during the first three months. The cause may never be found or it may spring from a variety of causes, such as a minor infection. However, there may be more potentially dangerous reasons, so always get any bleeding or spotting checked out.

Breast soreness One of the classic early signs of pregnancy, sore, sensitive or unusually tender breasts can be relieved greatly by a professionally fitted maternity bra. You will find that this symptom usually eases after the first trimester.

Fainting You may feel slight faintness alongside morning sickness and a general feeling of being under par. However, if faintness is persistent or regular, or you actually faint or feel like you are going to, then you should drink plenty of water and consult your family doctor without delay.

Fatigue Tiredness is the frequent complaint of many pregnant women, particularly during the first trimester, when hormonal changes put the woman's body under unfamiliar strains. The simple answer is to make sure that you go to bed earlier and take naps whenever you

Headaches are a regular occurrence for many pregnant women, and may accompany the general feelings of being unwell that often occur in the first trimester. Acupressure can be especially helpful in esing symptoms, but always seek out professional advice about using this.

can. However, fatigue can be a symptom of anaemia, so extreme tiredness should be always be checked out properly by a doctor.

Headache Troublesome headaches are another symptom that can accompany general under-par feelings in early pregnancy, as hormonal changes make themselves felt. If headaches persist for more than two days, you must consult your family doctor without delay.

Acupuncture can be a useful therapeutic tool in relieving headaches. Massage can prove very effective, because it relieves the muscle tension that causes so many headaches and also improves blood circulation. Chamomile tea soothes headache symptoms, as can lavender oil – just three or four drops on a compress, applied to the temples. Good homeopathic remedies to try include calc carb, arsen alb, and nux vomica.

Insomnia Many women have problems sleeping during pregnancy – at first because of bodily changes and perhaps early anxiety, and then later because the increasing bulk of your growing baby can make it difficult to find a comfortable position. Perhaps the most important strategy here is to establish a regular night-time routine – for example, have a warm bath and a milky drink at night and go to bed at the same time. Do not eat late at night and avoid salty, sugary, fatty and spicy foods. Do not drink tea or coffee at night, as the caffeine is over-stimulating; chamomile tea is a very soothing night-time drink. Getting into these good habits as early as possible during pregnancy will mean that you don't suddenly have to impose them later on.

Complementary therapies have much to offer where insomnia is concerned. Ask your partner to give you a gentle massage in the evening. Walk or swim regularly, early in the morning or during the day, perhaps at lunchtime. A medical herbalist, homeopath or acupuncturist may also be able to help.

Morning sickness This is the main symptom associated with the first trimester and includes general feelings of nausea and actual vomiting. Despite its name, this sickness is not confined to mornings – some women feel nauseous only in the evening, some only in the morning and some at intervals all through the day.

The precise cause of morning sickness is unknown, but is assumed to relate to hormonal changes. Start the day with dry toast and a cup of tea. Eat light meals and take small, frequent drinks. Avoid fats and fatty and spicy foods. Reiki may help, and you might also like to consult a medical herbalist or a homeopath – good homeopathic remedies include ipecac, nux vomica and pulsatilla (See also pages 88-89.)

Stretchmarks Marks caused by stretching of the skin as your baby grows are common during pregnancy, and may persist afterwards. Get into the habit of moisturizing this area as early on as possible, so that, when the skin starts to be stretched, it is supple and marking is minimal. To do this, massage the abdomen, thighs and buttocks regularly (and gently) with vitamin E oil.

Urinary infection This is common in pregnancy, but should always be treated without delay. Signs include the need to race to the lavatory, burning or stinging upon urination, a need to pass urine frequently, difficulty in passing urine or passing urine flecked with blood. See your doctor straight away if you have any of these symptoms or suspect the possibility of infection.

In order to allay infection, make sure that you always drink plenty of water. Cranberry juice is very effective at keeping the urinary tract healthy and able to stave off potential problems.

Urination, frequent This is something most women have to put up with in pregnancy and especially during the first trimester. It is typically caused by hormone changes and the growing uterus pushing on the bladder

Milky drinks taken before bedtime may help to ease the insomnia that so often accompanies early pregnancy.

and decreasing its size. Do not drink less as this can lead to an infected urinary tract. In fact, the frequent urination may actually be caused by a urinary infection – tell your doctor if you have any signs of this (see above).

Vaginal discharge Consult your family doctor straight away if you notice unusual or heavy discharge.

This long list may make it seem as though pregnancy is fraught with problems. However, the great majority of women do not experience any serious difficulties. Many symptoms, including nausea, will not last long. They can be uncomfortable but most have no serious effects.

SEEKING ADVICE

If you are worried by any symptom, do not hesitate to call or visit your doctor.

See your doctor straight away if you have:
- A high temperature (38.5°C/101°F or above).
- Swelling of the hands and ankles.

Seek emergency assistance if you have:
- Vaginal bleeding other than spotting.
- Severe abdominal pain.
- Excessive vomiting.
- Sudden swelling of the hands and ankles or blurred vision with a severe headache.

Common Qs and As

Q: My partner and I are expecting our first baby in about six months' time, but he does not seem as excited as I am. Should I be worried?

A: Many men do not fully appreciate the wonder of new life until the baby is actually born and named: in other words when the baby has a tangible identity. This probably sounds awful to the newly pregnant woman, but don't despair. Once the baby is born, the man is usually fantastically proud, wanting to show off his little girl or little boy to everyone.

Q: My mother and my mother-in-law keep dropping broad hints about our starting a family – and we ourselves have wanted this for a long time. Now I am pregnant, but I am loath to tell anyone until I am absolutely sure everything is all right. Both of us are finding the pressure hard to take. What should we do?

A: Carry on fending off their enquiries as best you can. They will understand once you get to the 12th week and tell them the happy news. A word of warning, though: don't let them take over your pregnancy with lots of well-meaning advice. Tell them you that want to do things your own way and remind them that you are receiving good antenatal care. When the baby comes along, remind yourself that it is your child, not theirs, and set boundaries if you have to. Go with your own instincts about what to do – or seek professional advice.

Q: We had not intended to start a family quite so soon and my pregnancy has taken us both by surprise. Now the weeks seem to be whizzing by and I feel as if I cannot quite catch up. What can I do?

A: How lovely not to have to plan when to start your family. Don't worry, you and your partner will soon be rejoicing in your good fortune. In the meantime, make a list of all the things that you think you would like to do before the baby comes. Consider whether all these tasks are essential – if not, eliminate them. Work out how you will achieve these, month by month, making allowances for the fact that you will be feeling tired, especially in the latter months of pregnancy. Consider what you can delegate to others, and what you want to do yourself.

Q: I am not sure if I want all the tests to do with antenatal care but I don't know what to say to the doctor.

A: One of the benefits of having the tests is to receive confirmation that there is nothing wrong with the baby. Another benefit is that some problems can be treated in the uterus. Alternatively, hospital staff may arrange to have relevant specialists on hand at the delivery if they know of a potential problem. They will also arrange for the baby's well-being to be monitored through the hours of labour and delivery, and, if necessary, they will perform a Caesarean.

You are not obliged to have any test – and some women feel strongly that they do not want to do so. The best thing to do is to talk over your feelings with your midwife or family doctor so that he or she understands your perspective and can advise you accordingly. You can take your partner or a good friend to the appointment if you feel you need extra support. It can also be helpful to contact natural childbirth organizations for a different point of view.

Q: We are expecting twins and don't know how to tell our two-year-old the news. We are also worried how he will react when the twins arrive, since he will inevitably receive less attention in the future than he has been used to. What do you advise?

A: Children can become very excited about the birth of a brother or sister, even if they subsequently feel rather jealous of them. It's a good idea to tell children about a pregnancy when it is advanced enough to be visible. Show him your bump and let him touch it. Explain that there is a baby inside – he might like to try to talk to it. Show him any scan pictures you have as well. As your pregnancy progresses, your son will enjoy feeling the baby kick.

The fact that you have anticipated problems after the birth is half the battle. Your little boy may feel somewhat eclipsed because twins do demand a lot of attention, and they usually attract wonder and admiration from friends and family.

You need to keep in mind your little boy's need to be admired himself, and express daily your love for him. Perhaps you could arrange for someone else to look after the twins for a short period each day so that you can concentrate on your little boy.

Two is not an easy age in any case, when your little boy will, quite naturally, start to express his independence. Signs of temper and disobedience are all part of this and will not necessarily be related to the birth of the twins. Chat to your health visitor about this when the time comes so that she can give you useful tips for your individual situation.

Q: I have a hugely demanding job and cannot imagine how I can cope with pregnancy and then look after a small baby while I continue to work.

A: First, you will be on maternity leave – perhaps for as long as six months or a year. Second, someone else will be doing your job while you are away. Third, you will find that the pregnancy hormones will have the effect of slowing you down. While it may seem unthinkable at the moment, you will find ways of reducing the work demands made upon you as time goes on.

Ultimately, you will be compelled to make some difficult choices. Will you give up your job and stay at home? Could you job-share? Would working part-time be an option? Could you return to work full-time six weeks or so after the baby's birth and have a childminder or a nanny? Could you get help in the home to help you to cope?

You will not know what is really right for you until after the delivery of the baby. For the time being, concentrate on your work and your pregnancy, and deal with any problems only when and if they arise.

Q: I am self-employed and will need to return to work quite quickly after the birth. How can I keep my clients happy in the last month of my pregnancy and in those first few weeks?

A: You will need to cut down the hours that you work for a few weeks before the delivery, and you will not be able to return for a few weeks afterwards. Tell your clients your situation when you are about six months pregnant, so that you can prepare them for your absence. It may be worth employing someone to cover for you, or to take over essential administration. Avoid becoming overtired; stick to early nights and catnap in the afternoon if you can.

The second trimester

> **"** Many women find that they are glowing with good health and vitality. **"**

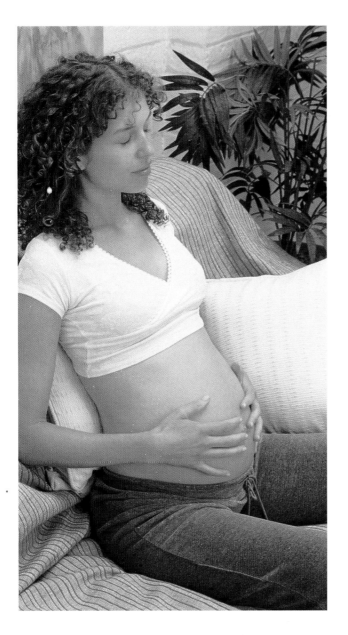

The second three months are often the best and the happiest stage of a woman's pregnancy. You are now past the early weeks in which the chance of miscarriage is high, and the 12-week scan is already behind you. This is the best stage at which to enjoy your pregnancy and start making plans for the birth.

By this time, most women are no longer suffering from sickness and the overwhelming fatigue brought on by the hormonal changes of the first few weeks. Better still, many women find that they are glowing with good health and vitality. You will most likely experience a growing sensation of well-being during the second trimester, and you may well look as good as you feel. Your eyes may shine, your hair may be thick and lustrous, and your skin may be clear, smooth and luminous.

This is an exciting period, too. You and your partner can see your body changing from week to week, and with each week passing you are better able to visualize your growing baby. You are likely to

As the second trimester progresses, you can watch your baby growing week by week. The extra weight may cause tiredness, so rest whenever you can.

be very physically aware of your pregnancy, but as yet the baby is not big enough to slow you down too much and prevent you from doing the things that you want to do. Enjoy it.

Continue to look after yourself as well as possible. Be aware that the steadily increasing size of the baby inside you is starting to place pressure on your spine. This may lead to backache and extreme tiredness if you don't take preventative steps. Check your posture at all times, standing tall and sitting with your back firmly upright and supported. Yoga will help to strengthen your back at this stage, and this is also valuable preparation for labour. Similarly, Alexander technique classes can provide many tips for relaxed but upright postures and movement.

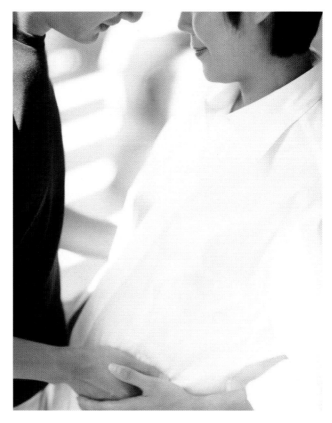

Top: For many women, the second trimester brings a wonderful sense of well-being, with morning sickness a thing of the past and a new lustre to skin and hair.

This is the time to enjoy your pregnancy to the full. Share the excitement and sensations of each new development with those closest to you.

Growth from twelve weeks

By the end of the third month of pregnancy (12 or 13 weeks), your baby has become a recognizable human being. All the body's structures and organs have formed. Your baby's arms and legs, fingers and toes have all developed, although they are still very small.

The baby's sexual characteristics are developing at this time. The boy's penis is emerging, while a girl's cervix, vagina, uterus and ovaries will already have formed. If the baby is a girl, she will at the moment have in her ovaries about 4-5 million eggs, a number that drops to 2-3 million by the time she is born.

The baby's heartbeat is stronger; it is not yet audible with a stethoscope, but it can be heard with a hand-held electronic device. The placenta has started to function, giving your baby the nourishment he or she needs. Your baby will start to practise breathing movements for the first time between weeks 12 and 16.

During the second trimester of your pregnancy, your baby will be developing at an astonishing rate. He or she will increase in weight from 10g to over 600g (¼oz to 1lb 5oz). This growth will be reflected in your growing size and in your continued need for rest.

At the start of the second trimester – which spans weeks 13 or 14 to around week 26 – the baby is still tiny and so you probably won't have a bump.

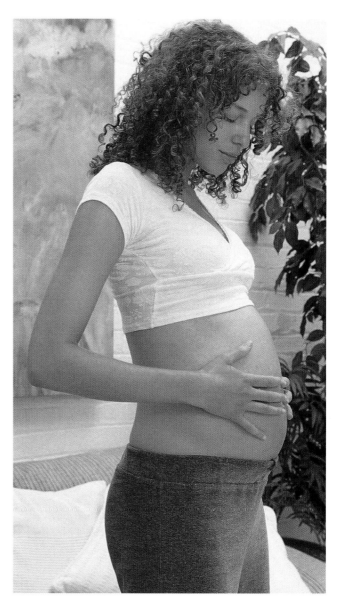

As your pregnancy develops, you will see your belly growing more noticeable. By the end of this second term, you will be quite obviously pregnant.

At week 12, your baby is about 60mm (2⅜in) long, measured from the crown of the head to the rump. He or she weighs about 9-13g (¼–½oz). He or she will have doubled in size in the last three weeks.

By now your baby is able to move his or her jaw and yawn. He or she can also suck and swallow – vital preparation for the life ahead. It is also around this time that the fingernails and toenails start to develop.

Week 13

The length of your baby, measured from crown to rump, will be about 65-80mm (2½-3¼in). If you include the legs as well, his or her length will be 100mm (4in). He or she will weigh about 14-20g (½-¾oz). The eyelids meet and fuse together. They will not now open again for several weeks. An ultrasound taken at this time may show that your baby now puts a thumb in his or her mouth. The baby's skin is transparent and rosy red in colour, because you can see the blood vessels beneath the skin. The skeleton is becoming stronger, hardening as cartilage gradually develops into bone.

Week 14

The baby now measures about 80–115mm (3¼–4¼in), crown to rump and weighs about 25g (1oz). The face is well developed with all the facial features recognizable. The cheeks and bridge of the nose appear, the ears move to a higher position on the head, and the eyes come closer together. As the baby develops more muscle tissue, he or she starts twisting and kicking and waving the arms within the amniotic sac. You are unlikely to feel your baby's movements because he or she still has plenty of space in which to splash around. A baby responds to gentle touch at this stage, and also moves away from threatening stimuli. During amniocentesis, babies have been seen to move away from the needle.

Week 15

Your baby is now a recognizable human being, but he or she is not yet capable of independent life. The baby weighs about 80g (2¾oz) and is 10cm (4in) long. His or her fingernails are developing.

GOING PUBLIC

Your pregnancy is bound to become obvious during the second trimester, not least because your bump is increasingly difficult to hide. You are past the most dangerous time for miscarriage, and will very probably have had the 12-week scan. This should give you the reassurance that your baby is growing normally. Now is the time to share your good news with family and friends, and to start making plans for the future.

EARLY SECOND TRIMESTER

The baby's rapid development is sustained by a constant supply of nutrients, drawn from the mother's blood supply via the umbilical cord, and a network of blood vessels in the placenta.

WEEK 14

uterus
spine
umbilical cord
fetus
placenta
amnion
amniotic fluid
cervix
bladder
vagina
rectum

Week 16

Your baby is now growing and gaining weight very quickly, He or she has grown to about 16cm (6in) in length and weighs about 110g (3¾oz). The baby is now moving around a great deal, although you are still unable to feel these movements. The baby's head is able to turn, the mouth open and the chest and stomach move up and down as if he or she were breathing deeply. The baby can also yawn and stretch, and even frown.

There is a growth of fine hair, known as lanugo, all over the baby's body. The head still looks very large compared with the rest of the body. The placenta is now completely developed. The baby's tiny toenails are forming.

Week 17

A baby now weighs about 150g (5oz), and the reproductive organs are fully formed. The baby passes water containing waste products every 40-45 minutes. Much of this waste passes through the placenta and into your own circulation. You then excrete it through your urine and sweat.

Weeks 18-19

By now your baby weighs about 200g (11oz). Between now and the 20th week, you may become aware of the baby's movements, which will feel like soft ripples. The arms and legs are well formed, and he or she does a lot of kicking, bumping, twisting and turning within the amniotic sac. The baby is able to move quite freely within the sac, and is lying in salt water, which gives extra buoyancy. The wall of the uterus is springy, so the baby can push against it with the feet, hands or head, then bounce off it.

Many babies are especially energetic in the evening when their mothers are more relaxed. You are most likely to feel the first signs of life – a little kick – at this time.

One of the most exciting thoughts of all is the fact that your baby is now able to make simple facial expressions, such as pleasure and distaste. His or her tastebuds are starting to form.

Weeks 20-23

The baby now measures 25cm (10in) in length, and he or she weighs between 260g and 280g (9-10oz). His or her head is still large in proportion to the rest of the body: this signifies the brain's spectacular importance in all aspects of the baby's development. The teeth are beginning to form in the jawbone, and the hair is starting to grow.

By this stage, your baby will be completely covered in an oily layer known as vernix. The vernix comprises fatty

---

CONTINUING DEVELOPMENT

By the end of the second trimester, the baby is well developed, with hair, fingernails and eyelashes all in place. His or her movements have become increasingly energetic. The baby's eyes will open for short periods in the next month. He or she will be able to see light, and will be aware of different sounds.

WEEK 20

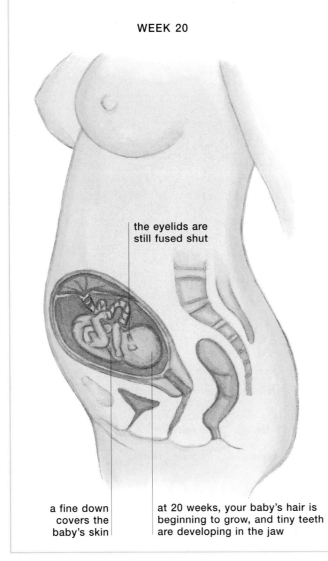

the eyelids are still fused shut

a fine down covers the baby's skin

at 20 weeks, your baby's hair is beginning to grow, and tiny teeth are developing in the jaw

WEEK 24

toenails and fingernails are fully developed

the baby has eyelashes and eyebrows

This detailed scan shows the baby's hands up by her face. She may be sucking her thumb at this stage in an instinctive action that helps prepare for feeding later on.

material and dead skin cells. This acts as a protective coating (in a sense, waterproofing the skin against the amniotic fluid). It remains present until the birth, when it helps to protect the baby during his or her passage down the birth canal and delivery into the outside world.

You may now be very conscious of your baby's movements, which feel like fluttering. At around this 20-week point, the key ultrasound scan – the mid-pregnancy one – is done. Most hospitals recommend this so that they can be well prepared for any problems that may arise at delivery time.

Week 24

The baby is well developed in most respects by now, but his or her lungs are not capable of functioning fully. A baby born at this stage stands a reasonable chance of survival, but would need to remain in an intensive baby care unit and be given assistance with breathing.

The baby is getting longer and is still quite thin. Creases are visible on the palms and fingertips, and the skin is red and wrinkled. The fingernails have completely formed by now.

> 66 If your baby was to be born at 24 weeks, he or she would stand a reasonable chance of survival. 99

The baby may be sucking his or her thumb and may be hiccuping a lot. He or she is learning to co-ordinate sucking and swallowing in preparation for feeding after delivery. The organs of balance inside the ears have developed and are the same size as an adult's. The baby will be able to hear sounds from within and outside your body from about week 21, although it is very unlikely that he or she will be able to make sense of those sounds yet.

The baby's eyes begin to open occasionally but they do not remain open until about week 27. He or she now has delicate eyelashes and eyebrows, and can perceive light through the abdominal wall. The baby is now about 33cm (13in) in length. He or she has been gaining in weight rapidly in the last few weeks. Now that you are six months' pregnant, your baby will weigh approximately 570g-630g (1lb 3oz-1lb 6oz).

Once the baby's weight starts to make itself felt, it can be all too tempting to slump, causing painful back problems. Always try to sit with your spine upright and your back properly supported.

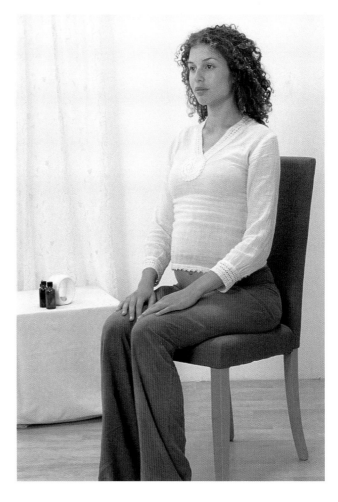

How your body is changing

In the early weeks of the second trimester, you will feel very aware of your pregnancy. It will become obvious to other people at this stage, but you can still disguise the small bump by wearing loose clothing if you wish. You may still be suffering with morning sickness but this will almost certainly wear off very soon.

Your body will undergo many complex changes during the second trimester. Some of the changes that started in the first three months of your pregnancy will also become much more noticeable in the next few weeks.

At the beginning of this trimester, your uterus is the size of a large grapefruit; the top of the uterus will be swelling out just above your navel by the time you reach the third trimester. Food takes longer to digest now – about twice as long as before you were pregnant – so you may feel congested or bloated.

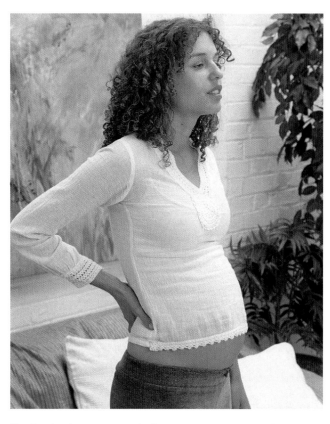

Backache is common during pregnancy, so make sure that your back is always well supported.

STANDING TALL
You can alleviate backache to some extent by maintaining good posture. Keep your shoulders back but relaxed. Avoid jutting your head forwards; keep it back and tuck your jaw into your chin.

This posture increases pressure on the spine.

Standing tall helps your back muscles.

COMMON SIGNS AND SOLUTIONS
Your clothes may start to feel uncomfortable, so choose trousers and skirts with elasticated waists. Wear loose sweaters, T-shirts or tunics on top.

Because your uterus is pressing against the bladder, you will probably feel the need to pass water urgently and frequently. Some women may need to wear an ultra-thin panty liner to catch any leaks. Your breasts will be much larger. You should be professionally fitted with a good bra in a larger back size and larger cup size.

You may be suffering from backache. This is very common during pregnancy, and is a result of your increased weight and altered posture, combined with the effect of the pregnancy hormones upon the muscles of the back. It can be a good idea to invest in a pelvic belt to give your back increased support. Practising yoga or Pilates on a regular basis can also significantly alleviate back pain, and it can often prove helpful to visit a chiropractor or osteopath.

Your heart is beating more strongly and faster than usual in order to pump an increased volume of blood around your body and into the placenta to feed the growing baby. There are more blood vessels in the vagina than before, and it will gradually become darker and softer. The nipples and surrounding areolae will be noticeably darker because of a general increase of pigmentation in your body. This increased pigmentation affects pregnant women in varying degrees, depending on their skin type and natural colouring. Women with pale skin will probably see very little change, while olive-skinned women may notice that their skin goes several shades darker everywhere, particularly around the nipples and areolae.

A dark line down the centre of the abdomen, known as the linea nigra, usually appears around the 14th week. It may be up to 1cm (½in) wide, and may stretch from the pubic hair to the navel. In some women, it reaches as far up as the breastbone. The linea nigra usually fades after delivery. If you have any birthmarks, moles or freckles, these too may darken during pregnancy.

Some women develop blotchy brown patches, called chloasma, on the face and neck. These will be intensified by the sunlight, so it is best to avoid the sun if you are affected. Chloasma usually fades after delivery, and disappears completely within around three months of the delivery of the baby.

Because of the complex hormonal changes taking place within your body, your skin may develop a healthy bloom. You can enhance this by regular walking, which will also strengthen all your muscles in preparation for labour. You may also notice how shiny and luxuriant your hair looks: this, again, happens for hormonal reasons. Once you have given birth, you will shed a lot of hair, but this is nothing to worry about.

STRETCHMARKS

Some women develop stretchmarks on their breasts, abdomen, thighs and buttocks during pregnancy. These develop for two reasons. The extra weight and bulk you are gaining causes the collagen bundles of the skin to stretch so much that they tear. The increased levels of hormones in the blood disrupt the protein in the skin, making it thinner and more delicate than usual.

Stretchmarks show as pale wavy stripes on the skin. They tend to fade a little after the baby is delivered, but they will not disappear altogether. For this reason, it is best to do everything you can to prevent them: daily massage with vitamin E oil or essential oils, and care with your diet, may help.

Try to avoid excessive weight gain and make sure that your diet contains foods that are rich in vitamins B, C and E, as well as zinc and silica. Silica is found in wholegrains, green leafy vegetables, potatoes, nuts and seeds. A healthy diet that includes these foods will help to maintain the elasticity of your skin.

LOOKING AFTER YOUR FEET

Your feet enlarge during pregnancy, partly because of extra fluid in the body and partly because of the extra weight you are carrying. Some women find that they go up a shoe size. The following steps will help you to care for your feet:

- Do not wear tight, rubbing footwear.
- Avoid wearing shoes with high heels while you are pregnant. A laced almost-flat shoe is the ideal choice.
- Do not wear knee-high tights (pop socks) when you are pregnant.
- Put your feet up on a footstool in the evenings. This will improve the circulation and allow any swelling to subside.
- Walk as much as and whenever you can to boost the circulation in your legs and feet.
- Avoid standing completely still, for example, when in queues. If you have to stand, keep your circulation moving by walking on the spot, and by flexing and circling your ankles.
- Have a footrest for your feet if you work for long hours at a computer or bench.

If you work sitting down, support your legs by using a footrest; you can improvise by using a firm cushion or a pile of telephone directories.

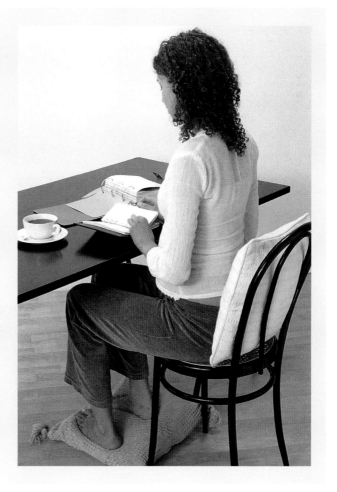

Emotional changes

As your pregnancy progresses, you will probably experience a mixture of emotions. Pregnancy hormones are likely to make you feel more emotional and excitable than normal.

You and your partner may be growing closer together as your pregnancy advances and you become more aware of the commitment now firmly established in your lives. You are likely to be making practical plans, such as where the baby will sleep, and deciding what you need to buy and what you need to do to your home.

By now you are likely to feel more confident about your pregnancy. The chances of miscarriage are greatly reduced and the early sickness and fatigue have almost certainly eased off, leaving most women with a sense of well-being and anticipation.

However, it is very common for women to feel happy one moment, and tearful the next. Many women run the entire spectrum of emotions, from confident, optimistic and relaxed to depressed, worried, irritable and weepy. Sometimes seemingly insignificant things may set you off.

Being pregnant and anticipating your future role as a parent can bring up difficult issues from your own childhood. You may have unresolved feelings, such as sadness, anger or guilt. At the same time, you may discover insights into your parents' feelings about you.

It is important that you express your emotions and work through any unresolved issues. Talking to your partner, a close friend or relative can often be all you need. Sometimes, it may be helpful to see a counsellor or visit a complementary therapist for extra support.

ENHANCING YOUR EMOTIONAL WELL-BEING

Most people will react positively when you tell them you are pregnant, but some may not. If someone shows a less than ecstatic response to your news, try not to let it affect you. A negative reaction is more likely to say something about that person than about your news. Some people have hidden issues about pregnancy or childbirth – for example, they may not be able to have children themselves – or they may simply not be that interested.

It can help you to deal with doubts and worries by imagining what a positive person would say if you were to ask for advice. For example, will I cope with childbirth? Well, hundreds upon thousands of women do. How will I

Holistic therapies such as t'ai chi and yoga emphasize the importance of relaxing the body. This can help you to carry the weight of your baby more easily.

manage without enough sleep? You will take catnaps and do less about the home than you have been used to doing. Will I be able to feed my baby? Breastfeeding does not always come naturally, but there will be people to help and advise you. At worst, the baby will not starve: you will simply bottle-feed her. There is not one problem that cannot be solved.

TIME TO THINK

During this time, it is good to allow yourself to relax and indulge in the dreams you and your partner have for your baby. You obviously want him or her to be happy and healthy, and we all hope for a world in which our children can grow up safely.

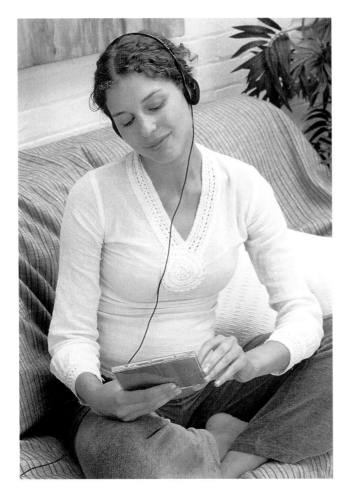

Spend time alone, just relaxing, whenever you get the chance. Enjoy listening to music, reading or simply sitting quietly and experiencing your pregnancy.

Take some time each day to allow yourself to get in touch with your feelings. Visualization can be very helpful: close your eyes and imagine the baby developing inside you. Bring to mind, too, a picture of how your own body is nurturing your growing baby.

Many parents-to-be feel that their baby is very real at this stage and begin to talk to him or her. There is good evidence to suggest that babies can learn to recognize their mother's voice before they are born. Communication need not be limited to talking. Play music, sing or stroke your belly. This can help you to form a bond long before the birth. Even if little of your communication reaches your baby, it can still have a profound effect on your emotions and enhance your psychological readiness for the most important role of your life.

HELPING YOUR PARTNER BOND

Encourage your partner to feel your baby moving and kicking by laying his hand upon your growing abdomen. The first time that this happens can be a very exciting experience. However, it is not unusual for a father still to feel a little removed from the pregnancy at this time. Certainly all the big changes seem to be happening to

> 66 It is very common to feel happy one moment, and tearful the next. Many women run the entire spectrum of emotions during pregnancy. 99

you rather than to him. He may even feel a little left out because of all the attention that you are attracting.

Your partner may harbour anxieties at the prospect of fatherhood, the changes it will mean for him and the changes that it will mean for your relationship. After all, you will soon be part of a family rather than a couple.

It is important that both of you have a chance to discuss your feelings, whether negative or positive. Left unspoken, they may lead to tensions in your relationship. You may be experiencing anxieties yourself about, say, the loss of freedom and your ability to accommodate both job and child. This puts you in a good position to show your partner understanding and support.

Many men do not express their feelings as freely as women. Do not worry if your partner seems to be preoccupied with readying the baby's bedroom, for example, rather than discussing his feelings with you. Be happy that actions speak louder than words.

Your partner may not want to spend hours discussing the pregnancy, but may show his excitement by getting the nursery ready for your baby.

Aromatherapy for pregnancy

It is important to take time to pamper yourself during your pregnancy. This can help you to adjust to the changes in your body, and will also enhance your emotional well-being. Aromatherapy can be an excellent feel-good therapy for the second trimester. Earlier, only a few oils are considered safe (some people think that no oils should be used), and in any case, morning sickness may make you dislike strong aromas. By 16 weeks, however, any nausea is likely to have passed and most women can use a greater range of oils.

Essential oils can be used to help alleviate a number of pregnancy-related complaints, notably stress and insomnia. They also have powerful effects on your moods. This is because scents are processed by the part of the brain that also deals with emotion and memory – making smell the most evocative of all our senses.

It is especially important that you observe basic safety precautions when using essential oils during pregnancy. Only use pure oils that you know are safe, and dilute them in a carrier oil before massaging into the skin or adding to

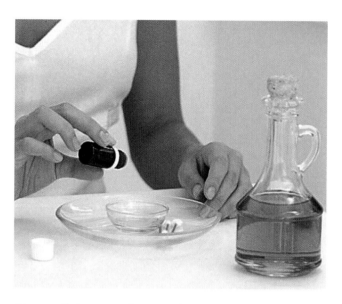

Always dilute aromatherapy oils before you apply to the skin. Choose a good-quality carrier oil such as almond, wheatgerm or sunflower.

the bath. Do not apply oils directly to the skin and never take them by mouth.

Many oils are not suitable for use during pregnancy; others should be used only at particular times or under the guidance of a qualified practitioner. Clary sage, for example, can be useful during labour but hazardous if used earlier. See page 230 for a list of the oils to be avoided during pregnancy. Seek professional advice if you are at all unsure about the safety of an oil.

DILUTING AROMATHERAPY OILS

Use a low dilution of essential oils during pregnancy – no more than 1 drop per 2 teaspoons (10ml) of base oil. Use a light vegetable oil, such as sunflower or wheatgerm, as a base. If using essential oils in the bath, dilute in oil or full-fat milk, then add to a warm (not hot) bath.

Do a patch test to check for sensitivity the first time you use any oil: apply a little of the diluted mixture to your inner wrist, then wait 24 hours. If no reaction occurs, the oil is safe to use. Your skin can become more sensitive during pregnancy, so do a patch test even if you have used the oil before conceiving. Stop using any oil if you develop a reaction to it.

USING OILS IN MASSAGE

You can use essential oils to enhance any of the massage sequences described over the following pages and elsewhere in this book. Experiment by blending different

SIX GOOD OILS

Essential oils are not suitable for everyone and it is a good idea to consult a professional aromatherapist for help on choosing oils, especially if you want to treat a particular problem. The following are generally considered safe for use during pregnancy.

ENERGIZING OILS

- **Mandarin** Refreshing, uplifting oil made from the ripe peel of the fruit.
- **Ginger** Warming, stimulating oil that can boost the immune system. It is good used in massages or footbaths, but should not be used in the bath.
- **Petitgrain** Uplifting, sweet-smelling oil made from the leaves of the bitter orange tree (neroli is made from the flowers).

RELAXING OILS

- **Ylang ylang** Exotic-smelling oil that has soothing properties. It is sometimes used to help to reduce high blood pressure.
- **Neroli** Soothing oil that also lifts the spirits. It has a rejuvenating effect on the skin.
- **Lavender** Versatile oil with calming and restorative properties, which is often used to treat insomnia and stress. Can be used from 16 weeks.

oils together: aromatherapists use up to five but as a novice, it is probably best to use no more than two or three at a time. Relaxing blends to try after 16 weeks include neroli and lavender, or ylang ylang and sandalwood. You may like to try rosewood, a gentle, calming oil that helps to steady the emotions.

Aromatherapy massage is often recommended as a means of preventing stretchmarks, although many doctors say that massage does not make an appreciable difference. If you want to try it, use a blend of mandarin and neroli diluted in wheatgerm oil. At the very least, this will have a moisturizing effect. Adding a little avocado oil to the mixture will increase its moisturizing properties.

OILS IN THE HOME

Use an aromatherapy oil burner to fill your home with relaxing or energizing scents. Fill the bowl with water, add a few drops of oil and heat. At night, try sandalwood, said to have aphrodisiac properties. Lavender is useful if you are having trouble sleeping (it also has antiseptic qualities). Lemon can be a good oil to burn if you are still suffering from nausea after 16 weeks.

For an aromatherapy room spray, add several drops of an essential oil to a spray gun filled with water, and spray several times around the room like an air freshener. Ylang ylang, mandarin and lavender make a refreshing blend that can help to relieve fatigue.

IN THE BATH

Aromatherapy baths can be a great way to relax at the end of the evening: add a few drops of diluted oil to a warm bath (do not add to running water).

For a quick booster when you come home from work, try soaking your feet in an aromatic footbath for ten minutes. Two drops each of ginger and mandarin makes

A vaporizer offers a subtle way to experience essential oils. Try burning oils in the bedroom before you go to sleep, or in the bathroom while you enjoy a long soak.

a warming blend, or try lavender and tea tree to soothe hot, tired feet. Add the oils, diluted in full-fat milk, to a large bowl of warm water.

To add another element to the footbath, add a large handful of marbles. As you soak your feet, roll them backwards and forwards for an easy mini-massage.

AROMATHERAPY FIRST AID

Most of the over-the-counter remedies for colds and stuffy noses are not suitable for pregnant women, but an aromatherapy inhalation can provide effective relief. Add a couple of drops of tea tree oil to a bowl of hot water, then place a towel over your head and breathe in the aromatic steam for a few moments.

Warm aromatherapy compresses are useful for soothing general aches and pains, while a cold compress can soothe a headache or any swelling. Dilute the essential oil in full-fat milk, then add to a bowl of hot or cold water (add a few ice cubes if using cold). Drench a clean cotton cloth in the water, wring it out and then apply to the affected area.

Try a cold lavender compress to relieve a headache, or a hot ginger compress for back pain.

Massage relief

We instinctively use touch to connect with each other, to nurture and to express love. This is why even the simplest form of massage can be richly comforting. Positive, gentle touch can also have a profoundly beneficial effect on our health. It is known to improve circulation, it relaxes the muscles, it helps the digestion, and it regulates the nervous system.

Massage is especially beneficial during pregnancy, provided that deep pressure is not applied to the abdomen or lower back. The number-one aim of massage is to relax mind and body, and so it can help to relieve the stresses and strains of daily living while you are pregnant. It can also help to alleviate many pregnancy-related problems, such as insomnia, circulatory disorders, high blood pressure, swollen legs and headaches.

HAVING A PROFESSIONAL MASSAGE

A professional massage can be a real treat. Choose a qualified practitioner who is experienced in treating pregnant women (your midwife may be able to recommend someone).

Most therapists work from a consulting room, which may be in their home. Some will come to your home, particularly if you find it difficult to get around. If you are having the massage at home, make sure you heat the

> **“ Even the simplest form of massage can be richly comforting. ”**

room well beforehand; your body temperature will drop after you have been lying still for some time. Your masseur should bring a massage couch and towels.

Before the massage, the masseuse will check whether you have any particular aches, pains or other health problems. He or she should also ask you for a basic medical history. It is important that you tell the masseuse

A head massage is particularly helpful for relieving tension commonly found in the upper back, shoulders and neck areas.

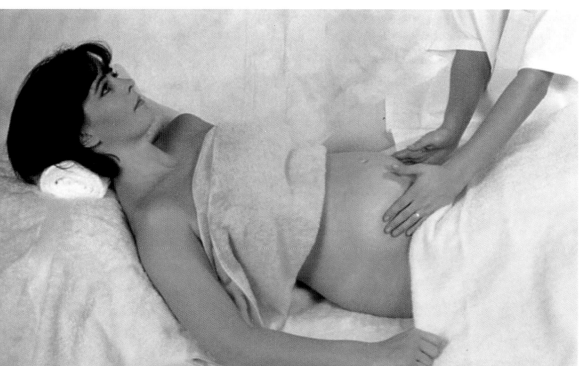

Go to a masseuse who specializes in pregnancy and antenatal massage so that you can relax in the knowledge that you are in good hands. Enjoy.

about your pregnancy and any health problems you have. You should tell the masseuse if you have varicose veins, since the skin over these should not be massaged.

You will be asked to undress and to lie on a massage couch, covered with a towel. You can keep your pants on if you prefer (although they may get covered in oil).

The masseuse will warm some oil in her hands and then spread it over the surface of your skin before starting the massage.

Most sessions include a full-body massage but your therapist may massage only certain areas of your body, depending on your needs. Each masseur will have a different way of combining the different massage techniques and of working around your body.

A full-body massage session usually lasts for an hour, but it may take an hour and a half if you are having a face and head massage at the same time. At the end of the session, you should be left to rest for a few minutes; close your eyes and relax. Don't plan to do anything strenuous afterwards – if possible, take the opportunity to put your feet up and relax for the rest of the day.

SEEING AN AROMATHERAPIST

Aromatherapists work in the same way as masseurs, but they add a blend of essential oils to the massage oil. Different oils will be chosen depending on your individual needs. It is important that you like the scent of any oils used so you will be asked to smell them before they are blended together. You can also ask your aromatherapist for advice on using essential oils at home. Check that any oils used are safe in pregnancy – you should therefore see an experienced practitioner who has experience of treating pregnant women because some oils can have a harmful effect.

MASSAGE AT HOME

You and your partner or a close friend can practise gentle massage at home. A simple massage can be a real help in soothing away general aches and in reducing tension.

Anyone can give a pleasurable massage. The key is to use slow, smooth strokes. Focus on what you are doing and ask the person you are massaging for feedback. You should not massage directly over a bone, and it is important not to apply deep pressure to the abdomen or lower back of a pregnant woman.

For a general massage, warm some oil in your hands; you want enough to give you a good slip, but not so much that your hands are dripping. Apply to the skin with plenty of smooth, stroking movements; these are very calming. Alternate between using your fingertips and whole hands. Then apply deeper pressure to release

Ask a friend or your partner to give you a quick massage to help relieve lower back pain.

areas of particular tension, making small circular movements with the tips of your thumbs.

It is often good to follow a back massage with a leg massage, but let your intuition guide you rather than following a set routine. Add a little more oil whenever you feel the skin starting to pull against your hands.

Back massage

Lower back pain is probably the most common complaint of pregnancy, but a massage can do a lot to relieve the discomfort. The best way of receiving a back massage when you are pregnant is to sit astride a chair, so that you are facing its back. Lean on a cushion and drop your shoulders to help release any tension.

As well as easing your backache, a massage can also give you a comforting sense of being lovingly cared for, which is in itself beneficial. You may like to have a shoulder massage at the same time – ask the person massaging you to adapt the self-massage routine described on the following pages.

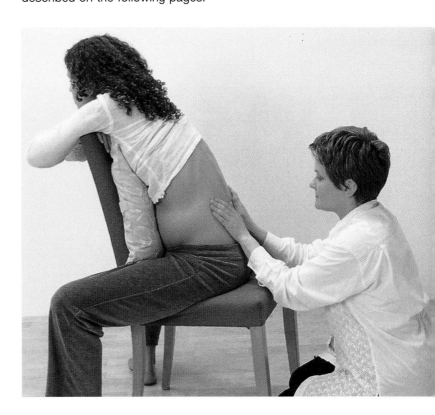

How to massage yourself

Self-massage can be very soothing and beneficial – and you can do it whenever you like. You can use it to energize yourself before an appointment during the day or to unwind in the evening before going to bed. Massage also feels good when performed in the bath. The following routines can also be adapted for partner massage.

Soothing tired legs

Massaging the legs is especially good if your legs ache after standing. It stimulates the circulation and soothes tiredness or swelling. Do not apply heavy pressure, and use very light movements on the inner leg.

1 Rest the foot of the leg you are working on flat, and bend the knee slightly so you can reach the lower leg. Stroke the whole leg with alternate hands, one on each side of the leg. Work up from the foot to the top of the thigh. Repeat five or six times, then work on the other leg.

2 Now use alternate hands to knead the thigh. Squeeze and release the flesh, working in a rhythmic fashion from just above the knee to the top of the thigh. Repeat this two or three times, and then work on the thigh of the other leg.

3 Stroke the thigh, working up the thigh from the knee and using both hands, with one hand following the other. You will enjoy the smooth, flowing strokes after the more energetic kneading. Now repeat on the other leg.

4 Make loose fists and lightly pummel the front and outside of the thigh. This movement will help to relieve any stiffness. Pummel up the thigh a few times, and then repeat on the other thigh.

5 Using the tips of your fingers, stroke the area around the kneecap. Hold the thigh steady with your other hand. Now stroke gently behind the knee, then continue the action up your thigh. Repeat on the other leg.

6 Knead the calf muscle using both hands, alternately squeezing it and releasing it. Then stroke the area gently, with one hand following the other one up the back of the leg. Repeat on the other leg.

Shoulder massage for tension-relief

Tension tends to accumulate in the shoulders, causing aching shoulders, stiff necks and headaches. This quick massage should help to relax your muscles. It is particularly beneficial if you work at a computer.

1 Stroke the left hand down the right shoulder, working from the neck to the elbow. Do three times. Repeat on the other side.

2 Use your fingertips to make small circles on either side of the top of the spine. Use firm but not painful pressure.

3 Making the same circular movements, work up the neck to the base of the skull. Keep the fingers either side of the spine.

4 Squeeze and release the flesh on your shoulder and at the top of your arm. Repeat the movements on the other shoulder.

Feel-good facial (self-massage)

A face massage can get rid of headaches, as well as relieving fatigue and anxiety. Use a good-quality face oil to prevent any dragging of the skin. Do all the movements at least two or three times – more if you like.

1 Put your hands over your face, fingers on forehead. Hold for a few moments, then slowly draw them towards your ears. Do not pull the skin.

2 Use your thumbs and the knuckles of your forefingers to inch gently along the jaw line. Begin just below the chin and work out to the ears. Pinch near the bone.

3 Slap the backs of alternate hands under the chin. This is a good stimulating movement, and it may help to prevent a double chin.

4 Stroke your hands, one after the other, up your forehead. Work from the bridge of the nose to your hairline. Close your eyes as you do this.

5 Place both index fingers on the bridge of your nose and stroke firmly upwards, then gently across. This may help to reduce any frown lines.

6 Using the fingertips of your index and middle fingers, make circular movements all over the forehead. Press firmly but do not drag the skin.

7 Using your fingertips, stroke your forehead gently, working from the centre to your temples. Finally, press them firmly against the temples.

Treating ailments at home

Some women glow with health throughout pregnancy, but most experience minor ailments at one time or another. The majority of these health problems are not a cause for concern, but they can cause considerable discomfort. Both indigestion and constipation, for example, can be painful and irritating.

You should avoid taking medication in pregnancy if at all possible. Some natural remedies offer a safe and gentle way of relieving discomfort. They can also help to balance mood swings and strengthen the emotions.

The following remedies are generally considered safe to take during pregnancy. Even so, not every treatment will suit every pregnant woman. It is therefore a good idea to seek advice from a qualified practitioner who is experienced in treating pregnant women. You should discuss health concerns with your doctor. Always tell your doctor about any natural remedies that you are considering taking.

HERBAL TEAS

Most herbal remedies should be taken only under the direction of a medical herbalist, but some are gentle enough to be used as self-help remedies. These include dandelion, lemon balm, meadowsweet, fennel and lime flower teas. They are available in tea-bag form from health food shops and some supermarkets, or you can make your own infusion (see box). However, do not drink herbal tea in excessive quantities – three cups a day is the usual recommended limit. Popular choices include:

- **Lemon balm or meadowsweet tea**. These can help to ease indigestion, which most pregnant women experience at some time or other. Sip a cupful after

Fennel helps with digestive problems such as constipation and also exerts a calming effect.

each meal. Lemon balm also helps to calm the emotions, so it can be also a useful tea if you are suffering from stress or anxiety.

- **Fennel**. This is a calming herb that also works on the digestive system and acts as a mild laxative, so it can be helpful if you suffer from constipation. Infuse 5ml (1 tsp) of crushed seeds in a cup of boiling water, strain, and drink at bedtime. Drinking a cup of hot water with a slice of lemon before breakfast can also ease constipation. You should also be drinking plenty of fluid – at least eight glasses of water a day.
- **Lime (linden) flower tea**. This can help to relieve anxiety and stress, which in turn can improve your sleep. It may be helpful for stuffy noses. Chamomile is another good stress-reliever and sleep promoter.
- **Dandelion tea**. This is useful if you are feeling bloated. It works as a diuretic, so it helps to remove excess fluid from the body. It is also a good source of iron, so it can be useful if you are anaemic.

TEAS TO AVOID

In general, do not drink one type of herbal tea repeatedly – a varied selection is key. Ask a herbalist which herbs to avoid or use in moderation during pregnancy as some encourage uterine contractions and should be avoided totally or taken only in the final stages and at the birth.

Always study the contents lists on bought teas and avoid any bought or home-made teas that contain the following: celery, cinnamon, cohosh, mugwort, nutmeg, pennyroyal and sage (sage is also to be avoided if breast-feeding). Raspberry leaf tea is a well-known uterine tonic and stimulant that helps to prepare the uterus for birth. As such, it must not be taken until the last six to eight weeks of pregnancy (one or two cups a day is a good dose) and during labour. There are many less common herbs that may be found in some teas, which is why expert advice should always be sought (see also page 228).

> ### MAKING AN INFUSION
> Place about 5ml (1 tsp) of dried herb in a cup or ceramic teapot (do not use an aluminium or tin teapot). Add a cupful of boiling water and leave to infuse for five to ten minutes. Strain, then sip slowly. To save time, make up enough for three cups and store in a vacuum flask to drink that day. Or let cool, and store in the refrigerator.

Homeopathic remedies are usually stored in dark bottles. This helps to prevent them deteriorating.

HOMEOPATHIC REMEDIES

Natural, usually plant-based medicines, homeopathic remedies are so highly diluted that only the minutest amount of the active ingredient remains. They are generally considered very safe in pregnancy but, like any remedy, they should be used with care.

Homeopathic remedies are widely available from pharmacies and health food shops, and they are commonly used for self-help. However, it can be very difficult to choose the correct remedy for your individual circumstances without specialist knowledge. It is therefore a good idea to seek advice from a qualified, professional homeopath – who will have trained for several years – rather than trying to diagnose and prescribe for yourself. Not all women require the same remedy, even when they are suffering from what seems to be the same problem. The homeopath will also bear in mind the fact that your unborn baby is receiving treatment as well as you.

Common homeopathic remedies for pregnancy-related ailments include:

- Nux vomica, carbo veg, pulsatilla or sulphur for indigestion and heartburn.
- Aconite, belladonna, natrum mur, bryonia or sepia for headaches.
- Bryonia, natrum mur, nux vomica or sepia for constipation.
- Nux vomica, hamamelis, aesculus or sulphur for haemorrhoids.
- Calc fluor or hamamelis for varicose veins.
- Calc fluor to improve the elasticity of the skin, thus helping to prevent stretch marks.

BACH FLOWER REMEDIES

These gentle flower- and plant-based remedies are highly diluted and are safe for use in pregnancy. They can be very helpful for dealing with difficult emotions, such as anxiety. Flower remedies are preserved in brandy, so you should take them in water. Simply add a couple of drops to a glass of water and sip throughout the day.

Bach Flower Remedies, like homeopathic ones, are highly diluted. Just add two or three drops of your chosen remedy to a glass of water, and take sips throughout the day.

There are 38 flower remedies to choose from. The following may be of greatest help in pregnancy:

- Olive to counteract lack of energy and fatigue.
- Walnut to help with adjusting to change.
- Red chestnut to relieve anxiety about your baby's well-being.
- Crab apple if you are feeling negative about the way that you look.
- Mimulus to help with anxiety about the birth or the effect that pregnancy is having on you.
- Rescue Remedy to use in moments of panic and general tearfulness.

Yoga for the second trimester

Pregnant women tend to feel more energetic and healthy in the second trimester, but the baby's increasing weight can alter your sense of balance and lead to poor posture. Yoga encourages you to stand correctly and also works to strengthen the back muscles, preventing backache. Yoga also encourages good breathing and improves the circulation, so that fresh nutritious blood reaches your baby. It is a good idea to attend specialist classes for pregnant women during the second trimester. You can also practise simple postures at home.

Centring down

Getting your legs, rather than your lower back, to support your increasing weight and bulk is probably the most important postural adjustment that you can make during your pregnancy because it will save you from backache. Stand tall with your head erect and chin tucked in naturally. Tuck in your tail bone (coccyx). Now extend up through the spine, relaxing the tension from your upper body. At the same time, bend the knees and imagine your weight dropping downwards through the legs.

1 Stand tall, feet apart. Bend your knees to take your weight down. Press your palms together at throat level, elbows out. Inhale, opening up your back ribs as you do so.

2 As you breathe out, stretch your arms forwards and bend deeply in the knees. Keep your upper body erect. Hold a moment, then breathe in again. Repeat several times.

Tiger stretch and relax

This exercise is a good way to relieve lower backache. It also helps sciatica, in which back pain extends down the leg. You will need to balance firmly on strong wrists and hands as you raise your leg parallel to the floor.

1 Go on to all fours, with hands below your shoulders and a cushion under the knees. Extend the spine (do not dip your back). Slowly lift your right leg parallel to the floor and extend it back to release any tension. Point your toes.

2 Let your leg sink to the floor and relax it. Maintain your balance and the strength in your spine, but drop your right hip. Shake your leg loosely from hip to toes to release pressure on the sciatic nerve. Repeat on the left.

Swing and release

In this vigorous exercise, the palms are pressed firmly together to strengthen the arm muscles and the muscles by the upper spine. Strength in these areas makes it easier to maintain a good upright posture.

1 Stand with your feet a comfortable width apart and your knees bent. Bring your palms together and bend forwards from the hips so that your fingertips touch the floor. Breathe out in this position.

2 Stretch the arms forwards, pushing the palms together. Breathe in deeply, raising your head, arms and trunk up and to your right, and turning the upper body gently to your right. Hold this for a few seconds, pressing your palms together and feeling your muscles engaging along the arms and upper spine.

3 Breathe out through the mouth, making a "HAH" sound, and drop back to the starting position with your knees bent. Keep your hands together and strong. Breathe in and out to relax in the starting position. Then breathe in again deeply to repeat the upward stretch and turn to the left. Repeat a few times.

Modified positions for deep relaxation

It is important to relax after doing any yoga routine. As your baby grows, lying on your back will no longer be comfortable. It will also restrict circulation, so it is not a good idea, particularly from 30 weeks onwards. Instead of lying flat on your back, either bend your knees and place a cushion or blankets under your hips, lie on your side or lean forwards over a bean bag. You can even relax deeply while sitting up, as long as you are well supported and your legs are not hanging down. Take time to find a comfortable pose for you.

1 Place a bean bag underneath your legs and a cushion under your hips. Your raised legs will improve the blood flow to your heart and should also reduce swelling and aching in the legs. Raising up the hips helps to take strain off the lower back.

2 Push the bean bag against a wall for extra support and recline against it so that you are as comfortable as possible. Sit with your knees bent and out to the sides and add cushions underneath to open up your hips and expand the whole pelvic area.

Pregnancy and your sex life

The most commonly asked question about making love in pregnancy is whether or not it is safe. Experts say that it is – and there is no evidence to suggest that it might not be. A pregnancy is actually much more robust than some of us believe. Some consultants even say that it is safe to go riding – something that women are usually advised to avoid. They maintain that if the pregnancy were to be lost in this way then it was going to be lost in any case; in other words, that the pregnancy was frail. So, one need not fear causing miscarriage through the act of lovemaking.

The next big question is whether or not both you and your partner feel like making love. Some women go off sex during their pregnancy while others enjoy sex more than ever before. Similarly, some men find that their partner seems even more attractive when she is pregnant. Others are nervous of making love once their partner is visibly pregnant and prefer to wait until after the baby has arrived. However, for many couples the frequency of love-making does not change substantially whether or not the woman is pregnant.

You may find it easier to be on top when you make love with your partner, so that pressure on the abdomen is reduced and you have better control.

If you lost interest in sex early on in your pregnancy, as many women who suffer with morning sickness do, your sex drive will probably return later on. Some women find arousal easier and orgasm more intense during pregnancy. It may be that the pregnancy hormones are responsible for this, but general feelings of well-being and happiness may also be a factor.

GOOD POSITIONS IN PREGNANCY

Now that you are getting larger, you will probably need to experiment with different positions in which to make love. Lying on your back will probably not feel comfortable. Experiment with different positions until you find some that work well for you and your partner.

One good position to try is the spoons position, in which both partners lie on their sides. You lie with your back to your partner, who lies curled around you and facing your back. He can then enter you from behind without putting any pressure on your abdomen. You may also find it easier to use the doggy position, with you on

Pregnancy can often have an impact on your sex life, but it is not necessarily a negative one. This is the time to experiment with different positions to find the most comfortable. The spoons position, where you lie with your back to your partner, is a good option.

your hands and knees and your partner behind you. Another good position is with the woman on top, when again there is no pressure on her abdomen.

IF YOU GO OFF SEX

If your sex drive has diminished, try to show your partner love and affection in other ways. Of course, your partner will respect your wishes but he may feel rejected or alienated all the same. Showing that you love him is all the more important at this time. Reassure him of your feelings in thoughtful ways. Give him a glorious pampering massage, cook deliciously for him, send him a card, email him during the day if he is at work.

IF HE GOES OFF SEX

Lovemaking necessarily involves respecting one another's wishes. You may naturally find it disturbing if your partner rejects you sexually while you are pregnant, particularly if your sex life was very active beforehand. Try talking to him when he is neither tired nor busy and explain how you feel. Ask him to talk about he feels, too.

Show your partner that you cherish him in ways that are unrelated to sex. For a start, make sure that you are paying him as much attention as you are paying your pregnancy and your unborn baby. It may be that your partner has started to feel a little left out while you are, inevitably, receiving a lot of attention.

It may help if you cast your mind back to what your partner found attractive about you when you first met. Find ways to subtly recreate that picture – what did you wear? where did you go? what did you eat? You may find that focusing on your partner and his needs helps to rekindle the sexual attraction between you.

Massage can be a wonderful way of achieving physical closeness, and relaxing together.

Show your partner that you are as interested in him as ever. Make time for him and have fun together.

Routine antenatal care

Many pregnant women find that the regular monitoring and tests carried out during pregnancy cause anxiety. Sometimes the anxiety can be so great that it can outweigh the benefits of good antenatal care.

It is important to remember that antenatal care is a well-established and thoroughly researched form of preventative health, with the interests of the mother and the baby at the fore. It is now more than ten times safer to have a baby than it was 100 years ago. However, you always have the right to veto any test or procedure that you do not feel is appropriate for you.

Most women find it helpful to be fully informed and to take time to think through the significance of each test, the possible consequences and any associated risks. Make sure that you discuss any medical concerns with your family doctor or hospital consultant. You may find it useful to take notes at such consultations and discuss the matter further with your partner, a close friend or relative. If you feel unsure about any test, ask for more information and for more time in which to consider your options.

MEDICAL TERMS

Doctors may use the following terms when talking about your baby:

- **Fetus:** 8 weeks to birth (before 8 weeks, the term is an embryo).
- **Neonate:** from birth to 4 weeks.
- **Baby:** from birth to two years.
- **Infant:** first year of life.

The arrival of your baby may still seem a long way off, but you will soon be able to greet him or her.

ROUTINE MONITORING

Your weight, blood pressure, urine and blood-sugar level will be checked at antenatal appointments – changes here can give early indications of common problems.

Weight

Your weight may be monitored throughout the pregnancy in order to judge the baby's growth, the estimated delivery date, and the amount of amniotic fluid, although very regular weight checks are now less common at many clinics as some doctors feel they are not so important. There are known disadvantages to starting a pregnancy overweight: for example, there is a stronger likelihood of pregnancy-related diabetes and high blood pressure as well as the increased risk of a difficult labour and

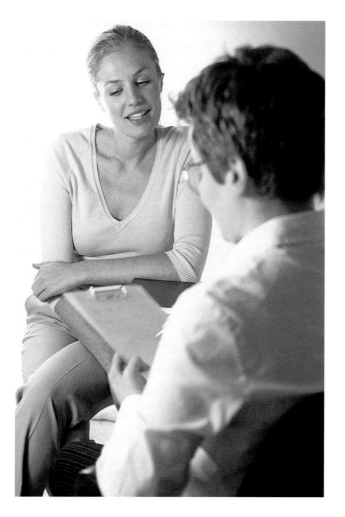

Antenatal check-ups are a good opportunity to discuss any anxieties you may have, however small they seem.

> **❝ It is now more than ten times safer to have a baby than it was 100 years ago. ❞**

delivering a large baby. In addition, anaesthetic complications associated with a Caesarean section are increased. These complications can sometimes occur if you gain excessive weight during your pregnancy.

Blood pressure

Your blood pressure is checked regularly. If it is too high, it is easily brought down with medication that does not harm the developing baby. High blood pressure is a typical sign of pre-eclampsia. If left untreated, it can develop into eclampsia, which can be life-threatening to the pregnant woman and the baby. In its fully developed stage, eclampsia is characterized by high blood pressure, severe headaches and fits. The symptoms of pre-eclampsia are high blood pressure, swelling of the ankles and hands, protein in the urine and sudden weight gain.

Urine

You will be asked to provide a urine sample at antenatal appointments. This will be checked for various substances: protein, sugar, bile, salts and blood. Urine tests are used to detect a number of conditions that could adversely affect your pregnancy, such as kidney disease, diabetes and infections in the urinary tract, such as cystitis.

For this test to be performed as efficiently as possible, you need to provide the hospital with a 'mid-stream' urine sample. To obtain this, first pass a little urine into the lavatory in the normal way, then contract your muscles to halt the flow for a couple of seconds. Resume the flow, allowing some of the urine to pass into the specimen bottle. Then remove the bottle and finish passing water.

Blood

Your blood sugar levels are checked to see whether pregnancy diabetes has developed. Your blood may also be checked for a number of other conditions, depending upon your individual medical history.

CHECK IT OUT

As soon as you tell people that you are pregnant, you are likely to find yourself on the receiving end of a lot of advice, particularly from women who have already had children. It can be very helpful to talk to women who have experienced pregnancy. However, do bear in mind that antenatal procedures and our understanding of what constitutes good pregnancy care are continually changing and developing. Always check any advice with your midwife.

A multiple test stick is used to check your urine at each antenatal appointment. The colour of each pad is held against a colour chart to ensure that levels of protein, blood, bilirubin, glucose, ketones and acidity are normal.

Talking to your mother or another older woman about your pregnancy can help allay doubts and fears. However, be wary of following out-of-date advice.

Tests and procedures

As part of your antenatal care, you will be offered various tests to check that your baby is healthy. Some tests are standard and offered to all women; others are recommended only if the risk of a problem is higher than average. No test is compulsory: it is entirely up to you whether or not you have any procedure. However, most hospitals recommend the routine tests.

Ultrasound

Pregnant women are usually offered their second routine ultrasound scan at around 20 weeks. This important scan is used to assess the baby's growth, to confirm the estimated date of delivery and also to check that the baby is developing in a normal way.

At the scan, the baby's head can be seen clearly in outline and its diameter can be measured on the ultrasound screen and correlated with the known average. Earlier in the pregnancy, it may be difficult to measure the head and later on, each baby will develop its own shape and size. At this point, though, most babies' heads are roughly the same size. Once the diameter of the head is measured it is plotted on a graph and equated to a known value so that an accurate estimate of the delivery date can be made.

The baby is checked in all respects including the heart, the limbs, the spine and the head, which provides the opportunity to look for any abnormalities such as spina bifida, kidney, brain and heart defects. Some defects detected at this time can be treated *in utero* (in the womb) before the baby is born. Others may require medication or surgery after the baby has been born.

DON'T FORGET
The two golden rules to keep in mind when thinking about antenatal care are:
- Antenatal care is an effective and well-established form of preventative health.
- It is always your choice, for yourself and for your baby, as to which tests and procedures you do or do not have.

Nuchal screening

This more detailed ultrasound scan is carried out between about 11 and 14 weeks, and can indicate the likelihood of a Down's baby. It is described on page 108.

Chorionic villus sampling

This test is usually performed within the first ten or so weeks of pregnancy. It is a way of detecting the likelihood of the baby being affected by Down's. See page 108.

Alphafetoprotein test

The substance alphafetoprotein (AFP) appears in your blood in varying levels throughout the pregnancy. Between about 15 and 18 weeks the level is fairly constant in most women (before or after this time the level is very variable). A higher than normal level at this time can indicate that the baby could be suffering from a defect of the spine, such as spina bifida, or another abnormality of brain development. A low level of AFP may be found in Down's syndrome babies.

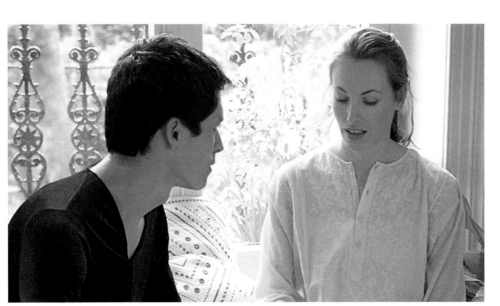

People often have strong feelings about amniocentesis, and it is important to discuss these fully, with your partner and with the hospital consultant, before you come to a decision about the test.

The non-invasive AFP test may be done before amniocentesis: if AFP gives a good result, you may feel that amniocentesis is unnecessary. However, AFP tests are being done less often as ultrasound can be more accurate.

Bart's test

This test – known as the 'triple screen' in the US – involves taking a blood sample from the mother at about 16 to 18 weeks and measuring three hormones that are commonly secreted in pregnancy. The hormones are AFP, oestriol (which indicates how much oestrogen is circulating in the blood; spelled estriol in the US) and HCG (human chorionic gonadotrophin, present in high levels in pregnancy).

The Bart's test is essentially a screening test for fetal abnormality, the commonest of which is Down's. A very high result indicates the risk of a Down's child but it does not absolutely diagnose a Down's baby. The advantage with this test, like the AFP, is that it is non-invasive and you may feel it renders amniocentesis unnecessary.

Amniocentesis

This test is usually carried out around 16 weeks. It involves a sample of fluid being drawn from the amniotic sac using a needle. Ultrasound is used to guide the needle to the correct place. The fluid is then analysed to determine the likelihood of Down's syndrome and other fetal abnormalities. The test and its implications are described in detail over the following pages.

Fetal blood sampling (cordocentesis)

This procedure (called PUBS or Percutaneous Umbilical Blood Sampling in the US) involves taking blood from the umbilical cord and analysing the baby's blood cells. Like amniocentesis, it makes use of ultrasound to guide the needle to the correct location. Cordocentesis can be performed from the 18th week to determine the baby's condition and to identify inherited disorders such as those detected by amniocentesis.

The advantage of cordocentesis is that results are available within a week, while amniocentesis usually means a wait of up to three weeks. Cordocentesis may be used if a late ultrasound scan indicates a problem or if the alphafetoprotein test reveals a level of protein that is too low or too high. It is also useful when it is vital to know the baby's blood group before birth, as in cases of congenital forms of anaemia, or if the baby's blood needs to be tested to determine whether he or she has developed an infection – for example, of the toxoplasmosis organism.

Like amniocentesis, cordocentesis carries a small chance of causing miscarriage (it may be 1-2 per cent) – discuss this with your consultant. Rhesus-negative women will be given a protective injection of anti-D immunoglobulin after this test in case any fetal cells are disturbed, which would increase the risk of antibodies developing.

Test samples are sent to the hospital's laboratory for analysis and interpretation. You may have to wait several weeks for some results.

Fetoscopy

This procedure is used only rarely and involves inserting a fibre-optic tube into the uterus through a cut in the abdomen. A microscope camera can be attached to the end of the tube so the fetus can be photographed. The fetoscope can also be used to take a sample of tissue, which enables diagnosis of several blood and skin diseases that amniocentesis cannot detect. In some centres, certain fetal conditions can be treated before delivery by means of fetoscopy. For example, babies with excess fluid of the brain can have a shunt inserted to drain the fluid. Other conditions, such as urinary tract obstruction, can be treated, too.

Amniocentesis in perspective

Amniocentesis is an antenatal procedure that may be offered to women who have a higher than average risk of carrying a baby with an abnormality. It may be offered, for example, to women who have been in contact with the rubella virus in the first three months of their pregnancy. Amniocentesis may be offered to women in their late thirties, and will usually be offered to women over the age of forty as a matter of course.

WHAT AMNIOCENTESIS INVOLVES

Amniocentesis is normally performed at around 16 weeks, although it can be done a little earlier and up to a few weeks later. Ultrasound is usually used to locate the amniotic sac, the placenta and the baby. It is best not to have amniocentesis without ultrasound since this increases the risk of miscarriage. In addition, the test may not be successful if insufficient liquid is obtained.

You will need to have a full bladder to have ultrasound and you will therefore be asked to drink a pint of water an hour before your appointment (and not to go to the lavatory). A local anaesthetic may be applied to your abdomen and a fine needle is then inserted through it. You may feel some discomfort at this point.

The ultrasound picture is used to locate the best pool of liquid in the amniotic sac and to make the sure that the needle does not pierce either the placenta or the baby. This is particularly important in women who are rhesus-negative as the procedure may cause the fetal and maternal blood to mix, which will sensitize the mother in future pregnancies. A protective injection of anti-D immunoglobulin is given at the time of amniocentesis to a woman who has a rhesus-negative blood group.

> **" The vast majority of people are given good news after amniocentesis. "**

The needle is used to draw some of the amniotic fluid. The growing baby is not harmed by the needle because it swims around in fluid and tends to move away from any object that approaches it.

After the test, it is advisable to rest for the remainder of the day in order not to irritate the uterus and to prevent leakage of fluid from the tiny hole made by the needle.

The amniotic fluid is then analysed in a number of different ways to detect fetal abnormalities. The levels of AFP hormone will also be measured. The cells will be grown (cultured) in a laboratory and their chromosomes subsequently analysed.

AFP analysis results from amniocentesis come within a couple of days but the chromosomal results of an amniocentesis normally take up to four weeks, as it takes some time to culture cells.

IS AMNIOCENTESIS SAFE?

The main disadvantage with amniocentesis is that it carries a risk of causing miscarriage. Withdrawing the fluid can sometimes cause trauma to the uterus, which may then start contracting. Twenty years ago the risk of miscarrying a healthy baby through amniocentesis was one in 100. Improved procedures mean that it has now fallen to about one in 200.

The degree of risk depends to a certain extent on how experienced the doctor is in carrying out the technique: some doctors are more skillful than others. It also

---

WHO IS OFFERED AMNIOCENTESIS?

It is up to each individual woman, in consultation with her partner, whether or not she decides to have an amniocentesis. The test will usually be offered to the following women:

- All women over the age of 37, because there is an increased risk of Down's syndrome.
- Women with a history of a child born with Down's syndrome or with certain other chromosome abnormalities.
- Women in whom a Down's blood test has shown an increased likelihood of chromosome abnormalities.

- Sometimes, women who have had a previous child affected by spina bifida or hydrocephalus. However, sophisticated ultrasound techniques may mean that an amniocentesis is not necessarily recommended in such cases.
- Women whose medical history includes having a child affected by certain sex-linked diseases, such as haemophilia.
- Certain women with a family history of rare abnormality, following genetic counselling and possibly genetic testing of several or all family members.

Most hospitals will offer amniocentesis to older women, sometimes to the over-35s and usually as a matter of course to women over the age of 40.

depends on whether or not ultrasound is used to help guide the needle. If you are considering amniocentesis, you should ask your consultant the following questions before deciding to go ahead:

- Is ultrasound going to be used?
- Who is going to carry out the test: will it be the consultant or senior registrar or another doctor?
- What is the practitioner's personal rate of miscarriage? Is it higher than the average?

When deciding whether to have the test, weigh up the risk of miscarriage against the value of the information ascertained. A 20-year-old woman has a one in 2000 chance of bearing a Down's syndrome child and a one in 200 chance of miscarriage as a direct result of amniocentesis. She is thus likely to feel that the test is not worth the risk. On the other hand, a 41-year-old woman has the same risk of miscarriage from the test, but a one in

50 risk of carrying a Down's baby. She is therefore four times as likely to have a Down's child as she is to miscarry through having amniocentesis. In this situation, many women decide that they do want to take the risk.

THINKING AMNIOCENTESIS THROUGH

Amniocentesis is a useful test, which can offer you the peace of mind necessary to enjoy the rest of your pregnancy. It also provides valuable information for medical and nursing staff, so that they are more likely to know what, if any, abnormalities they are dealing with, and to be better prepared. The difficulties surrounding amniocentesis are:

- It could cause miscarriage and the unnecessary loss of a healthy baby.
- It could lead to a further dilemma – whether or not to terminate the pregnancy if the baby should be affected by Down's syndrome or another problem.

It is important that you and your partner share any concerns with your consultant, and ask any questions that you have before you come to a decision. Ideally, you will make a decision that all of you are happy with.

YOUR OPTIONS

The choices you have are as follows:

- Not to have amniocentesis.
- To have amniocentesis for information, even if you are certain that you would not terminate the pregnancy if you were carrying a Down's baby.
- To have amniocentesis, having already decided that you would terminate the pregnancy in the case of a serious abnormality.
- To have amniocentesis for information, although you are uncertain as to how you would proceed in the case of an abnormality.
- To have other tests that carry a lower chance of miscarriage, in order to assess the chance of carrying a child with an abnormality. You then have the option of proceeding to amniocentesis if the risk appears to be high. Other useful tests include nuchal screening, the alphafetoprotein test and Bart's test.

THE RESULTS

The vast majority of people are given good news after amniocentesis. The test shows that there is something wrong in about 3 per cent of cases. Nearly half of these concern Down's syndrome babies.

A termination may be recommended if the amniocentesis shows that something is severely wrong with your baby and his or her quality of life would be strongly affected. If amniocentesis identifies a less severe disability or an operable deformity, many women will continue with the pregnancy.

When something is wrong

If tests show that something is seriously wrong with the baby you are carrying, then you will be asked if you want to end the pregnancy. Terminating a wanted pregnancy is obviously a very difficult and complex decision to make. Only you and your partner can know what is the right choice for you.

Some people feel strongly that they would not terminate a pregnancy under any circumstances. For example, people who hold profound religious or humanitarian beliefs would probably decide against termination even if there was a serious problem with the baby. Women who believe that this pregnancy is their last chance of having a child may also be reluctant to terminate the pregnancy. Some parents feel that they are able and willing to care for a disabled child, whatever the extent of his or her problems.

Many couples would, however, consider termination the most feasible option if a test such as amniocentesis or chorionic villus sampling (CVS) showed that the baby was not developing normally. There are many reasons why a pregnancy may be terminated. These are just some of the common ones:

- The parents may know that they could not cope with a disabled child.
- The parents may believe it to be wrong to bring a child into the world if she or he would develop an incurable, untreatable disease.
- The mother's physical and mental well-being may be at risk. If the child is so severely handicapped that he or she will inevitably die later in the uterus or shortly after birth, the mother, and the father, may be saved some suffering by opting for a termination.
- The likely effect on the parents and other children in the family may seem too great. A severely handicapped child can exert a profound influence upon its family. He or she will need full-time care and this may strain the emotional, physical and financial resources of the family to a great degree.
- The child may suffer needlessly and die either in childhood or in early adulthood.

Everyone involved in maternity care knows that choosing to have a termination is the most distressing decision a woman can make. You will be given all the support that you need.

You may want to talk to your family doctor, the hospital consultant or your midwife more than once if you are contemplating a termination. Healthcare staff will understand only too well that you need to gather as much information as possible, and that you need to take time to make your decision. Rest assured that nobody will try to persuade you to have a termination if you really do not wish to do so.

TERMINATING A PREGNANCY

The procedure for terminating a pregnancy varies depending on whether it is performed before the end of the 13th week or after it. If you are considering having a termination after an amniocentesis, you will need to have a late termination.

Early termination

A termination performed at 13 weeks or earlier is a simple and quick operation, with minimal risks to the woman's physical health. It may be done following a test carried out early in the pregnancy, such as CVS.

Early terminations are carried out under general anaesthetic. The woman's cervix is dilated (expanded) so that the fetus can be removed by suction. You will usually be able to go home on the same day as the operation, but you will be advised to rest for 24 hours.

Late termination

A late termination is available to those women who wish to end a pregnancy after amniocentesis or other tests. At this stage of pregnancy, it is not possible to dilate the woman's cervix to the required degree without risking permanent damage to it. Because of this, many doctors prefer to use the technique in which the natural process of birth is imitated.

The woman is given synthetic prostaglandin in the form of a vaginal gel or pessary, or in the form of an infusion directly into her uterus, at regular intervals. This process is known as prostaglandin induction, and causes the woman to go through what is, in effect, a mini-labour. Her uterus starts contracting to expel the fetus, and in response to this, the cervix dilates. If the pregnancy is being terminated after 20 weeks, then an irritant substance may be injected directly into the amniotic sac around the fetus.

It may be some hours before the fetus is expelled, just as it is during labour and birth. The fetus is usually born dead. The woman then normally undergoes a procedure called dilatation and curettage (D and C) in which all the contents of the uterus are removed. This is done to ensure that no part of the placenta or anything else relating to the pregnancy remains.

You will probably have to stay in hospital overnight, and should rest at home over the days that follow.

THE RISKS

There are certain risks attached to terminating a pregnancy, and these risks are higher the later the abortion. Your doctor will explain these to you in detail, but they include:

- Infection in about 3 in 100 women.
- Prolonged bleeding in 4 in 100 women.
- Abnormal blood clotting in one in 200 women.
- Operative trauma, such as tissue damage or perforation of the uterus. This occurs in less than one in 100 women.
- Feelings of regret for what might have been. Most women will need time to come to terms with the end of a wanted pregnancy.

FEELINGS OF REGRET

In cases where the developing baby has, or is likely to have, severe abnormalities, having a termination may be the best choice for everyone. However, this does not mean that you will not mourn your baby. Ultimately, this may prove to be an event in your life that is never completely forgotten, never completely accepted.

It is extremely important that, immediately after the event, you give yourself whatever time you need to grieve and to fully explore and express your emotions. Talk to your partner about how you feel, and also encourage him to share his feelings.

You may wish to carry out some kind of closing ceremony or ritual to help you say goodbye. How you choose to do this is a personal matter, but you could visit a local church or religious centre of some kind, or simply go somewhere beautiful and say goodbye in your own way. Making a donation to a children's charity or perhaps planting a tree that will live for many years may feel like a positive and helpful thing to do.

FINDING SUPPORT

You and your partner may well need support from other people – don't feel that you have to sort out your feelings between just the two of you. Friends and relatives can be a great source of comfort, although they may be too close to the two of you and to the situation. If you prefer to see a counsellor, your family doctor will be able to refer you. There are centres you can contact direct that offer specialist post-termination counselling and also confidential helplines. Remember that such counsellors are happy to discuss your feelings about a termination even if it is years after the event.

A complementary therapist may also be able to offer support. Acupuncture and zero balancing – a therapy in which gentle touch is used to release difficult emotions – may go some way towards helping you to deal with what has happened to you. Reiki is another gentle and non-intrusive method of healing that might prove helpful.

Checklist of common problems

By the second trimester, women usually feel healthier and more confident about their pregnancies. You are likely to have more energy, and morning sickness has usually passed. However, you may still be affected by ailments such as constipation and indigestion.

The following solutions should help to relieve any discomfort, but also check the relevant safety advice in Section Four.

Some treatments may work better for you than others and you may need to experiment to find one that suits you. If any complaint persists, or if it troubles you, or you are not sure what it is, you should consult your family doctor. In any case, tell your midwife about the problem at your next antenatal check.

Back pain Many women suffer from back pain during pregnancy (and almost everyone is affected in the last months). However, there is a lot you can do to minimize the pain. First of all, make sure that you have a good, supportive mattress; if you do not, consider buying a new one. Be aware of your posture: check how you are holding yourself at regular intervals, and change your position if you are sitting awkwardly. Try yoga or Pilates, which can help to strengthen the muscles in your back and improve your posture.

For persistent back pain, see an osteopath, Alexander technique teacher or chiropractor. Flotation therapy, which allows you to relax in a supported position, can be a pleasing way to relieve back pain. Reiki, massage and acupuncture can also be good therapies to try.

Varicose veins Eat a healthy diet, that includes plenty of foods that are rich in vitamin E, such as wheatgerm, wholegrains, sunflower seeds and cold-pressed vegetable oils. Avoid standing still for long periods: walk on the spot or flex and rotate your ankles. Walk daily to help the circulation, and rest with your feet up twice a day, for 20 minutes a time. Brushing the skin daily with a soft-bristled brush can help – use long, upward strokes.

For temporary relief, apply commercially prepared witch hazel or aloe vera compresses to the affected area. Ask your doctor about wearing support stockings. Homeopathy, acupuncture and aromatherapy can be helpful. You may also draw comfort from the fact that varicose veins often subside after the birth.

Stretchmarks Eating a healthy, balanced diet that is rich in vitamin E, silica and other nutrients can help to

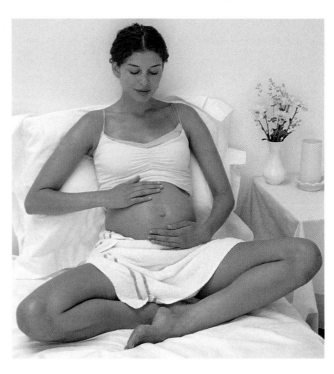

Massaging oil into the skin of your abdomen, using a circular clockwise motion, may help to prevent the formation of stretchmarks.

prevent stretchmarks (see also page 121). Massage the skin gently with a good-quality oil enriched with vitamin E to help maintain suppleness. Add a few drops of an essential oil such as neroli or mandarin to your massage oil. Marigold or lavender flowers can also be used. Soak the flowers in wheatgerm oil for two weeks, then strain. Apply the oil daily, rubbing it gently into the skin in a circular motion. A homeopath may prescribe calc fluor as a preventative measure.

Constipation Start the day with a glass of hot water with a little fresh lemon juice. Include plenty of wholegrains, fruit and vegetables in your diet, and drink lots of water. Avoid bananas and hard-boiled eggs, and do not eat late at night. Take more exercise, particularly walking, and try yoga – some yoga postures specifically work on the digestion.

For temporary relief, try massaging the abdomen with essential oil of ginger diluted in wheatgerm oil (see pages 124-7): use a smooth circular movement, starting on the lower left-hand side and working clockwise (apply light pressure only). Herbal medicine, homeopathy, acupuncture, chiropractic and osteopathy can all be helpful.

Haemorrhoids Piles are often caused by constipation, so follow the steps given. Try resting on your left side regularly; this can relieve pressure on the pelvic veins. Keep the area clean, washing with unperfumed soap after emptying your bowels. Cold, witch hazel compresses can help relieve itching. However, be sure to tell your doctor or midwife about the problem.

Headaches and migraines Eat regularly and make sure that you are drinking enough water – low blood sugar and dehydration can lead to headaches. Try to identify any migraine triggers, such as cheese, chocolate, citrus fruits and caffeine, and avoid them. Watch your posture: relax your shoulders regularly since tension here can cause headaches. A shoulder massage can provide temporary relief, as can applying a lavender-oil compress to your temples. Consider seeing an Alexander technique teacher, chiropractor, osteopath or cranial osteopath. Reiki, reflexology and acupuncture can also help.

Cystitis Urinary infections require immediate treatment: see your doctor if you have an increased need to pass urine, and burning or pain when you do so. Drinking plenty of water and two glasses of cranberry juice a day will help prevent and ease cystitis. Tea tree and lavender oils have a healing effect: dilute two drops of each in a base oil or full-fat milk and add to a warm bath. Do not use lavender if you are less than 16 weeks pregnant.

A homeopath may recommend remedies such as cantharis or apis mel, which can be taken alongside antibiotics. Reflexology and herbal medicine can also be useful as an adjunct to medical treatment.

Thrush See your doctor to check the diagnosis, even if you have had thrush before (other vaginal infections may also cause itching, redness and discharge). Many women

You may be able to relieve a headache by massaging the acupuncture points just above the bridge of the nose and at the external tip of each eyebrow.

find that it helps to avoid sugar and yeast, and to eat plenty of vegetables. You should make sure that you use unscented soap and bath products.

Live yogurt is a soothing natural remedy: apply to the affected area every two hours. Tea tree and lavender essential oils may help: try diluting two drops of each in a base oil or full-fat milk, and add to a warm bath. If you are less than 16 weeks pregnant, use tea tree oil only.

Indigestion Eat little and often rather than having two large meals a day. Limit fluid intake at mealtimes, and eat slowly. Do not bend or lie down afterwards, and make sure that you eat your evening meal at least two hours before bedtime. If indigestion persists at night, use more pillows to keep your upper body elevated. Try drinking lemon balm tea after meals, and ask your doctor about taking calcium-based indigestion tablets. Homeopathy, acupuncture, osteopathy, Alexander technique and chiropractic can all be beneficial.

If you suffer from heartburn at night, do not sleep on your back; sleep on your side propped up with pillows. Do not eat less than two hours before bedtime.

WHEN TO CALL A DOCTOR
Seek emergency assistance if you have:
- Vaginal bleeding other than spotting.
- Severe abdominal pain or vomiting.
- Sudden swelling of hands and ankles or blurred vision with severe headache.
- From week 22, no fetal movements for more than 12 hours.
- Breaking of the waters.
See your doctor if you have:
- A high temperature (101°F/38.5°C +).
- Swollen hands or ankles.
- Pain on urination.

Common Qs and As

Q: I am getting irritated by all the advice that I am receiving from anyone and everyone, and by all the tests that one is given during antenatal care. Is all this fuss necessary?

A: It is important to distinguish between well-meant advice from friends and family, and that from your doctor and midwife. Remember that friends and family may not be up to date – some of what you are told may not be correct. Antenatal care, however, is valuable. Today, it is the expectation of most women in the West that they will have a safe and successful pregnancy leading to the delivery of a healthy baby. This is in stark contrast to our grandmothers and great-grandmothers. Before 1935, one in every 200-250 pregnancies resulted in the death of the mother, most commonly from infection. These days you almost never hear of women dying in childbirth – thanks largely to regular antenatal monitoring and improved delivery procedures.

Q: My sister has been trying for a baby for three years. Now that I am pregnant she is avoiding me. What can I do?

A: This is a very difficult situation, particularly for your sister. It may help to be open about what is happening; perhaps you could tell her that you fully realize how painful it is for her to be around you while you are pregnant and that you understand how she is behaving. You could also reassure her that many couples do conceive after several years of trying, and encourage her to see her doctor for investigations if she has not already done so.

You may want and need your sister's support at this eventful time in your life, but it is probably best to let her decide how much she wants to be involved with your pregnancy. If she does remain distant, you may find that the situation changes when the baby is born, and your sister can enjoy her niece or nephew.

Q: How would I know if there was anything wrong with my baby?

A: The chief way of checking that everything is progressing well is through your regular antenatal checks: this is why it is so important that you attend them. If anything should be amiss, it can be quickly identified and treated.

If there were anything seriously wrong, your body would soon tell you. Be alert to the chief danger signs and symptoms, which are listed on page 145. Be aware, too, of your baby's movements. Should these stop for a period of 24 hours or more, you should consult a doctor without delay.

Q: I am five months pregnant and have only a very small bump. Is something wrong?

A: Women do vary in the size of their bump, and if you are of a slight build you are more likely to give birth to a baby who also has a slighter build. However, if you are worried, the best thing for you to do is to talk about your concerns with your antenatal team. They should be able to reassure you that everything is fine.

One of the great advantages of antenatal care and all the research that has gone before is that the hospital consultants will almost certainly know if anything is wrong. They will be able to tell if you are carrying what is known as a 'small for dates' baby. They will also know from blood and urine tests, as well as from the scans, if the pregnancy is not progressing as it should do.

Q: I feel uncomfortable about the whole idea of making love now that I am well into the pregnancy, and worry that some damage may be done. Am I being ridiculous? Exactly how safe is it?

A: There are certain circumstances under which sex must be avoided – in certain high-risk pregnancies or in the last trimester when expecting more than one baby, for example. Your doctor will advise and warn about this. However, in the majority of cases, experts feel that there is no danger at all in making love at any stage of the pregnancy, as long as you are not overly athletic.

You will find that you need to explore different positions as your size increases, in order to be as comfortable as possible. Also, be prepared for some loss of libido at certain stages due to hormonal changes or fatigue. Take time to explore non-penetrative options and always keep loving lines of communication open with your partner.

Q: I cannot decide whether or not to have an amniocentesis. I would be devastated if I lost the baby through having the test.

A: This is without doubt an extraordinarily difficult decision to make. You should discuss with your hospital consultant the risks of your particular case, bearing in mind your medical history and your age. Then give yourself and your partner time to consider how much you are personally at risk of carrying a baby with a serious problem such as Down's syndrome. If the risk is slight, you may be well advised not to have amniocentesis. If the risk is thought to be high or very high, you may prefer to have the test. However, if you knew that you would be devastated at the loss of any baby, whether or not he or she was impaired with a condition such as Down's, clearly it would be better if you did not have the test.

Q: If I had to terminate a pregnancy, how long would I have to wait before we started trying for another baby?

A: Medical opinion remains divided on this issue. The minimum wait is naturally until your periods return to normal or at least return to what was normal for you. After that, the general consensus is that you should wait for three or four months before attempting to conceive again. If you wait a little longer than that, both you and your partner will have that little extra time in which to recover both physically and emotionally after the termination. Some consultants advise six months but this is not strictly necessary.

Q: My doctor says that I need a course of antibiotics to clear up a severe attack of sinusitis. I am worried about taking medication when I am pregnant. Do you think that it is okay to take them?

A: You should obviously avoid taking any unnecessary medication during pregnancy. However, if the infection is severe, clearly it needs to be treated before it starts to affect your general health and energy levels. Any medication prescribed during your pregnancy will be given in the knowledge that you are pregnant and will be chosen accordingly. Always remind any prescribing doctor that you are pregnant, just in case he or she fails to refer to your notes and especially if you are not yet big enough for it to be obvious.

The third trimester

" It is important for you to make rest and relaxation a priority. "

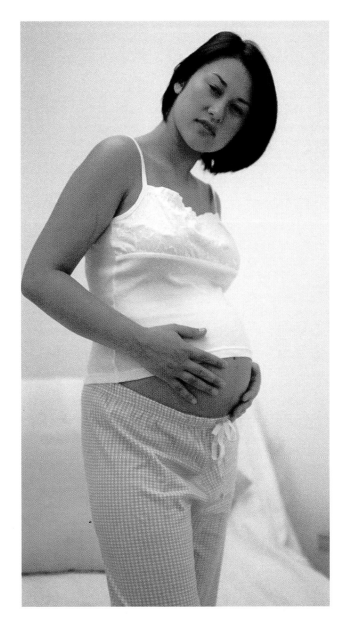

You are now embarking on the last trimester of your pregnancy, week 27 onwards. This is a tumultuous, exciting time for you and your partner. Now that your baby is fully formed, you may more easily be able to imagine him or her as a little person.

The normal length of time for a pregnancy is 40 weeks, but yours may last just 38 – less if the baby is premature – or it may run to 42. Once a pregnancy goes beyond 42 weeks, medical intervention may be recommended. If you are pregnant with twins (or more), you will almost certainly deliver early, usually at about 37 weeks.

During these last weeks, you may feel that you have been pregnant forever. You may feel slightly breathless when bending down. Your sleep may be interrupted when you turn over, by frequent trips to the lavatory, and by kicks from your baby.

It is important for you to make rest and relaxation a priority. Take a rest every day, and perhaps chat to

You may feel a greater bond with your baby in these last weeks. Now you can start looking forward to getting to know him or her in person.

your baby or play music as you do so. Complementary therapies can be particularly beneficial during the last three months. Good ones to try include reiki, yoga, massage, aromatherapy and Alexander technique. These will encourage you to relax, improve your posture and help relieve any backache that you may be experiencing.

Do not attempt to do any more than you feel comfortable with, but remember the value of exercise. A short walk each day will improve muscular fitness and at the same time boost your energy and prepare you for labour and the birth.

Top: You may feel increasingly disinclined to go out as your pregnancy progresses. Spending quiet evenings at home with your partner can seem far more appealing.

Sleep may become more fitful in later months. Get as much relaxation as you can, and take an afternoon nap to compensate if possible.

How your baby is developing

During these last months of your pregnancy, the baby will continue to mature, and he or she will also become much fatter.

Weeks 26-27
The eyelids open briefly for the first time at the end of the second trimester; they start to remain open from week 27. The iris of the eye is blue at this stage, and will remain so until a few months after delivery. The baby looks quite lean, and at 26 weeks weighs about 500g (1lb 2oz). Over the next few weeks, his or her body weight will more than double as more muscle and fat develops.

Weeks 28-31
At 28 weeks the baby measures 36cm (14in), and weighs about 900g (2lb). You will feel a good deal of kicking and fluttering at this stage. Your baby's breathing movements will have become rhythmic by week 30, but he or she may experience hiccups – which you will feel as small jerks – when amniotic fluid goes down the wrong passage.

If your baby were to be born at this point, there is a fair chance that he or she would survive. However, the lack of body fat means that the baby would have difficulty in regulating his or her body temperature. He or she would also experience breathing difficulties and would need to be placed in an incubator with a ventilator attached. The baby's immune system and liver functioning would still be weak, rendering him or her particularly susceptible to infection. Specialist care would be needed for several more weeks while the baby continued his or her development outside the uterus.

Week 32
Your baby is perfectly formed, with fully developed lungs. It has been shown experimentally that the baby can now focus on external stimuli – a needle, for example. From now until week 34, your baby is likely to turn so that he or she is head down, in preparation for the birth. Before this time most babies are in the breech position, with the head facing up. The baby weighs about 1.8kg (4lb).

THE FINAL STAGES
You will become much larger in the last trimester as your baby is growing rapidly. Your expanding uterus will press against your intestines and stomach, impeding your digestion, and on the lungs, causing slight breathlessness. The baby is fully formed at 36 weeks but needs to put on weight before birth.

WEEKS 27-31

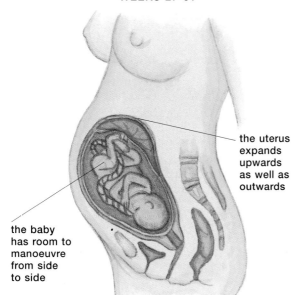

the uterus expands upwards as well as outwards

the baby has room to manoeuvre from side to side

By about week 27, your expanding uterus is halfway between your navel and ribs.

WEEKS 32-36

the uterus is high in the abdomen, and may compress the lungs

the baby is in a head-down position, in preparation for the birth

Between weeks 32 and 36, the uterus has expanded to fill the abdomen, extending almost up to the ribs.

Weeks 33-36

The baby is becoming plumper and gaining about 14g (½oz) of fat each day. Fat ensures that a baby can regulate heat and cold once they leave the controlled environment of the uterus. The fingers and toes have soft nails, which reach right to the ends. The hair on the baby's head may be as long as 2.5cm (1in) long and is very slippery to aid the baby's passage during birth. By week 36, the baby's skull is firm but not hard, because it will need to compress as the baby squeezes down the birth canal.

The baby is about 46cm (18in) long and weighs about 2.75kg (6lb). If this is your first baby, the head will soon engage – drop downwards into the upper pelvis – in preparation for the birth. If you have given birth before, the baby may not engage for several more weeks, and sometimes not until just before the labour.

Weeks 37-39

Your baby's nervous system is maturing, ready for birth. The layer of fat under the skin is now ready to regulate body temperature when the baby is born. The lungs are lined with surfactant, which resembles bubbles of foam. This keeps the lungs partially inflated each time the baby breathes out after she is born; without surfactant the lungs would collapse. The baby's heartbeat is about twice as fast as yours, about 110–150 beats per minute.

During these final weeks, you will feel a variety of movements as your baby turns over, moves his or her hands and feet, and even hiccups. These movements are often felt more when you are resting.

Other people may now be able to hear the baby's heartbeat simply by putting their ear to your abdomen. The baby will weigh about 3.1kg (almost 7lb).

Week 40

The baby's movements decrease from now on, because there is less space in the uterus for him or her to move around. You may miss these movements, although you may still feel strong kicks from the baby's hands and feet. When the baby is awake, his or her eyes are open a good deal of the time. In a boy, the testicles will almost certainly have descended. The baby may now measure about 51cm (20in) in length and he or she weighs about 3.5kg (7lb 8oz).

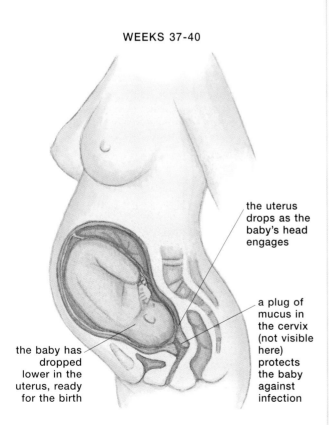

WEEKS 37-40

the uterus drops as the baby's head engages

a plug of mucus in the cervix (not visible here) protects the baby against infection

the baby has dropped lower in the uterus, ready for the birth

Some time from week 36 onwards, the head engages. The uterus drops lower, easing pressure on the lungs.

What the baby hears and feels

As recently as the 1970s, some people believed that babies were born both deaf and blind. However, we now know that babies learn to recognize the sound of the mother's voice several weeks before they are born.

The uterus is neither completely dark nor silent: babies discern light through the uterine wall, and they can also feel vibrations made by music and voices. They may learn to associate certain sounds with the mood of the mother, and may even develop preferences for particular sounds.

TOUCH

The unborn baby's sense of touch starts to function before the other senses. Experiments have shown that the fetus responds to touch on the lips as early as seven weeks. This responsiveness then spreads to the cheeks, the forehead and the palms, followed by the arms. By week 14–15, most of the body responds to touch.

It is difficult to assess whether or not an unborn baby can feel pain. However, increases in heart rate have been observed in fetuses following invasive tests such as fetal scalp blood sampling, and increases in movements have been observed during amniocentesis.

HEARING

Research has shown that a baby's sense of hearing begins to function before the birth. What a baby hears is a jumble of sound – perhaps a low rumble and the distant beating of the mother's heart – as well as the mother's voice, which the baby will recognize and respond to once he or she is born.

Your baby's ears begin to develop in the fourth week of pregnancy and they are reasonably well formed by the end of the seventh week. It is known that external sounds filter through to the baby, although they are likely to be changed in quality. The rhythms of the sounds, however, remain unchanged. Ultrasound pictures have shown that an unborn baby of 24-25 weeks will respond to a noise

> **" The uterus is neither completely dark nor silent: babies discern light through the uterine wall, and they can feel vibrations made by music and voices. "**

applied to the mother's abdomen. However, the external noise has to be quite loud to be audible over the noise of the mother's digestive and cardiovascular system.

In the last few months of your pregnancy, your baby will learn to register your voice, becoming familiar with the vibrations of your speech. The unborn baby's experience of speech patterns and vibrations may actually begin the process of acquiring language.

VISION

Experiments have shown that the visual sense is functioning in the uterus from 26 weeks. Babies will blink or close their eyes if a light is shone on the mother's abdomen. They will also train their vision by focusing on their own hands and feet, and on the umbilical cord.

A baby is likely to recognize the sound of the mother's voice as soon as he or she is born. It seems that babies start to learn while they are still in the uterus.

HOW MUCH DO WE KNOW?
New technology has given us great insight into how babies develop physically. However, we can only speculate about how much they perceive. One leading expert, Professor Peter G. Helpert, says that 98 per cent of what is said about fetal perception is guesswork and 2 per cent is proven fact.

Researchers have discovered that babies can remember sounds and tastes that they experienced in the uterus.

TASTE AND SMELL

It is impossible to distinguish between a baby's sense of taste and smell in the uterus, since both may be stimulated by chemical stimuli in the amniotic fluid. For this reason, researchers tend to investigate them together. We know that babies practise sucking movements in the uterus, in preparation for feeding after the birth, and it seems that they have a preference for sweet tastes. When saccharin is added to the amniotic fluid, an increase in swallowing is observed.

One study found that a newborn responded to an odour previously experienced only in the uterus. In this experiment, a mother was given capsules of cumin with meals for the last 12 days of pregnancy. After the birth, the newborn baby was exposed to cumin, lemon and clean air while his heart rate was measured to assess his responses. The greatest change in heart rate was noted when the baby was presented with cumin. Thus there is some evidence that the sense of smell starts to function before a baby is born.

LEARNING IN THE WOMB

Studies have provided some evidence that learning ability is present at about 22 or 23 weeks. It is thought that the sensory system develops sufficiently in the uterus to allow a developing baby to discriminate between different stimuli, and that the baby's memory is good enough to retain this information.

One study looked at the babies of women who regularly watched a well-known television serial, screened five times a week, during their pregnancies. Researchers found that these babies seemed to recognize the programme's theme tune. This suggests that an unborn baby is able to learn and remember familiar auditory stimuli in the uterus and retain this information over the birth period. Other later studies have confirmed the ability of the unborn baby to learn familiar auditory stimuli *in utero*.

The continuing study of fetal behaviour may in the future make significant contributions to the understanding of the development of mind.

DO BABIES THINK?

There is little doubt that babies' sensory systems are functioning, to a certain extent, while they are still in the uterus. The big question now is whether babies also have powers of perception. In other words, do they attach meaning to what they hear, smell, taste or feel? As yet, there is no way that we can know the answer to this question.

How your body is changing

You will experience both physical and emotional changes in the last three months. The often powerful emotions are nature's way of preparing you for all the changes and challenges ahead. Heightened sensitivity and the ease with which tears often flow are all signs that you are in an emotional state that will make you peculiarly responsive to your newborn baby. In this way nature ensures that you look after your baby, that you respond to cries, that you feed him or her, and that you keep the baby with you and protect him or her from others.

You and your partner may watch, curiously, as your body steadily changes in shape and size. During the third trimester, the changes become much more pronounced.

Towards the end of your pregnancy, Braxton Hicks contractions can cause discomfort, but they do not last long. Unlike labour contractions, they are irregular and do not increase in intensity. Putting your hands on your belly and breathing deeply may help to relieve them, and they usually stop if you have a bath or lie down.

There are five principal signs that help to indicate that your baby is well and progressing normally towards delivery. These signs are:

The baby's kicks

You will feel a lot of kicking. Many babies are lively at certain times of day, suggesting that they develop a regular pattern of sleep and activity. Babies are often most active when the mother is resting.

Breathlessness

It is common to be out of breath in pregnancy, particularly in the last few weeks. You may feel quite short of breath

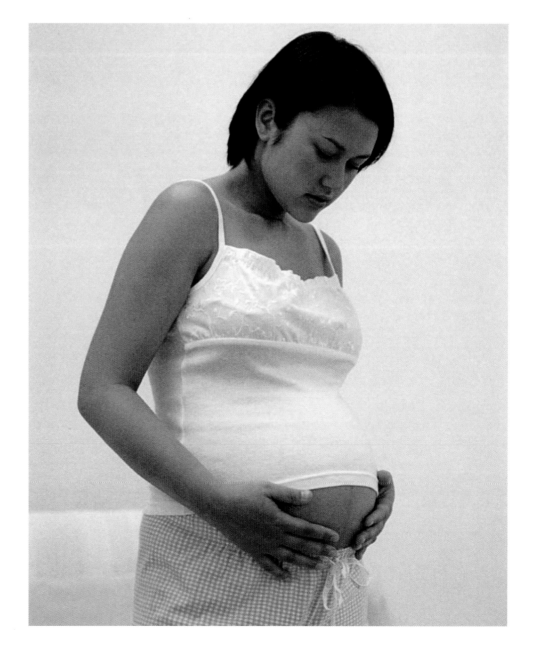

during even relatively minor exertion. This happens for two reasons. Your lungs are working twice as hard as usual in order to supply both you and the baby with oxygen, and the work of the lungs has been made harder because the baby is now so large that he or she is pressing up against your lungs. Rest assured that the baby will receive enough oxygen, even though you may sometimes find yourself panting with the effort.

Increased urine frequency

You will probably want to pass water often, and you may be caught short now and again. This happens partly because the baby is pressing upon all your internal organs, including your bladder, and partly because your muscles have become smoother and softer, in preparation for the birth, when they will be required to stretch to the limit. When you urinate normally, you relax your muscles. When you are pregnant, these muscles tend to relax of their own accord whether you want them to or not. That's what causes the feeling that you need to pass water, and what can cause slight incontinence, too.

Small and irregular contractions

'False labour' contractions can start from week 23, or even earlier, although some women do not experience them at all. They feel like a tightening in the abdominal area. Towards the end of pregnancy, these contractions are known as Braxton Hicks contractions and they become more pronounced, although they are still nothing like the contractions for labour. These 'false labour' contractions last for no more than 20 seconds or so.

When you go into labour, contractions will be more powerful and last for 40 seconds or more. Some specialists maintain that contractions occur throughout pregnancy in order to encourage the blood flow in the placenta, which brings oxygen to the baby.

Engagement

The baby's head becomes engaged in the upper part of the pelvis, usually after the 36th week. All through pregnancy, your uterus expands upwards in your body in order to accommodate the baby's increasing size. The baby is quite low down in your body during the first trimester; after this, he or she rises steadily upwards until week 36. Then, the lower part of the uterus expands, in preparation for the baby's birth, and the baby moves downwards a little.

The baby's head engages in the upper part of the pelvis ready for delivery just a few weeks later. You will experience this as pressure against the cervix (the neck of the uterus). Women who have had babies before may find that their baby's head does not engage so soon, not until the final week of the pregnancy or even as late as the start of labour.

Your increasing size and the frequent activity of the baby mean that you may need extra support to keep you feeling well. Natural therapies can be really helpful in relieving any sleeplessness, stress, tension, fatigue and anxiety that you might be experiencing. They can also help you to feel good about yourself, encouraging you to revel in your swelling size – after all, this is a sure sign that your baby is progressing well.

SUPPORTIVE NATURAL THERAPIES
A weekly session with an experienced therapist may help you cope better with the ups and downs that are often part of pregnancy. Acupuncture, aromatherapy massage and reflexology can all help you to maintain a sense of balance and well-being.

Small feel-good treats – such as soaps scented with essential oils, or gentle herbal home treatments – can lift your mood and relieve tension in the last weeks.

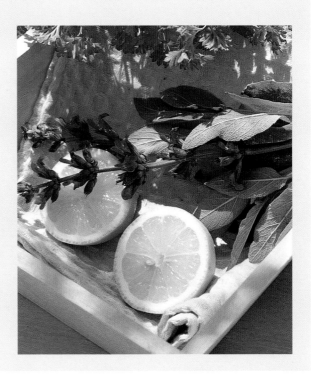

Emotional changes

The last few months of pregnancy are a time of great anticipation and preparation. Both emotionally and mentally, you are readying yourself to become a parent. Physically, your body is gearing up for the birth as well as meeting the needs of your rapidly growing baby. On a practical level, you are likely to feel a strong urge to create a welcoming home for your child.

Not surprisingly, many women find that they become more inward-looking during the third trimester. You may feel absent-minded or forgetful, or rather detached from the world. Work, family and socializing may become less important to you as your focus turns towards the birth.

However keen you are to have your baby, you may experience a real sense of boredom about the pregnancy, particularly in the last weeks. It may feel as though you have been pregnant forever. Now that the birth is near, you may long to get it over with, and start your new life.

> ❝ It is important that you allow yourself to express any recurrent emotions, doubts or anxieties that you have, so that you can deal with them and release the tension they create. ❞

A LIFE TRANSITION

The strong and fluctuating emotions associated with pregnancy may intensify in the final months, although many women find that they start to feel much calmer as the birth approaches.

Some women feel sad about the loss of freedom having a first baby entails, even if the baby is very much wanted. Many women find themselves worrying about something quite minor – such as where they will put the baby clothes or how they will find time to exercise after the delivery. Almost every pregnant woman feels anxious about the pain of labour and worries that she will not achieve the birth she is expecting.

All these feelings are normal and natural. However, it is important that you allow yourself to express any recurrent emotions, doubts or anxieties that you have, so that you can deal with them and release the tension they create.

Talk to your partner so that he can understand what you are going through and offer you support. This may encourage him to share any ambivalent or difficult emotions that he is experiencing. If you are on your own, talk to a close friend or relative. It can also be invaluable to share your experiences with other pregnant women or with mothers. Your midwife is another good source of support and reassurance.

YOUR RELATIONSHIP

Pregnancy is bound to affect your relationship. For many couples, a new closeness and tenderness emerges. Your partner may develop a new protectiveness towards you. At the same time, you may become aware of a new feeling of vulnerability and dependency – something that can feel very strange to you both.

The emotional turbulence of pregnancy can put pressure on the relationship, too. Your partner may miss the companionship you used to share and find it difficult to cope with mood swings; you may have unreasonable expectations of how much others can do for you, or feel disappointed that your partner does not seem as interested in your pregnancy as you are.

As with most aspects of pregnancy, it is helpful to cultivate a sense of acceptance and enjoyment about these changes. Continue to spend time alone together and to talk about your feelings.

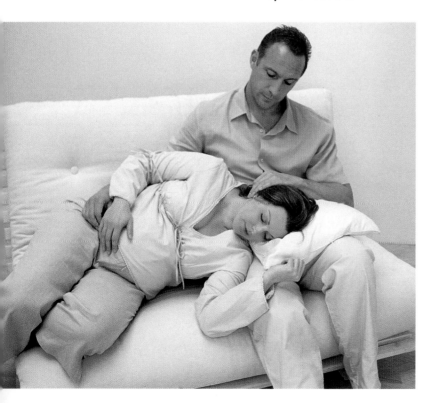

Couples often draw closer in the later stages of pregnancy, and men commonly feel a new sense of protectiveness towards their partner.

Talking to the baby regularly will help him or her to become familiar with the voices of both parents. You may even feel your baby respond with a little kick when you start speaking.

Physical closeness is also important. Massage can be a wonderfully sensuous way of retaining intimacy. Of course, making love will help you to explore any new feelings towards each other. Pregnant women often worry that their partner no longer finds them attractive, particularly in the later stages of pregnancy. However, you may find that your partner enjoys your new curves and voluptuousness. Some couples find that the tenderness pregnancy can evoke – as well as the need to experiment with new positions – brings a new element to their love-making. Other couples find it hard to contemplate the idea of having sex late in pregnancy.

There are no rights and wrongs here – and it is best to do what you feel most comfortable with. But if you both want to make love, sex can usually continue until the waters have broken, as long as the pregnancy is progressing normally. Check with your midwife or doctor if you are not sure.

THE FATHER-TO-BE

The third trimester can be an exciting time for fathers. The baby is becoming more and more visible and active, and may respond at the sound of the father's voice.

However, late pregnancy also has its challenges. Inevitably the attention is on the pregnant women and some men can feel rather isolated and redundant. This is a false impression: the woman needs their support and love more than anyone else's.

New fathers do have a lot to contend with – and this is something that is rarely recognized. If they are to be the main breadwinners for a while, they may well worry about how they will cope with the extra burden. In addition, men often grow nervous about how the baby will affect their lives. They might find themselves wondering if they will ever again be able to go out for a quiet drink once the baby has arrived.

Becoming a parent is a huge event and it is natural for fathers to have anxieties. Expressing these fears will make them seem more manageable, and will help fathers to support their partners.

As well as talking to their partners, father could try seeking out other fathers. It can really help to talk to someone who has been in the same situation. Another man is likely to have a similar perspective and may have dealt with the same feelings.

COUNSELLING
You may want to consider seeking help from a counsellor if your emotions become overwhelming and you feel that you cannot cope alone.

Rest, rest and more rest

You are bound to feel tired during pregnancy. The extra weight you are carrying – which can be as much as 13.5kg (about 2¼ stone) – means not only that fatigue sets in more quickly, but also that your muscles have to put more effort into making even small movements. Your body is also working harder than usual – your heart, for example, is pumping 25 per cent more blood around your system in order to meet the baby's needs.

Despite the fact that you need a lot of rest, you are likely to suffer from disturbed sleep. Your size can make it hard to find a comfortable sleeping position, while increased urination means you are likely to be getting up several times during the night.

It is important that you respond to your body's needs and relax as much as possible during the day. Relaxation helps you to maintain good health, and makes you better able to cope with mood swings. Your baby needs you to relax, too. When the muscles around your uterus are at rest, more blood and oxygen gets through to the baby – which helps him or her to grow.

BOOSTING YOUR RELAXATION QUOTA

If you are suffering from insomnia, herbal teas, gentle homeopathic remedies or aromatherapy oils can help. However, even if you are sleeping well at night, you still need to rest during the day. Doing the following may help.

- Have a nap whenever you are feeling tired. Don't be embarrassed if you need a short sleep if you are visiting friends or relatives. Most people understand that pregnant women need extra care and will be happy to accommodate you.
- Make sure that you have a sleep each afternoon. Be aware of when your energy dips – often between 2pm and 4pm – and set this time aside for a rest.

- Go to bed early. Cutting out television and late-night telephone calls can help you to prepare for sleep.
- Get up late at the weekend or any other day that you can. If you have had a restless night, eat breakfast in bed and try to doze afterwards.
- Make a point of getting out into the fresh air every day. Breathe deeply as you walk to increase the supply of oxygen around your body.
- Put your feet up whenever you can. Always sit rather than stand up.
- At regular points during the day, stop whatever you are doing and check how you are standing or sitting. Notice any awkwardness in your posture and move if necessary to adopt a more comfortable position. In particular, drop your shoulders down and slightly back, and relax any tension in your face by smiling a little. Take a few deep breaths.
- Don't push yourself in any activity, whether it is socializing, exercising or housework. Respect your body's limitations and be prepared to leave jobs unfinished if you need to.

QUICK RELAXER
A short relaxation or breathing exercise can be as energizing as a nap. This quick abdominal breathing exercise can be done anywhere – including on public transport or at work.

Rest your hands on your abdomen and breathe deeply, allowing your abdomen to rise on the in-breath and fall on the out-breath. Focus on your hands rising and falling to help you to concentrate. Continue for about ten breaths.

It can be hard to find a comfortable sleeping position when you are pregnant. Avoid lying on your back as this can put pressure on the spine, and can also impede the supply of blood to the baby. Try lying on your side, with your bump supported with pillows.

WORK AND REST

How long you continue to work obviously depends on financial considerations as well as on how you are feeling. Many women work during the last months of pregnancy, which can make it difficult for them to get enough rest. Finding a place to nap in your lunch hour, working at home sometimes, or changing your hours to avoid rush-hour traffic can all help.

Consider taking occasional days off sick: don't struggle into work if you are feeling poorly. Talk to your doctor if you do work that involves standing up for long periods, bending down or carrying things, or if you do shift work, which can disrupt your sleep patterns; you may need to change the way that you work.

All other things being equal, you should give up work as soon as it becomes too difficult to manage both your work and your pregnancy – your baby is more important than your job, after all. Ideally, you should stop working four to six weeks before your due date at the latest. This gives you time to prepare for birth and, who knows, the baby might come early.

Adopt a sense of moderation and balance in all that you do. For example, if you have to carry shopping and work files, spread the load between two bags.

Deep relaxation exercise

The starting point of this exercise is to tense the muscles in your body one by one. As you relax them, the psychological tension will dissipate and flow out of you, like water down a drain. You can do this in bed at night or whenever you feel you need to relax.

1 Lie down in a comfortable position (on your side or propped up against a pile of cushions). Breathe deeply a few times, letting your body sink downwards. Try to release any obvious tension from your body – in particular, drop your shoulders.

2 Squeeze your toes so that they are pointing inwards. Hold the tension for a few seconds, then release it. Press your heels downwards until you feel the stretch working the muscles in your calves. Hold, then release. Clench your thigh muscles, hold, then relax. Do the same with your buttock muscles.

3 Bring your focus to your abdomen. Take a few deep breaths, letting your abdomen sink downwards as you do so. Your middle area should feel heavy and warm.

4 Move on to your upper body. Draw your shoulders back and, breathing deeply, feel your ribcage expand. Release the tension as you breathe out. Make fists, then let go, and repeat. Hunch your shoulders, hold tight, release, then repeat until your shoulders feel relaxed. Pull your chin down towards your chest, hold, and then release.

5 Now work on your face. Purse your lips, hold, and relax. Grin, hold, and relax. Make a deep frown, hold, and relax.

6 Your body should be feeling soft and heavy. In this state, continue to breathe deeply and regularly for 10 or 15 minutes. If you like, you can practise some visualization at this point – imagine you are lying on the grass under a warm sun as you breathe.

Purse your lips for a few moments.

Grin like a Cheshire cat.

Make a deep frown, then relax.

Feel-good treats and therapies

Many women revel in the changes that late pregnancy brings, enjoying their new voluptuousness. However, others dislike becoming so much larger and heavier, particularly if their weight has been an issue before conceiving.

Pregnancy can certainly be a challenge to your self-image, and many women find it hard to cope with stretch marks, varicose veins and other visible ailments. However, it is important to develop a sense of acceptance and appreciation of your body in these last months. This will not only help you to enjoy pregnancy, but it will enhance your general feeling of well-being.

Touch is one of the best ways to maintain a sense of connection with your physical self. Try regular self-massage or enjoy massage with your partner. Gentle exercise, particularly walking, swimming and yoga will help you to feel good. Above all – treat yourself. Incorporating indulgent moments into every day and looking after yourself physically will help you to embrace your growing body. This, in turn, will help you to enjoy the journey towards motherhood.

LOOK GOOD, FEEL GOOD

Making an effort to look good can often improve the way you feel. Try these quick fixes.
- Get your hair cut. Having a good haircut is one of the quickest ways to make yourself feel attractive. This is probably not the time to go for a radical style – choose something that you know suits you.
- Have a manicure. Even if you don't usually worry about how your hands look, late pregnancy can be a great time to spoil yourself.
- Buy something new to wear. By now, you are probably heartily sick of all the maternity clothes you

Late pregnancy is one time when you can enjoy being lazy without feeling guilty – after all, your baby needs you to rest. Go to bed for the afternoon with a glossy magazine or paper, and indulge yourself.

have bought so far. Women often feel guilty about spending money on clothes they are going to wear for only a few months, with the result that they make do with two or three outfits throughout their pregnancy. However, one new outfit can lift your self-esteem and help you to feel happy about the way you look.
- Wear clothes in natural fabrics, which are softer and more comfortable than manmade materials. Colour therapists often recommend green or blue as good colours to wear during pregnancy because they have a calming effect. Yellow can also be a good choice since it can lift the spirits. But, most importantly, choose clothes in a colour that you feel good in.

PAMPER YOURSELF

Late pregnancy is a good time to indulge yourself. Set some time aside to do things that you really enjoy – such as meeting a friend for a long catching-up session, reading a novel, going for a walk in the park, or one of the following:
- Buy yourself a large bunch of flowers and put them somewhere you will see them often.
- Book a meal in a favourite restaurant for you and your partner. Enjoy spending a romantic evening together as a couple. Book the table for the earlier part of the evening so that you can still get a good night's rest.

Enjoy small extravagances, such as buying yourself a bouquet of beautiful fresh flowers.

- Spend an afternoon or a whole day in bed. Forget about chores, preparing for the baby or working. Enjoy getting up late, reading the papers or a book or just dozing for a day.
- Go to the cinema, theatre, opera or ballet. It will be much more difficult to organize nights out once the baby is born, so make the most of these last weeks. Go to an afternoon or an early-evening show if you usually feel tired later in the evening.

NATURAL THERAPIES

A treatment with a qualified complementary therapist can boost your energy and help to relieve some of the discomforts of late pregnancy. The following can also be deeply pleasurable to receive:

- **Reflexology** Few things are more relaxing than a foot treatment. Find a professional reflexologist who specializes in treating pregnant women – some points can stimulate contractions of the uterus.
- **Reiki** You can receive reiki sitting up and fully clothed. It is gentle, soothing and non-invasive. The practitioner places his or her hands on or just above different areas of your body. You may feel a warm or tingling sensation as healing energy flows through the practitioner's hands to wherever it is needed.
- **Shiatsu** This Japanese massage is given on the floor, and you remain clothed. It can be deeply relaxing,

Take the time to look after yourself in the evening: have a warm bath, wrap yourself in a robe and apply a mask or deep moisturizer to your face.

and acupressure points may be used to relieve common symptoms such as fatigue. See a practitioner who is experienced with pregnancy. Tell them if you have any varicose veins, as direct pressure should not be applied to them. Abdominal work and heavy pressure on the legs should also be avoided.

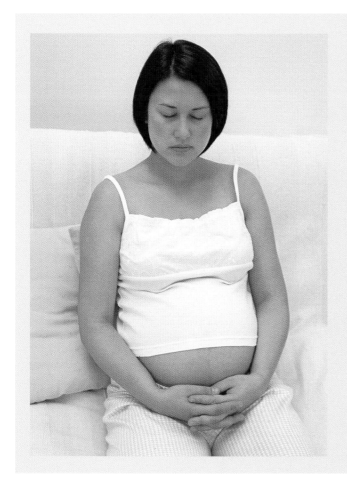

POSITIVE THINKING

If you are finding it hard to embrace the physical changes of pregnancy, try doing this exercise for five or ten minutes. It will work best if you do it daily.

Sit in a comfortable position, ideally with your back straight. If you have back problems or are feeling tired, prop yourself up against a pile of cushions. Take a few deep breaths, allowing your body to release any tension.

Silently focus on an affirmative phrase about the physical changes you are experiencing. Your affirmation should be a short, positive phrase in the present tense. Make up your own or try one of the following:

I am growing more and more beautiful every day.
I welcome and embrace the changes in my body.

Continue to breathe deeply as you repeat the affirmation over and over. Don't worry if you don't feel what you are saying is true – just keep on silently repeating yourself. Eventually, the message will sink in.

When you are ready to finish, bring your attention back to your breathing. Now, slowly open your eyes. Remain sitting quietly for a minute before you get up.

Positive affirmations can shift negative feelings about yourself and help you to enjoy your pregnancy more.

Perineal and breast massage

assage of the perineum and breasts is both pleasant and beneficial during the last trimester. Regular massage of the perineum, the area between the vagina and rectum, may help to reduce the chance of tearing during the birth. Massaging your breasts will help to prepare them for breastfeeding. You need not use oil to massage these areas, although you may well find it easier to do so. Use pure, plain oils such as wheatgerm, olive or almond oils, avoiding any that are contraindicated during pregnancy. If you want to use any oils not mentioned below, then consult an aromatherapist first.

PERINEAL MASSAGE

The perineum has to be strong to support the contents of the abdomen, especially as your baby grows heavier. At the same time, however, the perineum will also have to yield and stretch in order to let your baby pass down the birth canal. Nature provides for this change in texture by releasing "loosening" hormones that soften the ligaments. You can also help to improve elasticity in this area by self-massage. Massaging gently can greatly increase the comfort and ease with which you give birth, and possibly prevent a tear or the need for a surgical cut (episiotomy).

It is truly amazing just how quickly the normally tight tissues in the perineum and vagina will stretch with regular massage. The more that you are able to pre-stretch these tissues before the birth, the better you will return to your original shape after it.

During the last weeks of pregnancy (starting around 36 weeks), massage the perineal area once a day for around five or ten minutes, always doing so with great care and sensitivity. Ideally, perform the massage after soaking in a warm (not hot) bath, to soften the area, and when your bladder is empty. If using oil, wheatgerm is a good choice, and aromatherapists recommend adding a few drops of lavender to the oil.

HOW TO MASSAGE THE PERINEUM

When you start practising perineal massage, use two fingers, oiled if you wish. Insert the two fingers into your vagina up to the first knuckle, progressing to the second

For massage of the perineal and vaginal areas, make sure you are in a relaxed and comfortable position. Lying on your side against a bed or beanbag is a good position, as is squatting or half-kneeling with one leg up.

knuckle with practice. You may like to use three or four fingers, and apply a little more pressure, once you are used to the technique. Now use a light touch to explore the layers of tissues along the back wall of your vagina and the skin that separates your vagina and anus. It is this area that will be most stretched during the birth of your baby and is most prone to tearing.

As you press against the back wall of the vagina, against the spine, breathe deeply. You will experience a tingling sensation and will feel the muscles under your fingers as they engage on the breath out. As space is gradually created, move in further and exert a little more pressure, using your breath to help you, but you should never take this kind of massage any further than feels totally comfortable.

You will probably find that nothing much seems to happen at first, but soon your perineal tissue starts to give and then begins to stretch. You will be amazed how much you can stretch it, simply by breathing out into the areas under your fingers.

MASSAGING THE BREASTS

Up to around 36 weeks, regular massage of the breasts is a wonderful way of bringing a combination of tone, strength and elasticity to the tissues here, in readiness for breastfeeding. Remember to avoid the nipple area. If you decide to use oil then almond oil is a good choice. Calendula cream is also gentle and safe. Like perineal massage, breast massage is best done after a warm and relaxing bath.

To massage the breasts, use your entire hand, with your fingers kept together. With each stroke, start with the heel of your hand and take the stroke through your fingers. Keep the pressure even and smooth; do not jab or press harshly.

In order to understand the technique, you need to imagine the ducts that carry breast milk rather like the spokes of a wheel, radiating out from the central spoke – your nipple. The milk travels down these ducts to the

When massaging the breasts, either massage through clothes or directly on to the skin. As well as massage, you may find that exposing your breasts to the elements from time to time will feel especially pleasant.

nipple, and your massage should also work from the outside of the breast towards the nipple. Do this slowly around the whole of each breast, working in a clockwise direction. Many pregnancy books compare the breast to a clockface, and recommend starting at 1 o'clock, working from the outside in to the nipple, then repeating this at 2 o'clock and so on.

MASSAGING OTHER AREAS

While you are in a relaxed mood, with suitable oils at the ready, it is a good idea to extend your massage to other areas of the body. A facial massage is always enjoyable (see p129) and you could also try gentle massage of the abdomen, in order to help prevent stretch marks. During the latter weeks of pregnancy, massage down the sides of your belly. Work from the ribs to your navel, with both hands and using circular strokes, and continue down over your hips and thighs. Using plenty of oil feels especially pleasant when massaging the abdomen.

SAFETY POINTS

Take great care with perineal or vaginal massage, and never deliberately stretch out or pull these very delicate tissues.

Do not perform breast massage after about 36 weeks. When massaging the breasts, always proceed gently and avoid massaging the nipples themselves. However, a very gentle tweaking of the nipples can be appropriate once your due date has arrived. This tweaking is said to stimulate production of the hormone oxytocin and so may help to bring on labour.

Yoga for the third trimester

You will find that your baby is sensitive to your moods, shares your enjoyment and joins in with many of your activities. So the more that you dance around and stretch, and open and tone your body, the better he or she will like it. Your centre of gravity lies deep within your pelvis. The opening up of your hips and pelvic area, plus all the activity, will encourage your baby to find the very best position to be in as birth approaches. Putting aside time each day for a few minutes of energetic yoga dance, followed by a perineal stretch, is a great way to prepare for labour with your baby and it will also help release tension. Don't forget that all these rotating, twisting and opening movements of the hips should be done with knees bent. Keep breathing deeply all the time.

Knee circles

This is a balancing exercise that shakes out your hips and legs as you get into a knee-swinging stride. It is a loosening and strengthening movement, which helps to boost the circulation and is also good for lifting your mood. If you feel wary about trusting your balance, try placing one hand against a wall for support. Keep your arms, shoulders and neck relaxed. The raised leg is also kept as loose as possible throughout, and the knee circles should be done smoothly and lightly. Before you start, stand erect and breathe deeply for a few moments.

1 Raise your left leg, bending the knee. Stand on your right leg, with your arms spread out to the sides to help your balance, and your spine erect. Now swing your left knee up in front of you as high as is comfortable.

2 Bring your left knee to the side to open your left hip and so make more room in the abdomen and pelvis.

3 Swing the left leg slowly round behind you and kick back with your left foot. Finally, swing your knee forward, then straighten your left leg and place your left foot firmly on the floor. Repeat the exercise with the right knee.

Pushing the sky

In this empowering pose, you are pushing your palms up into the sky. The aim is to lift and strengthen your upper body, and to make space in your lower body as you flex your thigh muscles. Use your diaphragm and breathe deeply, so that you involve all your abdominal muscles in the action.

1 Stand with feet wide and toes pointing outwards so that you can bend your knees deeply and hold this position comfortably. Keeping the spine erect and coccyx tucked in, raise your arms. Push up further with first one palm and then the other. Turn your palm upwards if you can. Feel a lengthening stretch up through each side of your body in turn.

2 Keep your arms raised directly over your head. Push both hands upwards while bending the knees further and dropping into a semi-squat. Do this on an outbreath, feeling a lengthening stretch through your middle as you do so.

Standing twist

This is a good position for easing tension in the neck and shoulders, and it also acts as a counter-pose to the strong sideways stretch of the Knee circles. Breathe deeply and twist through the whole torso.

Seated perineal stretch

A low stool and several cushions are useful props for this gentle perineal stretch, which is good preparation for the birth. Place one cushion on the stool and the others under your dropped knee as required in Step 2. The breath is very important when you are stretching the yogic way – otherwise nothing happens, or you simply stretch a little in the groin area. Remember to move gently and slowly.

Place your right foot on a low stool, thigh parallel to the floor. Raise your arms and open the elbows to expand the chest. Place your palms behind your head, neck erect. Breathe in. As you breathe out, turn the head and shoulders to the right. Let your chest follow, but keep your lower body steady. Come back to the centre, change legs and repeat on the left.

1 Place a cushion on a low stool and sit astride it, with your knees wide and feet firmly planted on the floor. Stretch up through your spine by pressing the palms of your hands against your spread thighs. Breathe normally but evenly as you do this.

2 Press into your right foot and drop the left knee back and down on to two firm cushions. This is a good stretch for the perineum and the left groin. Clasp your hands. Inhale as you push the palms away, pressing further into your right foot. Push out further as you exhale and lift through the spine as you inhale. Do this several times. Change legs and repeat.

Hip-openers in water

Here are some good yoga exercises to do in the swimming pool. The buoyant water supports your weight, making it much easier to stretch and move around. In these exercises one leg is raised to rotate and open the hip, involving all the lower back muscles on that side as well as the pelvic muscles. They both prevent and relieve lower backache, particularly sciatica or inflammation. Start with the small knee circles, then proceed to the wider hip circles. Do them very slowly, with your leg moving as much water as possible.

Knee circles

For this exercise, face the wall and hold on to the bar or edge of the pool, or face the pool and rest your arms on a woggle (long float) in front of you. The same exercise can be done facing the pool and supporting yourself on the bar or edge from behind, or on a woggle under your arms and behind your back. While facing the wall, the main stretch is in the lower back; facing the pool a greater emphasis is placed on opening the pelvis.

1 Start in a standing position. Bend the knee of your standing leg slightly. Lift your other leg up from the pool floor, bending your knee as you do so. Keep your upper body relaxed.

2 Move your knee to make small smooth circles in the water. Keep your whole body relaxed and feel the resistance of the water. Change legs and repeat the exercise.

Hip circles

Start in a standing position, facing the wall and holding on to the bar or the edge of the pool, or resting your arms on a woggle in front of you. Keep your standing leg a little more bent than for the knee circles, to allow for a wider opening of your other leg as you engage your hip in the rotating movement.

1 Lift one leg, bending the knee. Slowly circle the hip and knee, feeling the resistance of the water as you do so. Make small circles at first.

2 Gradually increase the size of the circles by pushing your raised knee back. Exhale each time you open out the knee. Repeat on the other side.

3 Move away from the side of the pool. Make larger circles, stretching the leg out to the side, then bending it again to come back to the centre. Do this a few times. Breathe deeply, using your abdominal muscles.

4 Now extend your raised leg back behind you before bringing it back. As you become fitter, extend your leg higher towards the surface of the water, straightening your standing leg.

5 Move so your back is facing the side of the pool or place a woggle under your arms for support. Make circles with your leg, opening the hips wide on each side while keeping your back straight.

6 Supporting your extended arms on the bar, pool edge or a woggle, work both your hips at the same time, using a wide backstroke movement with your legs.

7 Now stretch the legs out in front of you, inhaling as you do so. Bend the legs in as you exhale. Keep the upper part of your body as relaxed as possible.

8 Complete the routine by bringing both legs together and making a rotating movement. Do small circles at first, then gradually increase the size of the circle, breathing deeply all the time. With practice, your circling will start to become smoother and more regular.

Antenatal care

The three cornerstones of antenatal care at this stage of your pregnancy are: attending antenatal checks; going to antenatal classes; and looking after your general health.

ANTENATAL CHECKS

Most women attend their antenatal clinic every month until about the 28th week, fortnightly until about week 36 and then weekly until the birth. During your antenatal visits, the following routine checks will be carried out:

- Weight.
- Blood pressure, to detect pre-eclampsia.
- Urine, to detect signs of pre-eclampsia and diabetes.
- The baby's heartbeat.
- The size of your abdomen, in order to monitor the baby's continuing growth.
- Your hands and legs for any sign of swelling, which could indicate pre-eclampsia.

Your blood pressure

Pregnancy brings about enormous changes in blood volume and pressure, partly because your heart is beating much faster and more frequently than usual and partly because of hormonal changes in the blood vessels. Your blood pressure will usually return to normal within a few days of the birth.

High blood pressure early in pregnancy can indicate a number of conditions, including kidney disease and diabetes. In later pregnancy, raised blood pressure alone does not usually signify problems, but high blood pressure combined with swelling of the ankles or feet, pronounced weight gain and the appearance of protein in the urine are signs of pre-eclampsia, which develops in about one in every 20 pregnancies.

What is pre-eclampsia?

Pre-eclampsia is not yet fully understood, but it is believed to be due to abnormalities of hormone secretion, kidney secretion, or the production of abnormal substances by the placenta. Mild pre-eclampsia is usually simple to treat: rest may be all that is needed. Left untreated, it can progress to eclampsia, which is a dangerous complication of pregnancy.

An eclamptic fit dramatically reduces the oxygen supply to the unborn baby, and can also be life-threatening to the mother. If a fit occurs, the baby will be delivered immediately either by induction or by emergency Caesarean. You may not notice any symptoms if you have pre-eclampsia, which is one reason why

A severe headache accompanied by blurred vision or flashing lights could be a sign of pre-eclampsia.

antenatal checks are so vital. The symptoms of this condition can include:

- Severe headache.
- Visual disturbances such as flashing lights or blurring.
- Vomiting.
- Severe pain in the upper abdomen.
- Feet, ankles or hands swelling up suddenly.

Seek immediate medical advice if you develop any of the symptoms listed above during your pregnancy; you must call an ambulance if any of them are severe.

    If you or your partner are in any doubt about an aspect of your health, your baby's health or your antenatal health care, seek professional advice.

The 32-week scan

You will probably have had a scan around week 20 of your pregnancy. If you are receiving specialist antenatal care because of an identified risk factor in your pregnancy, you may have another scan at about 32 weeks. This allows the accurate measurement of the baby's head and abdomen. The information obtained from the scan at this stage of development is more precise than that obtained from a physical examination.

LOOKING AFTER YOUR HEALTH

During the third trimester, you should still be eating healthily every day, taking some exercise and avoiding smoky atmospheres and alcohol. It is especially important at this stage that you make every effort to keep stress at bay and make sure that you get plenty of relaxation, rest and sleep each day. This will stand you in good stead not only for the birth itself, but also for dealing with your newborn baby once he or she arrives.

If you or your partner are in any doubt about an aspect of your health, your baby's health or your antenatal health care, never hesitate to seek professional advice. The family doctor, your midwife, your hospital, and your antenatal class teacher are there to answer any questions that you may have.

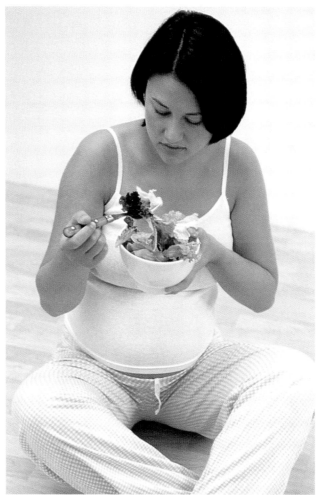

Look after yourself and your baby by continuing with a healthy lifestyle – the food you eat and the amount of exercise and relaxation you get are all important.

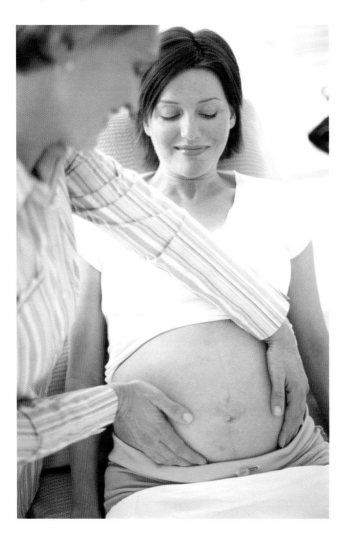

WHEN THE BABY COMES EARLY

A pre-term baby is one that arrives or has to be delivered for medical reasons up to three weeks before the estimated date of delivery. A premature baby is one that has arrived more than three weeks early. He or she has an increased chance of respiratory problems in the first few days, and may need special care. Drugs can be given to activate the baby's lungs artificially to speed them towards maturity. These work only if administered early in the third trimester (about weeks 29-33), and are given only if doctors are about to deliver the baby. Once the baby is born, he or she can be put on a ventilator to assist with breathing. The baby also needs to be kept very warm while he or she builds up the fat reserves that would normally have built up by delivery.

During each antenatal visit, the midwife will feel your abdomen to check the increase in the size of your uterus, and therefore the growth of your baby.

Antenatal classes

The various kinds of antenatal classes are quite distinct from antenatal care, which you receive in an antenatal clinic. While the clinics concentrate mainly on your health and that of your baby, antenatal classes cover the practical and emotional aspects of pregnancy and labour. Classes usually cover a wide range of topics, from sex during pregnancy to pain relief at the birth.

Many women find antenatal classes helpful. You are not only given valuable information, but the classes also provide an opportunity for you to ask any questions that you may have and to swap experiences with other women at the same stage of pregnancy as you. Women often forge friendships at antenatal classes that continue long after the birth of their babies. These can be a good source of support during the first months of motherhood.

Antenatal classes are known by various names: for example, parentcraft, childbirth education classes or preparation for parenthood. Active birth classes – which encourage the use of yoga – may also be available. Classes are run by different organizations, such as the health authority, charities and independent teachers. Your doctor or midwife will tell you about the different classes on offer, and you can choose a system that suits you.

The classes usually run weekly for five to six weeks, perhaps eight weeks, and you attend them during the last couple of months of pregnancy. Most classes actively encourage male partners to come along, and offer specific advice for them. However, you can also go on your own or take a friend or relative along with you.

Antenatal classes help you understand exactly what happens during pregnancy and childbirth. Here a teacher uses models of a baby and a pelvis to demonstrate the breech (feet or buttocks first) position.

You will learn simple exercises to relieve backache and to prepare your body for the birth. You can then practise these regularly at home with a friend.

WHAT ANTENATAL CLASSES COVER

Antenatal classes will always include an opportunity for you and your partner to ask any questions that you may have. The classes will usually also cover set topics each week, which will include all or most of the following:

Pregnancy

- Diet, health and fitness in pregnancy.
- Caring for your teeth and gums.
- Bathing in pregnancy.
- Posture and back problems.
- Maternity clothing.
- Relationships and sex during pregnancy.
- Talks for partners covering pregnancy, the birth and fatherhood.
- How the baby grows – the developmental milestones of the unborn baby.
- Coping with common discomforts such as piles, constipation and back pain.
- Exercises, including pelvic floor exercises, to help you prepare for the birth and to prevent problems such as stress incontinence.

The birth

- Breathing exercises for labour. In antenatal classes, you are taught how to change your breathing deliberately during labour, adjusting to the changing characteristics of the contractions. This can help you to manage your labour and cope better with the pain. Synchronizing the breathing with the signals that are received from the uterus demands total concentration and it is important to practise the techniques regularly beforehand.

Many classes will include special advice for your partner or a friend, who will then be able to assist you and provide support in labour.

- A visit to the maternity ward and labour ward. This will help you to understand the technology of birth: medical terms will be explained and you'll have an opportunity to see some of the equipment. You'll also get a chance to see what options are available in your particular unit (for example, water births), and to become familiar with the wards and labour suite.
- What you will need for a home birth.
- How to recognize the signs of labour.
- What happens during labour.
- Options for pain relief during labour.
- Breech births.
- Medical intervention, such as induction, Caesarean section and assisted deliveries.

After the birth

- Breast and bottle-feeding.
- Caring for the nipples when breastfeeding; coping with other associated problems, such as mastitis.
- What you will need after the birth for yourself – maternity bras and other clothing.
- What you will need for the baby – equipment and clothing.
- Basic baby-care skills – including how to change a nappy and how to bath a baby.
- How to recognize postnatal depression.
- Advice on contraception after delivery, because you can become pregnant quite quickly after the arrival of your baby. It is best to delay conceiving again for at least nine months after the birth.

Checklist of common problems

Your baby almost doubles in size during the third trimester, and your body has to stretch and grow to accommodate it. Not surprisingly, most women feel heavy and uncomfortable during this stage of pregnancy.

It can be difficult to find a comfortable sleeping position, so you may feel very tired. You may also suffer from breathlessness, since the expanding uterus presses up against the lungs, or from circulation problems, such as swollen ankles.

Make sure that you get plenty of rest during the day, especially if you are sleeping badly at night, and put your feet up regularly. If you are suffering from other minor ailments, complementary therapies can often help to relieve them. However, always check the relevant safety advice in Section Four, and talk to your midwife or doctor before using any remedy.

You should report any symptoms you are experiencing to your midwife during your antenatal visits. See your doctor beforehand if symptoms are severe, persistent or concern you in any way.

Sleep is an excellent restorative. Make sure you get as much as possible in these last weeks of pregnancy. You need to be well rested for the labour.

Cramp Leg cramps often occur in late pregnancy. They may be caused by deficiencies of calcium and magnesium, so try eating more dairy products, sardines and green leafy vegetables (for calcium) and plenty of nuts and seeds (for magnesium). Vitamin B2, which is found in yogurt, lean meat and fortified breakfast cereals, may help. You should make sure that you drink plenty of water and take regular exercise. If you do get cramp, rub your calf briskly. Try flexing your foot at the same time so that the toes point upwards.

Stress incontinence Leaking urine can be an embarrassing problem, but it is one that many pregnant women experience. It is usually caused by weakness of the pelvic floor, which supports the neck of the bladder. To prevent stress incontinence, practise pelvic floor exercises several times a day: tighten the ring of muscles around your vagina and anus, as though you were stopping yourself from urinating mid-flow. Hold for a count of five, then release. Repeat five times or more.

You are most likely to leak urine when you are lifting, laughing, coughing or sneezing, so pull up the pelvic floor whenever you are about to do so. Regular exercise and yoga can also help to strengthen the pelvic floor.

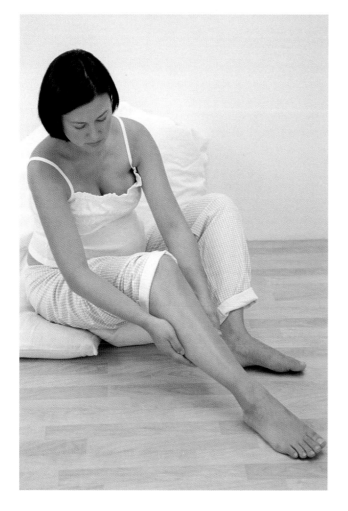

If you get cramp in the calf, rub briskly, then massage using a squeezing action. Make sure you get some gentle exercise – such as a half-hour walk – each day.

Backache Almost all pregnant women suffer from backache in the third trimester, and often earlier, too. The growing weight of the baby in your uterus alters your centre of gravity, and you may sit or stand awkwardly to compensate. An Alexander technique teacher can help you to adjust your posture, and chiropractic and osteopathy can also be very beneficial. Regularly practising yoga and Pilates often helps; ask your teacher to recommend specific exercises to do at home. A gentle massage should help to relieve discomfort. Chiropractic and osteopathy are also useful.

Pubic joint pain The pubic joint (symphysis pubis) softens in preparation for childbirth, which places strain on the spine and pelvis. This can cause pain in the pubic area, and sometimes in the lower back and groin as well. Tell your doctor if you are affected; he or she may refer you to a physiotherapist to be fitted with a support belt. Otherwise regular chiropractic or osteopathy sessions can be very helpful. Other therapies that may be useful include acupuncture, reiki, reflexology and the Alexander technique.

Shortness of breath As your uterus expands, it presses against your lungs, which can cause breathlessness or exacerbate respiratory problems such as asthma. Practising abdominal breathing will help to improve your breath control, as will yoga, Pilates and the Alexander technique. If the problem gets worse when you lie down, use pillows to prop yourself up. If you suffer from asthma, try eating more oily fish; fish oils seem to protect against attacks. Homeopathy, aromatherapy, acupuncture, reflexology and reiki may help with both asthma and shortness of breath.

Indigestion and heartburn These problems can get worse in the third trimester, when the growing uterus presses on the stomach. Eating little, often and slowly is the simplest way to prevent them, and you should avoid eating spicy foods. Sipping a cup of lemonbalm or meadowsweet tea after meals may help. If you suffer from heartburn, make sure that you do not bend or lie down for at least an hour after eating.

Itchy skin Hormonal changes during pregnancy can lead to skin problems, particularly during the third trimester. If you have dry, itchy skin, try eating more oily fish, nuts and seeds. Moisturizing your skin with an evening primrose lotion can help, or you may like to use essential oil of lavender or chamomile well-diluted in a carrier cream or base oil. Herbal medicine or homeopathy may also be useful – a homeopath may prescribe sulphur or kali arsenicum. See your doctor if the itching becomes severe.

Water retention Pregnant women often experience mild swelling (oedema) of the ankles, especially during the third trimester. If you have swollen ankles, rest with your feet up for at least 15 minutes twice a day. Regular leg massage – working up the leg – and drinking dandelion tea can be useful. You may also find acupuncture helpful. If you have severe swelling and a headache, see your doctor at once.

High blood pressure Your blood pressure will be checked at every antenatal visit; high blood pressure accompanied by fluid retention and protein in the urine indicates pre-eclampsia. This condition can affect your pregnancy so it is important that you follow any advice given by your doctor. You can help to maintain a healthy blood pressure by taking regular exercise and eating a nutritious diet that includes oily fish and plenty of raw fruits and vegetables; you should also follow a low-salt diet. Reducing stress and practising relaxation techniques, meditation, yoga or t'ai chi is often helpful. You may also like to try herbal medicine, aromatherapy, colour therapy, reiki or reflexology.

For immediate relief of itchy skin, use a cream containing evening primrose oil. Increasing the amount of oily fish that you eat should also help.

WHEN TO CALL A DOCTOR
If you experience sudden or severe symptoms, you should contact your doctor or the emergency services without delay. See page 145 for a list of danger signs in pregnancy.

Common Qs and As

Q: If I have a row with my partner or my mother, will my baby be affected or harmed by that? Will he or she know?

A: Your baby certainly won't 'know' that you are having an argument in any real sense of the word. He or she will have no means of placing what is said in a meaningful context and assessing it. However, your increasing heart rate and anxiety level will transmit to your baby in some way.

It is best to try to avoid becoming very stressed when you are pregnant, and it will help all of you if you can learn to handle disagreements calmly, through discussion and negotiation and compromise. Once your child is born, he or she will certainly be upset by rows, long before he or she is able to speak.

Q: I am so huge now, I feel quite otherworldly – as if this is not me – I just want it to be over and see my baby.

A: Many women feel like this towards the last few weeks of their pregnancy, and you are probably experiencing entirely normal feelings. However, it is worth discussing these feelings with your doctor just in case your feelings of depersonalization are associated with depression or acute anxiety. Depression can happen before the birth as well as after it, and it is best treated sooner rather than later.

Q: I don't know whether I will be able to handle the loss of privacy that giving birth entails. I am a very private person and am worried about the pain, the unknown nature of it all. All my friends seem to have coped better than I think I would.

A: Your question raises a number of issues. First, it would be a good idea to confide your fears and feelings to your family doctor and to the midwife in charge of you so that they can appreciate how you will feel in any given situation. They may well reassure you that many women feel this way. You will also be able to choose not have medical students present for the delivery.

Second, you may well imagine that all your friends have coped better than you think you would. However, this may be supposition on your part. Have you talked to them? Have you asked them if they felt nervous? You may find it helpful to discuss with them how they coped with the pain and loss of privacy.

Third, your own self-esteem may be an issue here. Are you usually confident? Do you often suffer from feelings of lack of confidence or low self-esteem? Experiencing the birth of your baby is without doubt something you can do. It does not matter if you scream or weep – medical staff will have seen other women do the same thing. You should also remember that people will be there to help and comfort you. Rest assured that you will receive the professional assistance and support you need.

Fourth, remember that this is just one day of your life, and you will get through it. Try to see the labour and delivery as a means to an end... seeing your very own gorgeous baby.

Q: I am seven months pregnant but I don't feel the emotional bond with my baby that other women talk about. Am I abnormal?

A: Not at all. Some women do feel rather detached from their pregnancy, almost as if the baby is growing within them irrespective of the woman herself as a person. Fathers-to-be also often do not bond with their baby until the actual delivery.

However, most parents do feel a surge of love for the baby once he or she is born. The hormones take over and allow you to feel the nurturing, protective love that is normal in parenthood.

If you have any remaining worries after the birth of your baby, be sure to discuss them with your family doctor or your health visitor.

Q: Now that I am pregnant, everyone seems to think they can touch my stomach. I really hate being stroked and prodded by strangers but don't know how to stop this happening. What can I do?

A: This is an entirely understandable reaction on your part and something expressed by many pregnant women – it is as if people believe that the bump is public property rather than part of your body. Short of staying at home, there is not a lot you can do, except to explain gently that your pregnancy is very personal to you and that you would prefer not to be touched.

Q: How will I know when to go to hospital?

A: Memorize the warning signs for labour and get your partner or best friend to do the same. They are:
- Breaking of the waters.
- A pinkish show of mucus tinged with blood.
- Contractions becoming regular and pronounced and lasting for some 40 seconds or more. (False labour is characterized by irregular contractions lasting less than 20-30 seconds.)

Ring your midwife if you are in any doubt about whether or not labour has started.

Q: What happens if I am caught short – say, if I am on a train or bus – when labour starts? Should I be taking any measures now?

A: Labour usually takes some time – and remember that even trains stop. Babies have been delivered in cars, buses, planes and on ships, but obviously one would prefer this not to happen. So, have a fully charged mobile phone with you at all times. From week 38, try to avoid any long journeys away from home and the place where you have chosen to have the delivery. If you are expecting twins, be cautious from week 35 onwards.

Q: I have started to worry that my partner may be away when the baby comes – he travels a lot, at short notice, for work – and am feeling panicky about what to do if he is.

A: In this situation, you may prefer to have a close friend or relative staying with you, or on stand-by, for the final stages, so make sure you have someone lined up now. If you do not have a friend or relative living close by, talk to your neighbours, who will probably be helpful, and alert your family doctor and midwife to the situation. They may be able to tell you of local back-up services.

Countdown to birth

"" The most important thing to do is to focus
on, and prepare yourself for, the labour. ""

Seeing your new baby for the first time is an entirely magical, joyful and breathtaking moment, an event that you will remember for the rest of your life. Now this moment is just a few weeks away.

As you wait, the most important thing you can do is to focus on, and prepare yourself as much as possible for, the labour and delivery, and for the first weeks of your baby's life. All other considerations – work, socializing, doing the housework – should take second place to this.

You are much larger now and may feel constantly tired. It is more important than ever to focus on rest and relaxation. Avoid becoming overtired because it will be difficult to catch up – once the baby has arrived, your sleep is likely to be repeatedly interrupted. Take a rest in the early afternoon if you can. Drink plenty of water every day in order to expel the toxins from your body and help to reduce general feelings of fatigue.

Practice makes perfect. Experiment together with different positions for the labour – standing, squatting or kneeling – so you know what to try when the time comes. As you practise, make sure you don't push or exert any downward pressure.

Feed yourself well, regularly and healthily. This will stand you in good stead for the demanding hours of labour and the delivery itself. Gentle activity and antenatal exercises are important in these last few weeks – try to get at least some exercise every day. It is also helpful to prepare mentally for the birth – through breathing, relaxation exercises and visualization, as well as enjoying periods of quiet contemplation each day.

On a practical level, you will probably already have decided on a room or space for your baby. You may be enjoying decorating it and providing for the baby's needs. Creating a welcoming space for your child can be a thrilling experience, and it is a real opportunity for you and your partner to share in the preparations in a practical way.

Top: You may find that this is a particularly comfortable resting position during the very late stages of your pregnancy. Place some padding, such as a pillow or two, under your upper leg in order to relieve pressure on the abdominal blood vessels.

Set aside some time each day to sit and relax and be with your unborn child. This can help the mother-child bonding process.

Your birth plan

Giving birth is the most personal and intense experience of a woman's life. It is natural that you will want to make it as comfortable and stress-free as possible. Women often have different approaches to giving birth, and midwives and hospitals are now happy to accommodate your preferences where possible.

A birth plan is a note of exactly what you want to happen during and after the birth. Your plan will include details on the type of pain relief you want and who you want to be present. It will also specify whether you want to have your baby at home or in hospital.

Birth plans are highly individual: what suits one woman is not necessarily right for another. It is easy to become overwhelmed by all the options that are open to you, but writing a birth plan can help to clarify your thoughts and preferences. It will also help to highlight any areas where you are unclear about what is possible. You will be able to discuss every aspect of the birth with your midwife. Remember that your midwife is there to help you make the right decisions for you.

Discuss your birth plan with your partner or anyone else you wish to be present at the birth, so that everyone is aware of your wishes. However, bear in mind that circumstances can change. Maintaining a flexible attitude will help you cope if your labour doesn't quite go to plan.

WHAT IS ON A BIRTH PLAN?

Birth plans vary from country to country and from hospital to hospital, but your plan is likely to include:

- Where you want to give birth.

Writing a birth plan encourages you to think seriously about all the options available. This can help you to identify what is really important to you – for example, having your aromatherapist present and ensuring that you have access to an epidural if you need one.

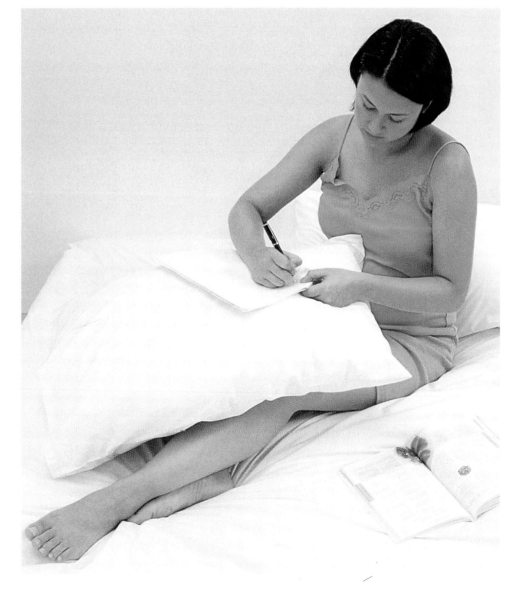

- A note of who you would like to be present (partner, friend, family member, acupuncturist, hypnotherapist).
- What position or positions you hope to adopt for labour and delivery.
- Your feelings about monitoring the baby.
- Your feelings about induction.
- Your feelings about episiotomy.
- Details of what pain relief you want, if any.
- Whether you want the baby put to your chest straight after delivery and before he or she is cleaned up.
- Whether you intend to feed by breast or by bottle.
- How you feel about staying in hospital after the birth.

A FLEXIBLE PLAN

Remember that a birth plan is a list of your preferences rather than an agenda of what is actually going to happen. Labour and delivery can take a different direction in individual cases, acquiring a momentum of their own. Whether or not your birth plan is followed will depend on what happens before, during and after the birth.

Some women prefer not to write a birth plan at all – and it is fine to turn up at the hospital without one. Equally, many women change their mind about certain things. For example, most women would wish to avoid an episiotomy. However, if the baby becomes severely distressed (short of oxygen) and needs to be delivered quickly with forceps, an episiotomy may have to be performed. Equally, some women decide they want to give birth with no pain relief at all. However, it is not possible to predict the degree of pain that may occur nor how easily you will be able to cope with it. In some cases, the woman changes her mind and asks for pain relief.

The birth plan, then, is provisional. It does not commit you to a particular course of action: you may deviate from it if you wish to do so. Medical and nursing staff will also be prepared to deviate from the plan if necessary to preserve your health and the health of the baby.

Include on the birth plan details of anything that you wish to take into the delivery room – from a birthing ball to soothing chamomile oil or homeopathic tablets.

WHO TO HAVE AT YOUR BIRTH

Most women want someone who they know well to be at the birth – this is usually, but not necessarily, the father. Your birth partner can offer valuable emotional support, act as an advocate with medical staff, and also do simple things to enhance your well-being, such as rub your back or pour you a glass of water when you need one.

Think carefully about who you want to be at the birth, and discuss this with your partner. Most men want to be at the birth of their baby, but a few do not feel able to support their partner in this way. It is usually better to ask a friend or relative to come with you rather than trying to press-gang an unwilling partner.

You may also like to consider asking a complementary therapist to be present for part of your labour. An acupuncturist, for example, may be able to stimulate certain points to ease labour pains, while a homeopath could prescribe remedies for weak contractions or distress.

If you are having the baby on your own or if your partner is unable to be present, take a close friend or relative to support you during the birth.

Where to have your baby

The first decision you have to make when planning your birth is where to have your baby – at home or in hospital. Your personal feelings are very important, but you also need to consider any medical issues, as well as your facilities if you want to have a home birth.

You should discuss the issue of where to have your baby with your partner, who may have strong opinions either way. In particular, if you want to have your baby at home, it is important that you have your partner's support.

HAVING A HOSPITAL BIRTH

The majority of women prefer to give birth in hospital, where there are the medical resources available to deal with any complications that may arise. You will also have access to the complete range of pain relief if you give birth in hospital, and advice and support will be on hand after the birth. The norm is to have a natural (vaginal) delivery, attended by a midwife rather than by a doctor.

However, doctors will be available should you need medical assistance to deliver the baby.

If you deliver normally, you may be encouraged to go home between six and 48 hours later. Women and babies who are unwell after delivery often need to stay longer. The community midwives will continue your care at home for up to ten days, extending to 28 days if necessary.

HOME BIRTHS

Some women feel more relaxed about the prospect of giving birth in their own environment. One of the advantages of having your baby at home is, of course, that you are the boss. You can watch television in the early stages of labour. You don't have to see anyone that you don't want to see. You can eat when and what you wish. You can have the music and the lighting of your choice. In addition, you can have as many people in the room as you wish.

BEING PREPARED FOR HOSPITAL

Have a small case or bag packed a few weeks before your estimated date of delivery, so that you are well prepared should the baby come earlier than expected. Have the bag packed at 35 weeks if you are expecting twins or more. You will need most or all of the following:

- Dressing gown.
- Slippers.
- Two nightdresses (which open down the front if you plan to breastfeed).
- Comfortable loose clothes, such as big T-shirts, track pants, skirts.
- Underclothes, including socks and a nursing bra if you want to breastfeed.

- Sanitary towels for after the birth.
- Something to read.
- Sponge bag, containing toothbrush and toothpaste, deodorant, flannel, soap, shampoo, cosmetics, tissues, skin cleanser, moisturizer, cotton wool, scent, wet wipes, nail varnish remover, comb.
- Essential aromatic oils plus electric vaporizer, flower remedies and homeopathic remedies.
- Herbal teas (for example, chamomile or raspberry leaf tea for the labour).
- Facial water spray.
- Address and telephone book.
- Phone card and coins for the telephone (you are often not able to use a mobile phone in a hospital).
- Music and portable stereo.
- Bottled water.
- Snack foods to eat during labour (dried fruit, nuts and raisins, bananas, grapes, carrot sticks, crackers, cheese, yeast extract, cereal bars).
- Sleep suits for your baby.
- Lightweight blanket or shawl.
- Mittens, woolly hat and outdoor suit for the baby.
- A correctly fitted new car seat for your baby to travel home safely.

Don't forget to take one or two outfits to the hospital for your new baby to wear.

Giving birth at home gives you greater control over your environment. It also means the first sights, sounds and smells a baby encounters are those of his or her home.

However, there are disadvantages to home births. The biggest drawback is that you will not have immediate access to specialist medical care if something goes wrong. This is the main reason that many doctors are uncomfortable about the idea of a home birth.

Another consideration may be any other children who live with you. It may prove difficult or distressing for them to hear you in labour, although there is no doubt they will be thrilled when they see the newborn baby. You may wish to arrange for your children to be looked after by a relative or a close friend while you are in labour.

If you give birth at home, it can be more difficult to let go of responsibility for household chores. Make sure that there is someone to look after you who will take over the running of the home. You will not want to answer the telephone or the doorbell within a few hours of giving birth to your baby. There will also have to be someone to clear up and change the bed linen.

DOCTORS AND HOME BIRTHS

Many doctors understand some women would prefer their baby to be delivered at home. However, they often discourage home births, particularly if there has been any indication that complications may ensue or if you are in a higher-than-average risk category.

If there is a problem during a home birth, valuable time will be lost while arrangements are made for an ambulance to collect the woman and drive her to the hospital. If the complications are serious, this delay could prove life-threatening to either you or your baby.

You may find that your own family doctor will not accept you for antenatal care if you choose to have a home birth. If this is the case, your midwife should be able to put you in touch with another doctor. The delivery will be undertaken by one or two midwives.

Can you have a home birth?

You have the right to give birth at home. However, if this is your first child or if you are in a high-risk group, a hospital birth will be recommended. The following women are actively discouraged from giving birth at home:

- Women over 35.
- Women expecting twins or more.
- Women expecting their first child.
- Women who had a difficult labour with their first child.
- Women who have had a Caesarean delivery, a stillborn baby, or one who died shortly after birth.
- Anyone who has a serious medical condition that could affect the outcome of the pregnancy and delivery, such as high blood pressure, heart disease, diabetes, significant heart murmur or kidney disease.

WHAT YOU WILL NEED AT HOME

You don't need a lot for a home birth, but the following are essential:

- Adequate heating – the room should be around 20°C (under 70°F).
- Telephone – so that help can be summoned in an emergency.
- Anglepoise lamp so the midwife can see in a dim light.
- Sheets and towels – these should be clean but preferably old so that it doesn't matter if they are stained.
- Clean nightdress for after the birth.
- Sanitary towels.

These items will be helpful:

- Chair and a low stool.
- Several cushions and a large bean bag.
- Natural sponge.
- Mineral water and fruit juice.
- Essential aromatic oils and vaporizer, flower remedies, homeopathic remedies.
- Herbal teas.
- Snack foods to eat during labour (dried fruit, nuts, bananas, grapes, carrot sticks, crackers, cheese, yeast extract, cereal bars).

Giving birth in water

Whether you are planning to give birth at home or in a hospital, you may wish to opt for a water birth. Midwives have long known that taking a bath can help with relaxation and pain control in early labour. Since the 1980s, an increasing number of women have chosen to spend long periods of their labour in water and to give birth in it. Water births account for approximately one in every 200 births in the UK, and they are also growing in popularity in the United States.

Supporters say that women who spend their labour immersed in warm water benefit in many ways.

- Warm water is naturally soothing and comforting. The pool provides a private space for the labour, which can help the woman to feel more in control.
- Water's buoyancy supports a woman's weight, making it easier for her to relax and change position.
- Water helps to support the pelvic floor and soften the perineum, making women less likely to tear or to require an episiotomy.
- Contractions are less painful because the body is less tense – your body releases pain-killing endorphins when it is in a relaxed state.
- When pain is reduced, women find it easier to concentrate on their breathing, which can help to shorten the labour.
- The father can get in the pool too, making the birth more of a shared experience.

Babies are usually lifted out of the water as soon as they are born, either by the mother, father, midwife or doctor, so that they can breathe. However, the family can usually stay in the water after the birth in order to bond.

ARE WATER BIRTHS SAFE?

Water births are controversial, and many doctors do not approve of them. However, the *British Medical Journal* conducted a study of all the water births that took place in the UK between 1994 and 1996. It found that the mortality rate for the babies was no greater than that associated with conventional births. There have been no major studies of water births in the United States, and the American College of Obstetrics and Gynecology does not take a stand on the practice.

There has been only limited research into water births, so it is impossible to be entirely sure of the risks. One problem is that it is difficult to maintain the water temperature: if it is too hot, it may cause the baby's heart beat to increase. Another concern is that the baby may be

> **Midwives have long known that taking a bath can help with relaxation and pain control in early labour.**

at risk of drowning. Supporters of water births say this is not possible because the baby does not breathe until he or she comes into contact with the air. However, one report from New Zealand suggested that a few babies have suffered respiratory problems as a result of inhaling water. Many women choose to get out of the water for the actual delivery because of this concern.

If you are considering a water birth, you need to discuss the benefits and risks with your midwife early on. Antenatal classes can be a good source of information, and you may find it helpful to seek out other women who have given birth in this way. Ask your antenatal teacher, search the Internet and look for local support groups.

CAN I HAVE A WATER BIRTH?

You should be able to have a water birth if your pregnancy has been straightforward and so long as no complications are envisaged. Many hospitals have birthing pools, so in theory water births should be possible in most areas.

In practice, however, the pool may not be available when you need it. For example, it may be being cleaned or in use by another woman. It may be available only if your labour coincides with the shifts of a specific midwife.

If you are having a water birth at home, hire the pool a few weeks before your due date. It is a good idea to fill the pool for a trial run beforehand.

Some hospitals actively discourage women from having a water birth, even if they have the facilities to provide one. Asking these questions should let you see how likely it is that you will be able to have a water birth at your hospital:

- How many women use the birthing pool each year?
- How many women actually give birth in the pool?
- How many midwives are trained to attend water births?
- Will the pool be available when I go into labour?

If you feel that staff are not keen on facilitating a water birth, talk to your midwife. There may be good reasons for this, and it may be that the hospital does not support the practice. If so, you may want to consider having the birth elsewhere. However, make sure you will be assisted by a qualified midwife who is experienced with water births.

WATER BIRTHS AT HOME
If you are having a home birth, you can hire your own pool. Ask your midwife for details of local companies who rent out pools. Make sure your midwife is happy and confident about facilitating a water birth. If not, ask for a referral to someone who is.

You will need to hire the pool for several weeks, so that you can be sure that you have it when you go into labour. Make sure that your floor can take the weight, and that there is plenty of space around the pool.

The father may want to get into the birthing pool to share the first moments of his baby's life, or even to cut the umbilical cord, under instruction from the midwife.

WHEN WATER BIRTHS ARE UNSUITABLE
Water births are not recommended if the baby is in the breech position; if you are expecting twins; if the baby is more than two weeks early; if you have an infection or other medical condition, or if there is meconium (the baby's first bowel movement) in the amniotic fluid.

It is also important that women do not get into the pool too early in their labour. You should wait until you are at least 5cm (2in) dilated, otherwise the relaxing effects of the water can slow labour down.

STAY FLEXIBLE
If you are planning a water birth, remember that labour does not always go to plan. If complications occur, you will need to get out of the pool so that medical assistance can be given. Also, bear in mind that the main aim of a water birth is to facilitate relaxation and well-being: don't turn getting one into a stressful event.

Preparing for the birth

Many women feel a growing sense of confidence and ease as the due date approaches. However, there can still be moments of anxiety about the birth ahead. You may also have times when you feel very bored – these last few weeks can seem to last forever. Fluctuating emotions are normal in pregnancy. However, it will help you to cope with the birth if you are feeling as emotionally strong as possible. Try to deal with any fears you have now so that you can concentrate on your labour when the time comes.

If you have specific worries, get as much information as you can about what lies ahead. If you are not sure how you will cope with the pain, for example, look into the different methods of pain relief that you can have. Don't rule anything out – even if you are keen to have a natural birth, it can be reassuring to know that you have access to medication if you need it.

MENTAL PREPARATION

Take some time each day to contemplate the birth. Visualization can be very helpful: try to picture yourself in labour, adopting your preferred positions. Imagine yourself coping with the contractions – you may like to think of them as hurdles that you are leaping over or as powerful surges that are bringing you and your baby closer together. Think of your pelvic area opening and expanding, so that the baby passes more easily down the birth canal. Imagine your baby's arrival, and the joy that you will feel on seeing him or her. Think of the birth as an empowering rather than a worrying experience.

PHYSICAL PREPARATION

In general, you want to feel as fit and healthy as possible. Get plenty of sleep and relaxation, so you start your labour feeling rested and mentally alert. If you are still working, consider starting your maternity leave (ideally you should leave work by week 34-36 so that you have time to prepare for the birth). Drink plenty of water to help your body expel any toxins. Eat healthily and regularly; you will find it easier to digest your food if you eat little and often. Eat plenty of complex carbohydrates, such as wholegrain bread and rice, in order to stock up your energy reserves. Make sure you eat iron-rich foods and protein each day, and include a wide range of different fruit and vegetables, to be sure that you are getting a full spectrum of nutrients.

Practising yoga or Pilates will help to enhance your suppleness and general health. It is also a good idea to practise your preferred positions for the labour, and to take a short walk each day to maintain your fitness.

BREATHING EXERCISES

Controlling your breathing will help enormously at the birth. You will be taught breathing techniques at your antenatal classes, and you should practise these in advance. What you are aiming to avoid is the 'over-breathing' that results when we are tense and panicky – sucking air into our lungs and letting out short, sharp gasps. This will soon exhaust you, and fail to give yourself and your baby plenty of oxygen to cope with the birth.

Any breathing exercises you are given will focus on keeping your breathing steady and rhythmic. The in-breath should not be longer than the out breath; if anything, aim for the reverse. Try these simple exercises:
- Breathe in through your nose and out through your mouth, keeping your mouth soft. Try making a noise such as "Aaaaaaah" as you breathe out.
- As you breathe in, count slowly to three or four. Then do the same as you breathe out.

When it comes to pushing the baby out, you may automatically hold your breath as you push. This can hurt

Do not lie flat on your back at this stage of pregnancy. Prop yourself up on plenty of cushions and place another pillow or two under your knees. Alternatively, lie on your side with your uppermost leg resting on a cushion.

your throat, and you should never hold your breath and push for as long as possible, which is sometimes advised, as this is tiring and oxygen-depleting. The better option is to take a deep breath as you feel a contraction starting, then breathe or blow out slowly as you push down.

If you feel the urge to push before the cervix is fully dilated, help to stop yourself from doing this as follows: give four short pants as a contraction arrives, then a quick in-breath, followed by four more pants. Breathe normally between contractions.

NATURAL THERAPIES FOR THE LAST WEEKS

A traditional herbal preparation for labour is raspberry leaf tea (see page 130), while perineal massage helps to improve the stretchability of the skin (see pages 162-63). It can be very helpful to see an acupuncturist who specializes in pregnancy. Specific points can be used to strengthen the emotions and help you to prepare for the birth. Your acupuncturist may also be willing to teach you and your partner about acupressure points to press during labour.

Practise breathing techniques learned at antenatal classes every day, so that they become automatic.

NATURAL REMEDY BIRTH KIT

The following natural remedies may be helpful to you during labour. Check with a qualified practitioner to ensure that you take remedies that are suitable for your individual needs. You should also discuss with your midwife any remedies you wish to bring into the delivery room, and they should be incorporated into your birth plan.

Essential oils

A mixture of 10 drops clary sage, 10 drops lavender and 5 drops jasmine in 100ml (3½fl oz) base oil makes a good massage oil for the lower back during labour; it can help to promote strong contractions as well as encouraging you to stay calm. Useful oils to burn in a vaporizer may include frankincense (for pain and hyperventilation), lavender (for anxiety), rose (for fear and doubt), ginger (for weariness) and chamomile (for irritability).

Herbal teas

Teas that may be helpful during labour include raspberry leaf (to promote regular contractions), chamomile, lime flowers or lemon balm (to induce relaxation), cramp bark (to release tension) and ginseng (to boost energy). Check that there are tea-making facilities in the delivery suite; if not, take two flasks of hot water and a cup.

Flower remedies

Gentle flower remedies can be very comforting: place a few drops in a glass of water and sip at intervals. Try Rescue Remedy for fear and panic; olive for exhaustion; or cherry plum if you start to feel that you cannot carry on with the labour.

Homeopathic remedies

See a homeopath for advice about remedies that may be helpful to take before, during and after labour. He or she may recommend arnica (for bruising), caulophyllum (to encourage regular contractions), nux vomica (for backache) or hypericum (to promote healing).

Chamomile flowers are used to make calming tea or oil.

Your baby's room

One of the best ways that you and your partner can prepare for the arrival of your new baby is to get the nursery ready. Ideally, the baby will have a room of his or her own. However, if you are short of space, don't worry. You can create a welcoming area for your baby in a corner of your own bedroom.

Creating a nursery can help you to adjust to the idea that you are bringing a new life into the world – something you may still find difficult to believe. Sharing this process with your partner will help you to prepare together for the new baby who is to share your lives.

Many women worry that they will not be ready in time. If this is the case, remember that preparing a room is more for your benefit than the baby's. Your baby will not mind if your home is disorganized, as long as he or she is with you. In any case, he or she should sleep in your bedroom for the first few weeks.

A RESTFUL NURSERY

First and foremost, your baby's room should be a clean and light place to be. Enlist your partner or a friend to help you clean it thoroughly (or ask them to do it for you). Don't

> **"** Creating a nursery can help you to adjust to the idea that you are bringing a new life into the world. **"**

forget to clean the windows inside and out. This will let more light into the room, which will make it feel cheerier. Make sure curtains or blinds are in a simple, non-fussy style, and do not obscure natural sunlight.

It is worth installing a dimmer switch or including a low-wattage lamp in the room. This will allow you to tend to the baby at night, without flooding the room with so much light that he or she becomes wakeful. A dim light will help to convey the message that it is still time for sleep: the sooner your baby is able to associate darkness with rest, the better for everyone.

Use child-friendly, non-toxic paint to decorate the room; matt paint gives a softer effect than gloss. Nurseries are often painted in primary colours, but it's probably better to use a soothing, sleep-inducing hue, such as lavender or pale blue.

Your baby is not going to care about great interior design. But he or she will probably thrive best in a room that is light, airy and restful. You could hang a mobile over the cot: this will provide something interesting for the baby to focus upon in the months to come.

A rose quartz crystal is a beautiful addition to your baby's room. It is said to evoke a sense of comfort and love, and to promote restful sleep.

Consider having light-coloured wood flooring rather than carpet; it is much easier to keep clean. However, place a rug under the cot, just in case the baby has a fall. You'll also want a larger rug (with a non-slip underlay) for when your child starts to walk.

Keep the room as uncluttered as possible: a cot, a chair for you, a changing table and a storage unit is all you really need. A rocking chair is a great investment: it can help you to soothe the baby. Wherever possible, choose natural materials such as wood and cotton for your baby's room.

Position your baby's cot against a wall. Ideally, the cot should be in a position where you can see it easily from the door – this is so that you can readily check on your baby while he or she is sleeping. You should not place a cot directly under a window, since this may expose the baby to draughts.

FENG SHUI FOR NURSERIES

The Eastern art of feng shui is used to bring health and happiness to the occupants of a home. It involves promoting the flow of beneficial energy (chi) around each room, by removing any blockages and by adding enhancements ('cures'). Try the following to create a good atmosphere in your baby's room:

- Clean windows regularly. Open them for at least 10 minutes each day to allow fresh energy to enter.
- Keep the nursery free of clutter, which impedes the flow of chi (and can be a hazard).
- Cover up sharp corners, which cause an excess of chi. Incorporate soft, curving shapes into the room wherever possible.
- Include a few splashes of bright colour, such as red or orange, especially in dark corners.
- Hang a mobile over the cot – moving objects are said to promote the flow of chi, and this will also give your baby something to look at when he or she is lying in the cot.
- Plant a window box with healing herbs, such as lavender, basil or catnip. You could also place a green pot plant in the room (move it out of reach when the child gets older). Care for all plants well and replace them if they become unhealthy.
- Include a lucky charm in the form of an animal motif: bears and dogs both signify protection, the stork is a classic symbol of birth, and swallows represent joy and playfulness.
- Place a crystal in the child's room – rose quartz is associated with love and comfort (crystal healers sometimes use it to help cure sleeplessness).

CLEARING THE SPACE

In China, a nursery is usually cleared of stale energy before it is decorated, and again just before the baby arrives. If you want to do this:

- Clean the room thoroughly and open all the windows on a sunny day; this brings fresh energy into the room.
- Stand or sit in the middle of the room. Spend a few moments quietly breathing and focusing.
- Go to each corner of the room in turn. Ring a bell or clap your hands there – as you do so, imagine you are clearing out old, stagnant energy and making room for the new. Follow your instincts and repeat a few times if necessary.
- To finish, stand in the centre of the room again for a few moments. You may like to practise some meditation or visualization, or to say a little prayer for the well-being and happiness of your baby.

Clap your hands to drive out stale energy.

What your baby will need

Shopping is all part of the fun of expecting a baby. Unless you have already had a baby, you will need equipment for the nursery – a cot, a changing mat, a chest of drawers. You will also need a stock of clothes (remember that the baby will grow very quickly, so don't buy too many), nappies, toiletries and other items for the first few weeks. There are now plenty of natural and organic options available, so look out for these.

WHAT TO BUY FOR...

The nursery

- Cot with a drop-down side – make sure that you can drop down the side with one hand only (you may be holding your baby with your other arm).
- You may like to buy a Moses basket for the first four months or so. This is transportable so you will be able to move it around easily. It is a good idea to buy a stand to put the basket on at night. This means that you won't have to stoop to pick up the baby.
- Well-fitting new mattress for the cot and basket.
- Two cotton cellular blankets – these keep the baby warm, but not overheated.
- Linen, including cotton, fitted bottom sheets. Note that the baby will not need a pillow and must not have a duvet before the age of 12 months.
- Thick, dark curtains for daytime naps.
- Nursery thermometer – to monitor the temperature.
- A chair for you or your partner, or a small sofa.
- Changing table.
- A chest of drawers for clothes and nappies.
- Smoke alarm in or just outside the baby's room.
- Nightlight and baby monitor – check you have enough sockets.

The kitchen or utility room

- Kitchen paper and disinfectant spray and wipes for cleaning surfaces.
- Check that washing machine, tumble dryer, washing line, clotheshorse and pulley are working properly. There will be a lot more washing than you are used to once the baby arrives. Make sure that you do not use biological washing powders since these may irritate a baby's sensitive skin.

Feeding your baby

- Breast pads to catch leaks.
- Herbal nipple cream.
- Breast pump for expressing milk; for when you are somewhere where it would be difficult to breastfeed; this also allows your partner to feed the baby.
- Formula milk (organic varieties are available) and feeding bottles as standby.
- Bottle brush and teat brush.
- Sterilizing equipment (unless you just use boiling water). See pages 214-215.
- Bottle holders and carriers.
- Old towels to protect your clothes while feeding.

A manual breast pump

Sterilizing tank and tablets

Your baby's clothes

- Vests, body suits and sleep suits.
- Dungarees.
- Dresses.
- Cardigans – easier to put on than sweaters.
- Socks or booties.
- Mittens, if winter.
- Warm hat or sun hat, depending on the season.
- Muslin squares.
- An all-in-one suit for outdoor wear.
- Small lightweight blanket.

Playtime

- Music.
- Rattles and soft toys.
- A ball.
- Mobile (to hang above cot).

Bathing your baby

- Baby bath (choose from options that are used on or in an adult bath, and others that have their own stand).
- Natural baby soap, shampoo, lotion and oil, free from any harsh perfumes or colourings.
- Baby wipes for when you are out only (otherwise use water or lotion as the gentle, eco-friendly option).
- Cotton wool.
- Large tissues.
- Nappies and related accessories (see pages 216-217).
- Gentle herbal creams and oils for dealing with nappy rash (avoid using talc, see pages 216-217).
- Baby scissors or nail clippers.

Your baby's health

- Forehead strip thermometer.
- Basic first-aid kit and book.
- Gripe water.
- Herbal, homeopathic or conventional treatment for colic.
- Infant paracetamol syrup.
- Infant medicine spoon.
- Cough and cold treatments for infants.

A strip thermometer   *Homeopathic remedies*

Going out and about

- Car seat – this must be correctly fitted; do not buy second-hand.
- Travel cot (or you can use a Moses basket).
- Lie-down baby buggy with transparent rain cover, or a pram (some are fitted with a removable carrycot to use as a bed, initially).
- Pram or buggy accessories, such as linen, cellular blankets, rain cover, parasol.
- Bag that is large enough to contain everything you need for feeding and changing your baby.
- A changing mat that you can put down anywhere on a table or on a floor.
- List of useful telephone numbers, such as your doctor's and health visitor's.

Changing mat

Sources for everything you need

Getting ready for a baby can be expensive, but there is no need to buy everything new. Shop around, and consider all the following sources:

- Friends and relatives.
- Charity shops and good second-hand shops.
- Magazines and direct-mail catalogues.
- The Internet.
- Large pharmacies and supermarkets (which often sell baby items more cheaply).

Remember that you are likely to be given outfits by friends and relatives. A close friend or relative who has recently had a baby may offer to pass on clothes and equipment that are no longer needed, especially if they are not planning another child.

REMEMBER

- Do not buy second-hand electrical equipment.
- If you are given or buy second-hand goods, make sure that they have been painted recently and do not contain leaded paint.
- Check catches, locks and hooks for safety.
- All clothes and linen should be washable and suitable for a tumble dryer.
- Cotton and light soft wools are kinder to the skin than synthetics.
- Avoid lots of buttons.
- Make sure that clothes are big enough to contain a nappy (diaper).

Before the birth

As the birth approaches, your baby will be monitored as part of your continuing antenatal care. During the last month of your pregnancy, you will probably visit your antenatal clinic once a week for the usual blood and urine tests and weight check. In addition, your baby's heartbeat will be checked at each visit, and he or she will also be checked over to ensure that growth and movement are progressing normally.

You and your baby will be assessed for labour by the following criteria:
- Just how well the baby is likely to stand up to the testing rigours of labour and delivery – this is assessed by checking the baby's general well-being and heartbeat.
- Whether or not the baby is in the right position for a normal vaginal delivery.
- Whether or not the baby will be able to negotiate the birth canal – this is determined by assessing both the size of the baby's head and the size of the mother-to-be's pelvis.

A Caesarean section will be considered:
- If the baby's head is thought to be too large in relation to your pelvis.
- If he or she is in a position that will make it hard to navigate the birth canal.
- If there are likely to be any other complications during the delivery.

THE POSITION FOR BIRTH

When discussing the baby's position for birth, medical staff will talk about the lie, the presentation and the position. These all mean different things.

The baby's 'lie'

When doctors and midwives use the term 'lie', they are referring to the way that the baby is lying in the mother's body. This term describes the relationship between the spine of the baby and the spine of the mother – the north-south axis. The baby may be lying in a longitudinal (vertical) lie with the head up or head down, or across the mother's body in a transverse (horizontal) lie.

Nearly all babies before the 32nd week change the way they are facing frequently, so yours may be in the breech position when you have your antenatal check-ups: this is a longitudinal lie with the head uppermost and the buttocks down. After the 32nd week, most babies turn to the head-down position. About 3 per cent of babies,

however, remain in the breech position. Another 1 per cent of babies assume a transverse lie, in which the baby lies across the uterus. You can see all of these positions clearly in the illustrations.

Babies who are in a breech position or transverse lie may suffer some difficulties during a vaginal delivery, so special checks are made beforehand. In particular, it needs to be established whether or not the mother's pelvis is large enough to accommodate the baby comfortably. If the pelvis is not large enough, then a Caesarean delivery is advised. This is always the case with a transverse lie, but it may be that a breech baby is able to be delivered vaginally.

It is important to know if there is an underlying reason for the baby assuming the wrong lie. For example, the placenta may be in a position that makes it impossible for the baby to assume a head-down position, or there may be some other obstruction – such as a fibroid, for example – in the mother's uterus. In these cases, a Caesarean delivery will be carried out.

The baby's presentation

This describes what part of the baby is at the pelvic brim before the delivery – that is, the part of the baby to be born first. Most babies adopt what is known as the vertex presentation. In this posture, the baby's head is well flexed, with the chin on the chest. This means that the vertex (crown) of the head is the part touching the cervix and will be born first.

A tiny number of babies – no more than 0.3 per cent – present their face or brow first. These presentations are known as face presentation or brow presentation. Face presentations are able to be delivered vaginally, but only if the back of the baby's head is facing the mother's spine. Brow presentations, however, are always delivered by Caesarean section because the baby cannot fit into the birth canal.

The baby's position

A baby's position describes the way the baby is facing as birth approaches. If he or she is facing towards the mother's spine, the position is said to be anterior and labour is likely to be easier, although that is not always the case. If the baby is facing outwards, with the back of its head to the mother's spine, the position is said to be posterior. In this case, labour may be slower, and the mother is more likely to experience severe backache during labour.

YOUR BABY'S POSITION

It can be hard to visualize the difference between a breech, transverse and face presentation. These illustrations show the various positions that a baby can adopt within the uterus in the last days before birth. All of them are perfectly comfortable for the baby, and none should cause undue discomfort to the mother.

NORMAL POSITION

Here the baby is in the normal 'head-first' position, ready for the delivery. He or she is lying slightly to the right and is facing the mother's spine. The baby's chin is tucked into the chest, so that the narrowest part of the head will be born first.

BREECH POSITION

This baby is in the full, bottom-first breech position, with head up and legs crossed in front. Breech babies can have their legs extended up, so that their feet are in front of the face, or have one or both legs dropping down.

TRANSVERSE LIE

In a transverse lie, the baby is across the uterus. This means that his shoulder would come out first if a vaginal delivery were attempted. A baby can sometimes be encouraged to shift position, but, if this fails, a Caesarean section will be needed.

FACE-DOWN PRESENTATION

Here the baby is in the head-first position, but the neck is not tucked into the chest as in the normal position. Instead, the neck is extended so that the face is presented first. A midwife will assess whether or not a vaginal delivery is possible.

Going into labour

There are three main stages of labour: the cervix dilating (opening up) to let the baby through; the actual birth itself; and the delivery of the placenta. Much more about these stages is explained over the following pages.

Women can find it hard to judge whether or not they have gone into labour. If you are in any doubt, you can contact your midwife at any time. You can also ring the hospital if you are not sure whether or not you should go in. There are three signs that indicate that labour is imminent or has started:

- A pinkish 'show' of mucus.
- The breaking of the waters.
- Contractions that last for 40 seconds or more, becoming more regular and pronounced.

A 'SHOW'

The first sign that labour is imminent is usually the show. This occurs when the plug of mucus sealing the cervix is released. The show appears as a mucous vaginal discharge, which may be tinged with blood. It can happen several days before contractions start, or it may coincide with the breaking of the waters. It often goes unnoticed.

THE BREAKING OF THE WATERS

The membranes surrounding the baby can rupture at the start of labour, shortly before it or at the end of the first stage. This is known as the breaking of the waters, and it is painless. Once this happens, you should go to hospital, or call your midwife if you are having a home birth.

Normally, waters break with an unmistakable gush of liquid. Sometimes there is a less obvious breaking that may be confused with the incontinence that is common in late pregnancy. Contact your midwife if you are unsure. In some cases, the waters break spontaneously but labour does not start. Most hospitals will admit you if this happens because the baby is no longer protected from infection and labour needs to be induced. Occasionally, however, the hole in the membrane seals itself over and the pregnancy continues. Sometimes the waters may be ruptured by the obstetrician using a probe. This may be done when the birth is being induced, as it can encourage contractions to start.

Women may mistake the breaking of the waters for incontinence. Call your midwife if you think that you are in labour but cannot tell for certain.

THE WATERS
The term 'waters' refers to the liquid contained within the membranes. This amniotic fluid is a clear, yellowish liquid that contains the baby's urine and dead skin cells. Breaking the waters means breaking the membranes that surround and protect the baby in the uterus.

The baby depends for his or her well-being on the amniotic fluid. It has several functions:

- It enables the baby to turn and move his or her limbs easily.
- It serves to extend the uterus so that the walls do not exert any pressure upon the growing baby.
- It guarantees a constant temperature for the baby, which is the mother's body temperature.
- It absorbs the baby's waste products.
- It acts as a shock absorber, and so protects the baby from the impact if the mother falls or receives a jarring blow to the abdomen.

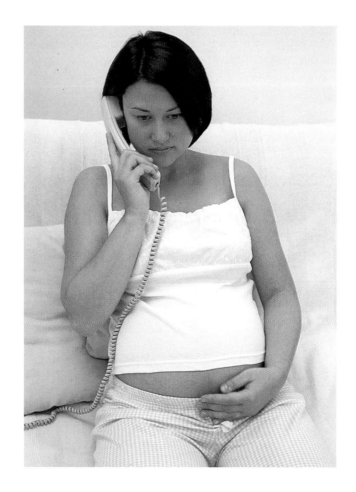

CONTRACTIONS

Many women experience small, irregular contractions throughout pregnancy. Towards the end of pregnancy these become more pronounced, when they are known as Braxton Hicks contractions. They can be painful but are irregular and do not cause the cervix to dilate – so you are not in labour. With Braxton Hicks contractions, the uterus may contract every 20 minutes or so for about 20–30 seconds. By contrast, the birth contractions felt during the first stage of labour last for 40–60 seconds, and become more powerful. This is the time to telephone the hospital to tell them that you are on your way. It will help if you have noted down the frequency and length of the contractions.

GOING TO HOSPITAL

Take your notes, birth plan and overnight bag with you. When you arrive at hospital, you will go through the normal admissions procedure and will then be taken to the labour ward, where your pulse, temperature and blood pressure will be checked and you will be examined externally and internally in order to judge the baby's position and see how far the cervix has dilated.

HOW LONG DOES LABOUR LAST?

	First birth	Subsequent births
1st stage	4–24 hours	2–12 hours
2nd stage	½–2 hours	10 minutes–1½ hours
3rd stage	10 minutes–1½ hours	10 minutes–1½ hours

When you go to the delivery room depends on how dilated you are, the baby's condition, and what space there is in the hospital. You may be allowed to make the delivery room a little more personal if you have arranged this beforehand – for example, plugging in a portable stereo or setting up an electric aromatherapy burner. These things should have been noted on your birth plan after discussion with the midwife, though there may not be time to carry this out if you are admitted as an emergency.

A team of midwives will provide all your medical care during labour, and will deliver your baby and check you are both well after delivery. Doctors are on duty for much of the day and night to assist if complications occur.

THE SIGNS AND STAGES OF LABOUR

As already explained, there are three signs that herald the start of labour, and three stages to labour itself. The three warning signs may occur separately or in combination. So, you may be in the first stage of labour, with strong contractions lasting 40 seconds or more, even though the waters have not broken. The artworks below show how the cervix widens during labour. Shortly before labour begins, the cervix starts to shorten in response to the contractions. A partially dilated cervix, encouraged by the pressure of the baby's head, indicates that labour is well under way. By the time the cervix has dilated enough to allow the baby's head through into the vagina, the second stage of labour has been reached – this stage lasts from when the cervix is fully dilated until the birth of the baby. The third stage of labour is the delivery of the placenta.

WHAT HAPPENS TO THE CERVIX BEFORE AND DURING LABOUR

Here the neck of the uterus – the cervix – remains closed. It is sealed by a plug of mucus, which protects the baby from infection. When this is released, labour is near.

The mucus plug is released before labour – this is the 'show', one of the early signs that labour is near or has started. When the contractions begin, the cervix becomes shorter.

The cervix now starts to dilate (open). This is the first stage of labour, which can last many hours. A normal rate of dilation is judged to be about 1cm (⅖in) an hour, but this varies.

As the cervix reaches full dilation (10cm/4in), ready for the baby to pass down into the vagina, you are in a brief period called the transitional stage, just prior to the second stage of labour – the birth.

Pain relief and monitoring

The key to having as fulfilling a labour experience as possible is to keep an open mind and to be well informed beforehand about the signs of impending labour, how your labour is likely to be managed, the type of pain relief you would ideally like and all the options available.

COMPLEMENTARY PAIN RELIEF

There are many natural, drug-free methods that can help to ease the pain of labour and birth. Some of these work by stimulating the release of endorphins, the body's natural painkillers. To use some of these methods, you may need to have a complementary therapist with you in the delivery room. If you do, then this should be noted on your birth plan, along with details of any natural remedies you want to use.

Make sure that any therapist treating or helping you in the delivery room is fully experienced in dealing with labour and birth. Also, any therapies that you use must be ones that you are already familiar with and have had some success with before, so you know what to expect

ORTHODOX PAIN RELIEF				
Method	**Stage of labour**	**How given**	**Does it work?**	**Side effects**
Gas and air	1st, 2nd	You breathe in from a mouthpiece	Up to a point – gives only limited relief from pain	May make you feel light-headed or drowsy. It is difficult to put your breathing techniques into practice while using mask
Pethidine	1st	Injection either into a vein in the arm or into a muscle in the buttock	Timing is crucial – if given too early, effects may wear off; if too late, can prevent you pushing and can affect baby	May necessitate forceps delivery if it affects your ability to push. May make you feel drowsy and/or sick. The baby may be drowsy and slow to breathe
Epidural	1st, and if Caesarean delivery	Injected into epidural space between spinal cord and backbone of lumbar region	Usually very effective but occasionally does not work	Chances of forceps delivery and episiotomy are higher if you have an epidural. Necessitates continuous fetal monitoring. You may feel numbness in legs for some time after delivery. May cause headache
Pudendal nerve block	2nd, if forceps delivery is indicated	Injection through wall of vagina	Not always	None
Transcutaneous Electrical Nerve Stimulation (TENS)	1st, 2nd	Electrodes attached to back, and a low-frequency current directed by mother	Not always	None – often recommended by complementary therapists
General anaesthetic	If Caesarean delivery	Injection	Yes	Recovery is often slow

and are confident that they may have some effect. Below is a list of some common drug-free approaches:

- **Positions** Moving around and trying different positions – leaning against your partner or a wall, for example – will often bring relief (see also pages 196-199).
- **Water** Immersion in warm water is often relaxing, as the warmth is soothing and the water helps to take the body's weight. Find out well in advance about birthing pool options in your chosen place of delivery.
- **Massage** Effective for relieving discomfort and promoting calm, massage can easily be done by your birth partner. Massaging the lower back can be especially effective. To promote relaxation, stroke gently but firmly with the flat of the hand, working towards the heart. Using lavender oil will help to ease pain, while mandarin will lift the spirits.
- **Visualization/meditation** Practise well in advance. Simple approaches include imagining a scene such as a peaceful, sunny beach as contractions begin.
- **Acupuncture** This can be used to control various aspects of labour, from calming fears to easing backache. For the latter, needles can be inserted at points in the lower back. Needles can also be attached to an electrical device called an acutens machine, letting you control the stimulation level yourself.
- **TENS** (Trans-cutaneous Electrical Nerve Stimulation). This straddles orthodox and natural approaches (see table opposite). It uses a small electronic device attached to electrodes placed either side of the spine. Electric current is used to block pain impulses travelling along nerves and to stimulate endorphins.

MONITORING THE BABY

With each contraction, the blood vessels supplying your baby with oxygen narrow, forcing the baby to hold its breath. Some babies cannot hold their breath for long and will become short of oxygen (distressed). If this happens for too long, they could suffer permanent damage or die.

During labour, the baby's heartbeat is monitored by the midwife, to detect any distress. In a low-risk pregnancy, a baby may be monitored for short spells by placing a Pinard stethoscope or an electronic ultrasound device on the mother's abdomen. In high-risk pregnancies, doctors may recommend continuous fetal monitoring during the latter part of the first stage of labour. There are two methods of continuous heart monitoring: external and internal.

In external monitoring, two belts are placed around the mother's abdomen. One holds the instrument that records the tightness and stretch of the abdomen during contractions, allowing the length and frequency of contractions to be measured. The other belt holds a transducer, which records the baby's heart rate. The belts are attached to a monitor, which records details of the baby's heartbeat and the mother's contractions.

Here, an ultrasound scanner has been strapped to the mother's abdomen to monitor her baby's heartbeat.

With internal monitoring, once the cervix has dilated, a fetal scalp electrode is passed up through the woman's vagina and the end-point (a probe with a clip on the end) is fixed under the skin of the baby's scalp or buttocks. This allows a continuous read-out of the baby's heartbeat. If it slows for more than a minute or two, medical intervention may be needed.

If there is any sign of distress, a blood specimen can be obtained through a prick in the baby's scalp – fetal scalp sampling. The specimen's acidity reveals the degree of distress. If it is extreme, then immediate delivery, probably by Caesarean, will be carried out.

DEALING WITH MONITORING

While monitoring is highly advantageous for the baby's health, the machinery needed can create a clinical atmosphere. It may also mean that the mother cannot move about freely during labour and often requires her to lie down at an angle that is somewhat unnatural and difficult for childbirth. Always tell medical staff how you feel about the monitoring process so that the most satisfactory compromise can be reached.

However, there are active birth positions that you may be able to get into when attached to a monitor. Adjust the bed head to a comfortable sitting position, usually around a 25° angle. Bend your legs alternately for about 10 minutes, placing the sole of the foot of the bent leg against the inner thigh of the straight leg. You could also kneel on the bed and lean against the angled bed head, using pillows for support. Another position is resting on your side with one bent leg above the other and a pillow between your knees. If possible, swap between these positions every half hour or so, to create a rhythm that helps to relieve contraction pain.

The first stage of labour

During the first stage of labour, you should feel free to follow your instincts and do whatever feels right for you. You may find yourself rocking or swaying during contractions. Many women like to take a bath, finding the sensation of water to be pleasantly soothing.

Move around and try out new positions until you find the one or two that seem most comfortable. Any of the positions shown here may be right for you.

A lot of women like to keep moving around during the first stage of labour, getting into their favourite position each time a new contraction starts. Take one contraction at a time, and breathe your way through it, perhaps using imagery to help you. For example, you could try to visualize your cervix opening out like a flower.

THE TRANSITIONAL STAGE

This is the term for the short period of time at the end of the first stage of labour, just before moving into the second stage. It is the shortest part of labour, but it can be very intense and contractions can feel even more painful and seem to be absolutely relentless.

You may feel discouraged and find yourself not wanting to go on for much longer without additional pain relief. You may also be very emotional and perhaps irritable or bad-tempered. Your legs may start shaking and you might shiver; you may even need to vomit.

You may also get an urge to push, or bear down, though you shouldn't do this until the midwife has examined you and has confirmed that your cervix is fully dilated. Panting a little may help you resist the urge.

Whenever you feel that you just can't go on, remember that your baby will be born soon. Keep telling yourself to hang on, stay calm, and all will be well.

GOOD POSITIONS IN TRANSITION

It is difficult to find a comfortable position when you are in transition. Any position that you have found helpful up to this point is suitable for use now. You may like to kneel forward over a pile of cushions, or you may prefer to stand, sit, squat, or be held in a supported squat.

If the cervix has not yet fully dilated and you feel the urge to bear down, try kneeling on all fours: put your head down against the floor and your bottom up in the air. This position uses the force of gravity to help slow the baby down, while the cervix continues to dilate. This position also takes pressure off your lower back.

HELPING SOMEONE GIVE BIRTH

Remember that labour can be a traumatic and difficult time for a woman, so be prepared to deal with any strange or aggressive behaviour without getting offended. If she tells you to go away, stand aside, but do not go too far away. However useless you feel, you do have an important role.

Simple actions such as sponging your partner's face and holding her hand can help a lot. Don't be surprised if she shouts at you – and at anyone else around.

- Try to help her to relax, especially between the contractions.
- Help her to cool down with a water spray or moist sponge if she's hot.
- Wipe away perspiration from her face.
- Encourage her by telling her she's doing fine, never criticize her.
- Be alert to her moods and adapt to them.
- If she feels sick and says that she wants to throw up, get her a bowl quickly.
- If her legs begin to tremble, hold her legs firmly and offer her a pair of socks in order to keep them warm and so help her circulation.
- If she has backache, massage her lower back and offer her a hot-water bottle.
- If she says she wants to push or she starts to grunt and make pushing motions, tell the midwife immediately.
- Once the midwife has told her that she is fully dilated and she can push, let the midwife guide her through the pushing stage. Always do what the midwife tells you.
- Drink lots of water to keep yourself hydrated.

SIT

Sit astride a chair, facing its back, with knees apart and your back straight. Put a cushion against the back of the chair and lean against it. In this position, your body is vertical yet completely supported, and your pelvis is kept open.

STAND

Stay upright and lean slightly forwards against your birth assistant. The downward force of gravity stimulates contractions and encourages the baby's descent. You may find it helpful to circle your hips. Your birth assistant can massage your lower back in this position, or rock you gently.

KNEEL

Kneel down and support yourself by leaning forwards against a nearby piece of sturdy furniture, over a pile of cushions or a big bean bag. You can also use a birthing ball for this.

SQUAT

Squat on a low stool or birthing ball. This position tends to intensify contractions, as well as allowing the pelvis to open widely. It also encourages the baby's descent.

KNEEL ON ALL FOURS

Kneel on all fours and rock back and forth during contractions. If they are very intense, kneel with your head against the floor and bottom in the air. Try moving your hips around, too.

LIE DOWN

You may feel like lying down, particularly if you are getting tired. Try lying on your side, with your 'bump' well supported on cushions. It is not a good idea to lie on your back for any length of time, although this is fine for when you are being examined.

The second and third stages

When the cervix is fully dilated (about 10cm/4in), you have entered the second stage of labour. The second stage can be over in minutes or it may take up to two hours. It ends with the birth of the baby. Second-stage contractions are typically very strong, with the whole body engaged in a massive involuntary urge to bear down. This is a reflex, caused by the baby's head pressing on the pelvic floor and the rectum. Even if you had read nothing about the birth, you would know instinctively when to take a deep breath, thus lowering your diaphragm and exerting pressure on the uterus, which helps to push the baby out. Some women find the second stage easier than the first, although it may be difficult, especially if the baby is large or there are worries about tearing.

BEST POSITIONS FOR BIRTH

Pushing is harder work if you are lying on your back, because you are pushing the baby uphill. An upright, or semi-upright, position is therefore best for delivery, as gravity will help your efforts. Your pelvis should be open, and your pelvic floor and vaginal opening needs to be relaxed. Many women move about and change position throughout the second stage of labour, eventually finding the best position for them for birth. The following positions, shown opposite, are all suitable for the delivery:

- **Lying down** This position is good if you are feeling exhausted. Lie on your side with your head resting on a couple of pillows. Keep your legs open by holding the knee – your birth assistant can do this for you.

- **Sitting** Here, the woman sits propped up with plenty of bulky cushions, with her knees bent and apart, and her head dropped forwards towards her chest. This position lets her see the baby being born. However, it is an unnatural position for birth and unhelpful for the baby, so it is not the best one to use.

- **Kneeling** Many women choose to give birth in this position. Kneel on all fours, leaning over a bean bag or large cushion. The midwife receives the baby from behind. A kneeling position eases pressure on the perineum, allowing the soft tissues to expand and stretch as the baby is born.

- **Squatting** This is often found to be a good position. You can squat either while being supported from behind by one helper, or while being supported on either side by two helpers. Squatting opens up the pelvis to its maximum, relaxes the pelvic floor and uses the force of gravity. If squatting with one helper, your helper should stand, or preferably sit, behind you in a firm and stable stance. He should support you by taking your weight on his arms. Surrender completely to the contraction, bending your knees and spreading your feet apart so that the pelvis opens. This position usually encourages a rapid birth and is particularly suitable if there is any reason to speed up delivery, as in cases of fetal distress or a long labour. It is also helpful in a breech birth.

YOUR BABY EMERGES

Pushing a baby out is hard work. Try to do so smoothly and gradually, so all the vaginal muscles and tissues have the chance to stretch in order to allow the baby's head through without tearing or necessitating an episiotomy.

The first sign that the baby is entering the world is a bulging of the perineum and the anus. More and more of the baby's head then appears at the vaginal opening, which is known as crowning, at which point you may feel a stinging sensation as the baby pushes against your vagina. This sensation can be eased by deep breathing, or if an attendant holds a warm compress against the perineum, helping the tissues to stretch. Sometimes the baby will be born very quickly at this stage, with its head and body coming out in one contraction. The birth may also take place more slowly, over a number of contractions. Typically, as the baby's head emerges, it will turn its head to one side. Your contractions may cease briefly here, giving those attending you the chance to check that the umbilical cord is not wrapped around the baby's neck and, if it is, to reposition the cord more safely.

Your next contraction should see the baby's shoulders emerging, and once these are out, the rest of the baby's body will follow on swiftly, usually followed by gushing amniotic fluid.

SPEED OF DELIVERY
How fast delivery occurs depends on your position and that of the baby's head, as well as its size. If it is slow and you are in a lot of pain, medical staff will help you breathe the baby out gently in order to avoid a tear. If it is felt that you are likely to tear badly, the doctor will perform an episiotomy.

LYING

SITTING

KNEELING

A SUPPORTED SQUAT

These pictures show four principal positions commonly adopted during the second stage of labour and delivery. The woman should be made as comfortable as possible with supportive cushions and allowed to swap between positions – she needs to find what is best and most comfortable for her.

YOUR BABY HAS ARRIVED

Caregivers will typically wrap the baby up and let you hold her immediately. Your baby may be breathing and crying as soon as he or she emerges, and may start to suckle virtually straight away.

If you are delivering twins, the procedures are the same. However, a twin delivery is more risky and complex, for the babies and the mother. There is an increased risk of fetal distress, and the likelihood of a Caesarean is higher with a twin delivery than with a single baby.

THE THIRD STAGE OF LABOUR

This stage occurs after delivery of the baby and is simply the expulsion of the placenta. When the baby is born, the uterus rests, but about 15 minutes later it starts to contract again, relatively painlessly, to expel the placenta and its membranes. You can help to push out the

Be prepared for a turbulent mix of emotions once the birth is over – relief, joy, shock, exhaustion and tearfulness are all perfectly normal reactions.

placenta yourself, both by squatting and also by putting the baby to the breast, which helps the uterus to contract. Medical staff will now carefully examine the placenta to make sure that absolutely all of it has been expelled, as leaving bits behind may lead to internal bleeding. Checks are then made for any large tears around the vulva area, which will have to be stitched.

Medical interventions

Sometimes births go slowly or other problems develop. Medical staff may intervene to hasten the birth if they think there is any danger to the mother or baby.

DELIVERY BY FORCEPS

Forceps can be used to facilitate a speedier delivery. They look rather like big salad servers and are sometimes used to help the baby out in the second stage of labour, when the cervix is fully dilated and the baby's head has come down into the mother's pelvis but is not descending any further. They may also be used in cases of fetal or maternal distress. The forceps are easy to apply and cause no harm to the baby if applied properly, although the baby's head may be marked.

Your legs will be put in stirrups and a local anaesthetic injected into the perineum. An episiotomy (cut) is then done, and forceps inserted into the vagina and the blades cupped round the sides of the baby's head. The idea is that the mother then pushes, while the doctor pulls. Once the head is delivered, the forceps are removed and you can push the baby out normally.

VENTOUSE EXTRACTION

More than one in ten deliveries now involve the use of ventouse ('vacuum extraction' in the US). Like forceps, it is used to help speed the delivery. A suction cap is attached to the baby's head and suction is used to pull the baby out gently with each contraction as you push.

There are no risks to the baby and no drugs need to be used. The advantages of this method over forceps delivery is that the cervix does not need to be fully dilated, and it is perceived as a lesser intervention. The mother still has to do a fair measure of the pushing so she does not feel quite so outmanoeuvred by technology.

The disadvantage is that it can take time to apply enough suction. The baby may have a small bump on its head rather like a large bruised blister, which subsides after a day or two.

INDUCTION OF LABOUR

Sometimes, labour may need to be artificially induced. This is done by breaking of the waters and by giving the mother drugs, vaginally or intravenously. An induction may be done for the following reasons:

- The baby is overdue and the placenta is becoming less able to supply his or her needs.
- Raised blood pressure in the mother.
- Pre-eclampsia.
- Rhesus incompatibility.
- Bleeding in late pregnancy.
- Diabetes.
- The baby has stopped growing.

EPISIOTOMY

An episiotomy is a cut in the perineum. A local anaesthetic is given first, and then a cut is made – using scissors – into the skin and muscle at the lower end of the woman's vagina. After the birth, the cut is stitched up. Some people believe that a natural tear heals faster than a cut. An episiotomy may be needed in an assisted delivery, or if the woman is likely to be severely torn.

Getting into a good delivery position will help minimize the chances of episiotomy. If you would like to avoid having one, you should discuss this well in advance with the medical staff who are taking care of you and include it in your birth plan.

CAESAREAN SECTION

A Caesarean is a major surgical procedure whereby both baby and placenta are delivered through a cut in the mother's abdomen rather than through the vagina. It may be done under general anaesthetic or after an epidural, in

A delighted father holds his baby after birth by caesarian section. It takes a mother a little time to recover from this operation – as with any major surgery.

which case the mother will be awake when her baby is delivered. It is possible to have your labour companion with you during this operation if you have an epidural, but not if you have a general anaesthetic.

There are two types of Caesarean section: elective (by choice) and emergency.

- **Elective Caesareans** These are planned during pregnancy, usually because there is a medical or obstetric complication which means that a vaginal delivery is considered unsafe. Occasionally, women choose to have their baby delivered by Caesarean because of a personal preference.
- **Emergency Caesareans** A Caesarean may need to be done following complications that occur during labour, when your baby has become distressed and needs to be delivered speedily and safely.

Reasons for a Caesarean

There are many reasons why a Caesarean may be done. They include the following:
- If the baby is large and the mother's pelvis is small, making normal delivery virtually impossible.
- If the baby is premature, small or particularly vulnerable to distress.
- Pregnancies in which there is more than one baby.
- Babies who are in a position – such as a transverse lie – that makes normal delivery impossible.
- Inefficient contractions – which mean that the labour does not progress.
- Placental abruption, in which the placenta detaches itself from the wall of the uterus. This usually causes pain and bleeding, and necessitates the immediate delivery of the baby.
- Placenta praevia, in which the placenta is lying across the cervix and would be ruptured if labour were allowed to continue, causing dangerous bleeding, (known as antepartum haemorrhage).
- When the mother has a condition such as high blood pressure, pre-eclampsia or diabetes.
- When the umbilical cord has prolapsed and is presenting before the baby, obstructing the delivery.
- When an induction has not worked.
- If there are tumours such as fibroids or ovarian cysts, which will obstruct the baby's delivery.
- If the mother has had a pregnancy that ended in stillbirth, or if she has experienced a previous complicated and difficult delivery.
- If the baby becomes severely distressed.

WHEN DOCTORS INTERVENE

Medical intervention in labour is becoming more common: about one in five births in the UK is by Caesarean delivery and the situation is similar in the USA. Some experts are concerned that medical staff can be too quick to intervene, and that some problems may resolve themselves naturally if allowed to do so. However, there is no doubt that intervention has saved the lives of many babies.

suction device

Assisted delivery may be necessary if the labour is progressing very slowly, if the baby becomes distressed or if the mother becomes so exhausted that she can no longer push. Here, a ventouse attached to the baby's head is used to help bring it out of the birth canal.

This woman is using a TENS pain-relief machine to cope with post-Caesarean discomfort. The stitched scar is from the operation.

Checklist of common problems

The last few weeks of pregnancy can be quite uncomfortable, and you may long to get the birth over with. Just remember that each day is bringing you a day closer to holding your baby. You may still be suffering from minor ailments, such as haemorrhoids or backache, at this stage. Natural therapies can often alleviate the worst of your symptoms and can also help you to cope with any tension. They may also help your baby to be better prepared for the birth – by virtue of you yourself being more relaxed.

Always discuss any natural remedies that you wish to take with your midwife – you will see her every week during the last month of pregnancy, so you will have plenty of opportunity to discuss any plans, anxieties or problems. If you decide to consult a complementary practitioner, make sure that you see only qualified therapists who are experienced in treating pregnant women. If you have any symptoms that are severe, prolonged or concern you, contact your midwife or doctor straight away. See page 145 for a list of emergency warning symptoms.

Breech baby   Most babies are in the buttocks-down (breech) position before 32 weeks but most will turn so that they are head-down for the birth. If your baby is in the breech position after 32 weeks, he or she may well turn spontaneously before the birth. There are also several natural methods that may help to encourage a breech or transverse baby to turn. Do not try any natural therapies if you are having twins or if you are ill.

- Take an hour-long walk each day. This may encourage your baby to move to the head-down position. Practising some yoga positions – such as 'the cat' – may also encourage the baby to move.
- Spend some time each day visualizing your baby moving into the right position. Make sure that you are feeling relaxed and comfortable when you do this – slow your breathing down and let go of any tension in your body first.
- The homeopathic remedy pulsatilla is sometimes used to encourage a baby to turn. Do not be tempted to self-prescribe; see a qualified homeopath to ensure that the remedy is suitable for you and that you take the correct dosage, and so that the homeopath can monitor the outcome.
- Moxibustion is a traditional Chinese method for turning breech babies. It is supported today by a variety of complementary practitioners, although it should be noted that doctors now do not attempt to

In moxibustion, a tiny amount of burning moxa is placed on different energy points on the body. In pregnancy, the points most typically used are located on the toes.

turn babies, as complications can result. Moxibustion involves lighting a stick of the herb moxa and holding it near acupuncture points on the outer corner of each little toe, or burning small amounts of the herb on the skin. The heat is said to stimulate the bladder energy channel, which is connected to the uterus. Moxibustion also has a general soothing effect. If you wish to try out moxibustion treatment, then you must seek the assistance of an experienced acupuncturist who is used to treating pregnant women, and do not attempt to do the treatment to yourself, or at home.

Late baby   Babies that are more than two weeks overdue are usually induced in hospital; induction may also be advised if your waters break early or you have high blood pressure. There are a number of natural methods that you can try if you have advance warning of an induction, but always talk to your midwife beforehand.
- Keep upright and keep moving around – activity can sometimes bring on contractions, but you should not overdo it.

❝ Natural therapies can often alleviate the worst of your symptoms and can also help you to cope with any tension you are feeling. ❞

- Make love. Having an orgasm can sometimes help to stimulate uterine contractions.
- Consult an acupuncturist: various points on the back can be stimulated, sometimes with electricity, in order to bring on contractions. You may need several treatments over the course of a week.
- See a reflexologist, who will work on various points on your feet.
- The homeopathic remedy caulophyllum is sometimes used to encourage contractions. However, you will need to see a qualified homeopath to ensure that this remedy is right for you, and so that your progress can be monitored.
- Try practising breathing techniques for relaxation, then visualize yourself going into labour. It can be helpful to do this daily.

Fear and anxiety Anxiety is a very common emotion for mothers-to-be. It is important that you discuss any specific worries that you have with your midwife. She may be able to put your mind at rest or advise you on any practical steps you can take. You might like to try the following suggestions:
- Practise relaxation techniques, such as yoga, Pilates, meditation or visualization. You may find it helps calm fears if you regularly visualize yourself and your baby surrounded by healing golden light.
- Consider complementary therapies, such as reiki, acupuncture or reflexology, all of which may help with stress or worry.

- Try Bach Flower Remedies, which are very gentle. Mimulus is good if you have specific, named fears, such as anxiety about the labour, while aspen is used for vague, unspecific fears. Red chestnut can be taken for excessive concern about the baby's well-being, and Rescue Remedy is excellent if you have moments of panic and tearfulness.
- Use essential oils such as lavender or rosewood, which can be very soothing in late pregnancy: use them in a burner or diluted in the bath or in a relaxing massage oil.

Bach Flower Remedies can be an effective natural way to relieve anxiety and fear. Keep them in a special box, separated out so each one retains its healing properties.

Instant calm

If you are feeling anxious or fearful, try this simple exercise to release tension and calm yourself down.

It serves to activate the energy channel of the heart, and it can feel very soothing and loving.

1 Hold your left arm straight out in front of you. Keep it loose rather than taut, and drop your shoulders to release tension here. Gently cup your right hand around the upper arm, just above the elbow.

2 Now, bring your forearm slowly towards your shoulder, until it rests upon your other hand. Breathe quietly for a few moments, focusing on your heart area, and feel a sense of release here.

Common Qs and As

Q: I felt my contractions starting and my partner took me to the hospital but they sent me home again, saying I wasn't ready yet. How could that happen?

A: It is possible to have contractions that mimic those of labour but are shorter and less pronounced. Once the hospital checks you out, they can tell immediately by how dilated your cervix is whether or not you have started true labour.

Q: I was planning a natural, drug-free birth but now my baby is going to be induced as I am two weeks overdue. I have heard that the contractions are more intense after an induction. Is that true?

A: Not necessarily. It depends on the individual woman, the reasons for the induction, how overdue she is, the drugs used, and how your particular hospital manages labour in respect of pain relief. It is better to induce a birth than to let the baby stay too long in the uterus, because there comes a point when the placenta can no longer nourish the baby.

Q: I had a very drawn-out, painful birth with my first child. My consultant has offered me an elective Caesarean. Do you think that this is a good idea?

A: It depends on the reasons why this has been offered. If the consultant knows that you are facing another lengthy and painful delivery, clearly it is sensible to elect for a Caesarean. If, for example, your pelvis and birth canal are too narrow to deliver a baby vaginally, the baby must be born by Caesarean. If, on the other hand, you are being offered a Caesarean to put your mind at rest, it may be better to try for a natural delivery first and only then to go for a Caesarean if there appears to be no other alternative. So, ask your consultant exactly why you have been offered a Caesarean, think it over, and base your decision on his or her advice.

Q: I am keen to give birth naturally and without pain relief. To me, it will not be a real birth if the doctors take control. How can I make sure that that this does not happen?

A: If everything goes well, you will not need medical intervention. You can give yourself the best possible chance of a natural birth by preparing well, practising your breathing exercises regularly, and by stating your wishes on a birth plan.

However, you cannot guarantee that your delivery will be straightforward. If anything does go wrong, you would be well advised to take advantage of all the skills and technology that modern medicine can offer. In the end, it is more important that your baby comes into the world safe and healthy than that you have the childbirth experience you hoped for.

Q: My underlying fears about coping with the financial aspects of having a baby are really crowding in on me now that the birth is imminent. How on earth are we going to pay for everything that the baby will need?

A: First of all, it is natural to start obsessing over certain worries once the baby is due, as this is a vulnerable time for you. Just focus on the fact that the most important thing for your baby is that he or she is with you. Your baby does not need much: just to be warm, fed and looked after. Think of positive solutions to any worries, such as asking your midwife if there are any outlets in your area where you can buy decent second-hand items.

Q: My partner seems quite relaxed about giving birth, but she has said she wants me to be there. I am not sure if I can handle this.

A: Many men feel this way. Some men really cannot cope and it would be unwise to try to persuade them. A few men have said that they never felt the same way about their partners once they had seen them giving birth. For other men, however, seeing their partner give birth is an absolute highlight of their life.

Explain exactly how you feel to your partner. It may be that when the time comes, you do feel able to be there. Alternatively, you could promise to be nearby during her labour, even if you feel unable to be in the room. You should also suggest that she takes someone else to support her through the labour. This will take the pressure off you, and you may then feel able to be there for some of the time.

Q: I have just broken up with my partner even though I am 36 weeks pregnant. I know that our decision to split is right for both of us but I am dreading giving birth alone.

A: You do not have to be alone. You can elect for one of your friends, a sister or another member of your family to be there with you. You could investigate the possibility and cost of a private room after giving birth for you and your new baby.

Try to arrange for extra help at home after the birth. Is there anybody who could come to help you for a couple of weeks after the birth? If not, it is a good idea to have at least one visit a day from friends or relatives. You should also tell your midwife your situation, as she may be able to arrange extra help.

Q: I have been asked to take part in a research project during my pregnancy and labour. Do I have to agree to this?

A: Many maternity units are committed to ongoing research projects to improve standards of clinical care. You may be asked to take part, but you do not have to. Many units are responsible for training doctors and midwives who need to conduct normal deliveries under close supervision by experienced midwives. You may refuse this option, but many women welcome the support that students can give them during labour.

Q: I am a single mother who is expecting my second child. I am worried that there will be prejudice about this from some of the other women on the delivery ward and from the nurses. How can I best cope with this?

A: Many women now have children when they are single: you are unlikely to be an unusual case. Nobody will be surprised if your birth partner is a friend or relative rather than the father.

You may find it helpful to discuss your anxieties with your midwife, and to note on your birth plan that you would like as much privacy as possible. Take a friend or relative to support you through the labour. Above all, remember it is your life and your baby: be happy and proud of the decisions you have made.

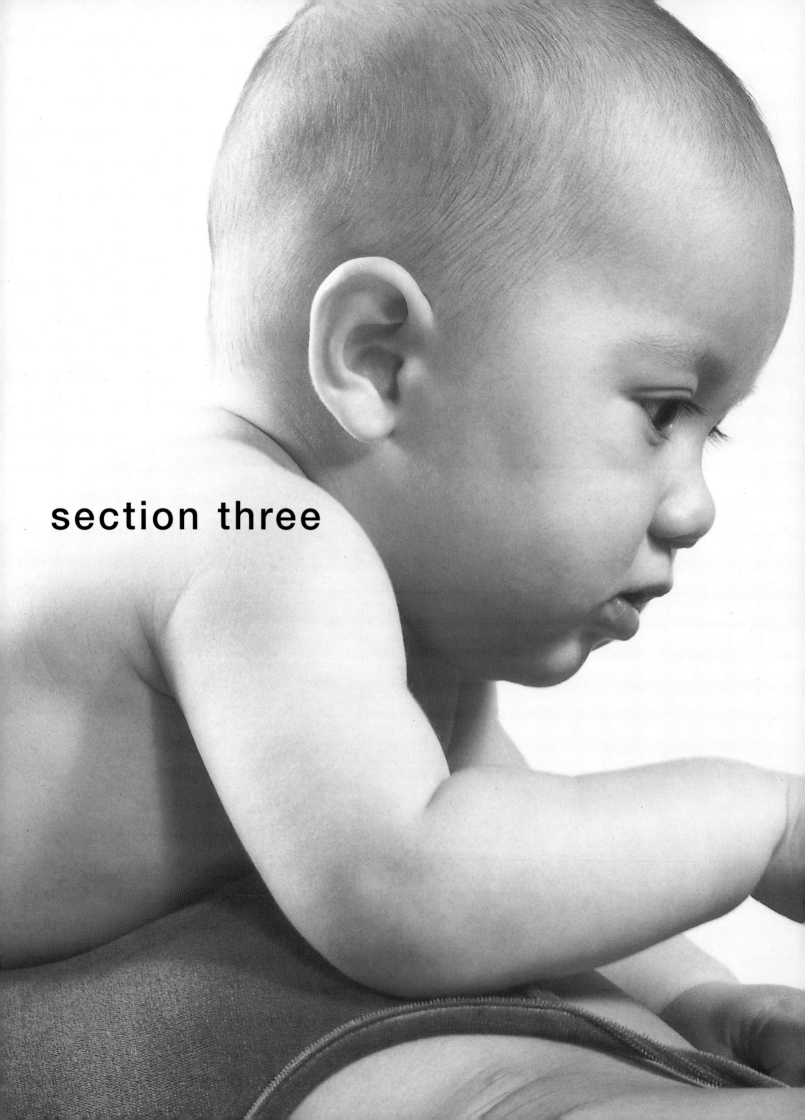

section three

you and your new baby

The first days with your baby will be among the most memorable of your life. This is a time of powerful emotions, of new discoveries, and of a growing understanding of the profundity of the love parents feel for their child. Many parents say that nothing can prepare you for the thrill of being with your newborn child. Your life will be turned upside down, but you will soon wonder how you ever existed without your child.

Caring for your new baby

> ❝ Your baby's needs are now the most important consideration in your life. ❞

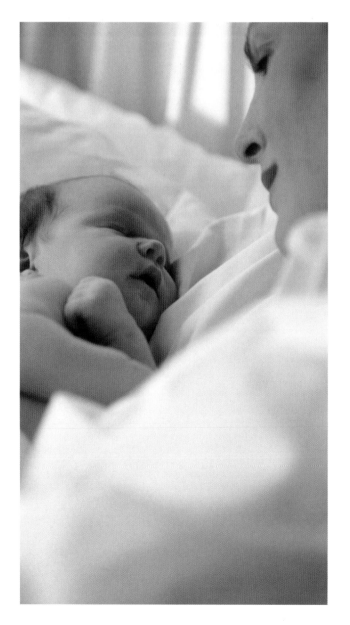

Your baby's feelings and needs are now the most important consideration in your life. When you offer your baby his or her very first feed, you are likely to experience a variety of emotions: joy, wonder, exhaustion and relief that all is well.

When you speak, your baby will recognize the distinctive rhythms of your voice, which he or she has heard for many months while growing inside you. He or she will be gazing at you, experiencing your smell, your look and the texture of your skin.

In turn, you and your partner are likely to spend many hours gazing at your baby, looking into his or her eyes, marvelling at the tiny fingers and toes, and the minute nails. You will be examining every curve of your baby's tiny body, every indentation, even the hairs on his or her head.

When you bath your baby for the first time, you may find that you naturally respond to his or her vulnerability with the gentlest touch. You will come to cherish the softness of your baby's skin and his or

Newborn babies cannot see very far. At first, they can see what is immediately in front of them, but very little more than that.

her natural helplessness, and you will want to do everything in your power to love and care for his or her various needs.

However much you love your baby though, you are likely to find that you experience some difficult emotions during these first weeks. Most women feel sad, anxious or overwhelmed at times – and everyone feels exhausted.

It is very important that you look after yourself as well as your baby. In particular, get as much sleep and rest as you can, whenever you can. Eat healthily and often, and try to get some fresh air every day. This will help you to cope with the inevitable challenges of looking after a small baby.

Top: Enjoying – and making time for – having plenty of interaction and fun together is enormously important for both parent and baby.

Your baby will enjoy the physical comfort of being breastfed, and breastfeeding helps you to know that you are doing everything possible to meet his or her needs.

Meeting your new baby

At long last you are being handed your baby. This is the moment that you and your partner have been waiting for. Whatever difficulties you have faced during the pregnancy, whatever kind of labour and delivery you have had, all that is now behind you. This is the moment to savour for the rest of your life – the very beginning of your child's life and the start of your lives as parents.

If you have delivered your baby in hospital, you will probably be left alone with your partner and the baby for a while. This will depend partly on how well you and the baby have stood up to the rigours of the birth. At some point, your pulse and blood pressure will be checked and your temperature will be taken. You will be able to take a bath. The baby will be weighed and measured in length and head circumference, footprinted and given a name band. She will also be assessed according to the Apgar score (see box below).

The umbilical cord will be clamped and cut when it has stopped pulsating after the birth and the clamped stump at the baby's navel will be left to drop off of its own accord within the next few days. A small blood sample

This is the moment that makes it all worthwhile – holding your lovely new baby. Medical staff will be sensitive and leave you alone with your baby as soon as possible.

> **❝ This is the moment that makes it all worthwhile – holding your lovely new baby. ❞**

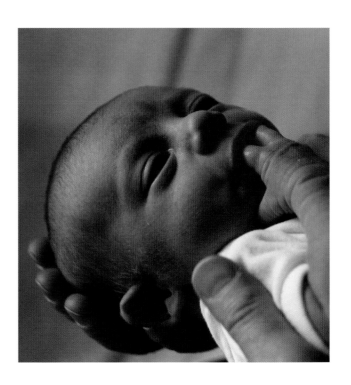

THE APGAR SCORE

Soon after the birth, your baby will need to be cleaned, weighed and measured. A name band will be placed around his or her wrist if you are in hospital. The baby's health will be assessed a minute after the delivery. This is done using the Apgar score in which five factors are checked. Points are awarded from 0 to 2 for each of the five factors. The baby who scores 10 is in good general health; if your baby scores less than ten, he or she may need special care for a while. The test may be repeated after five minutes.

SIGN	0 POINT	1 POINT	2 POINTS
Respiratory effort (breathing)	None	Weak cry, slow breathing	Good strong cry
Pulse (heart rate)	None	Slow, under 100 beats per minute	Fast, over 100 beats per minute
Colour (pallor)	Blue or pale	Pink body with blue fingers and toes	All pink
Muscular tone	Limp	Some flexing of fingers and toes	Active: fingers and toes flexing well
Response to stimuli (reflexes)	No response	Grimace	Cry

One secure way of holding your newborn baby is to cradle him in your arms, in the crook of your elbow, making sure that his head is well supported.

will be taken from the baby so that the Guthrie test can be done. This is used to detect phenylketonuria, a disease which causes mental impairment if left untreated. If the test is positive, the baby can be treated for the condition with complete success.

MARKS AND RASHES

When your baby first arrives, you may notice a few minor bumps and wrinkles caused by the journey down the birth canal. He or she may even have a little bruise and the odd spot, rash or area where the skin tone is blotchy, while some newborns have puffy eyes. The baby may have enlarged breasts and genitals caused by hormonal fluctuations, which will settle soon after birth. This is all very normal.

There are certain other skin marks that are more permanent. These include pale pink 'stork bite' markings on the face or neck that disappear within the first year; blue spots common on darker-skinned babies that fade away; and 'strawberry' birthmarks that start as red dots and may get larger within the first year, normally disappearing by the age of about five. Larger flat areas of red or purple known as 'port wine stains' are permanent – seek a doctor's advice about these.

INITIAL BONDING

Some new parents immediately experience a huge well of love for their newborn. Many women will have started the bonding process with their baby many weeks before giving birth, perhaps even from the first scan or earlier. For others, and for many fathers, too, the bonding process may take longer.

As you look at your baby in the first minute of new life, you will probably feel overwhelmed with emotion. You may find yourself simultaneously full of pleasure and weariness, curiosity and relief. Your baby will be looking at you, and taking in the smell of you. From this first day

of life, you, with your partner, are everything to this newborn person: warmth, shelter, comfort and security. It will take time for you all to be completely bonded to one another, but this will come.

HOLDING AND HANDLING

Many new parents are frightened of handling a fragile tiny newborn, but there is nothing to be afraid of, as long as you hold him or her safely and confidently – babies quickly detect if the person holding them is unsure of what they are doing and they feel more secure and more comfortable if they are handled with conviction.

Always lift your baby slowly and gently, avoiding any jerky movements. Make sure that your baby's head is properly supported at all times, as newborn babies cannot support their own heads for the first few weeks. Hold your baby close and bend right over when lifting, sliding one hand under their head, and the other under their lower back.

Newborn babies are monitored by medical staff to ensure that all of their vital functions are working well.

Feeding your baby

All the nutrients your newborn baby receives come from milk. The options are to feed from the breast or from the bottle. Bottle-feeding is done either by using made-up 'formula milk' (that is, milk that is specially suited to babies) or by using milk expressed from your breasts (see page 214).

Experts agree that breastfeeding is the best way to nourish your baby. They recommend that, ideally, you should breastfeed for at least six months, although some women find that they are unable to feed their baby for this long. Other women are unable to breastfeed at all for a variety of reasons, including illness or inability to breastfeed successfully or easily, and there are also those who simply do not like the idea of breastfeeding. For these mothers, bottle-feeding with formula milk is the only answer, and even breastfeeding women may want to use bottles from time to time for reasons of convenience – when they are out and about, for example.

The commonest formula milk is cow's milk that has been modified to make it suitable. About one in ten infants is allergic to cow's milk formula. Soya and hydrolysate formula milks offer an alternative, but they have less in common with human milk than cow's milk does. So, if you can persevere with breastfeeding, your baby will benefit.

Ultimately, how you feed your baby is a very personal decision. Talk through your feelings with nursing staff, who will be happy to advise you. They will give you plenty of help with feeding issues but in the end you have to decide what is best for you and your baby.

BREASTFEEDING

There are many advantages to breastfeeding, and paediatricians agree that it has the following benefits:

- Breast milk gives the baby protection from bugs, disease and allergy, such as eczema and asthma.
- Breastfed babies are less susceptible to stomach upsets and constipation.
- Breastfeeding helps to encourage the baby's facial development. It may also be responsible for the lower incidence of dental problems later in the baby's life.
- Breastfed babies are less likely to become overweight or obese later in life.
- Breastfeeding gives the newborn baby everything he or she needs and wants – physical contact with the mother, warmth and food. A crying baby usually finds breastfeeding more soothing and reassuring than bottle-feeding and is more easily consoled.

Breastfeeding is a skill that may need to be learned. Once you get the hang of it, feeding your baby becomes a pleasurable experience for you both.

- Breast milk is naturally sterile and the correct temperature – so mothers do not have the bother of making sure that bottle-feeding equipment is sterile and that the temperature of the milk is safe.
- Breastfeeding helps new mothers to get their figure back. Breastfeeding causes the release of a hormone, called oxytocin, which helps shrink the uterus.
- Breastfeeding reduces a woman's risk of developing breast cancer in later life.

What breast milk contains

Human breast milk contains all the nutrients your baby needs, in the right proportions. It has:

- Enough water to quench the baby's thirst.
- Protein for body building.
- Fat for energy and growth.
- Carbohydrate, in the form of lactose, for energy.
- Vitamins and minerals.
- Antibodies and iron-binding protein, which make the baby's intestine less vulnerable to bacteria and protect against a number of serious illnesses.

Breast pads, tucked inside your bra, are the answer to leaking breasts, which can be an embarrassment and may also lead to sore, cracked nipples. Both disposable and washable pads are available.

At the beginning of a feed, the baby gets foremilk, which has a high water content. When he or she continues to suck, the hindmilk comes: this is rich in calories and helps the baby to grow. You should therefore let the baby feed from one breast for as long as he or she wishes.

Getting used to breastfeeding

Breastfeeding can be difficult at the start – it doesn't always come naturally to the baby or the mother. It may take as long as a fortnight to establish breastfeeding and another month or so for a pattern to develop. It is important to accept that there will be no routine at first. Your family doctor or the hospital can arrange for you to see a specialist breastfeeding counsellor or midwife.

NATURAL SOLUTIONS TO BREASTFEEDING PROBLEMS

Many women experience problems with breastfeeding at some stage. Natural therapies can offer some gentle solutions.

- To increase the production of breast milk, try herbal teas, such as raspberry leaves, goat's rue, fennel, dill, borage, nettle, vervain or cinnamon. Do not drink more than three cups a day.
- If you are finding breastfeeding difficult, homeopathic remedies may help. Suitable remedies may include bryonia, phytolacca, conium and belladonna, but see a homeopath for advice.
- Cracked nipples may be relieved by the homeopathic remedy castor equi 30C. Applying calendula cream can help, but wash it off completely before feeding.
- Ease the discomfort of engorged breasts by placing savoy cabbage leaves directly on them (an ice-cold flannel or a bag of frozen vegetables wrapped in a flannel are other options).

Talk to your doctor or health visitor if you have any anxieties about your feeding technique or milk supply, or if you experience symptoms such as fever or swelling or redness of the breast.

How to get your baby latched on

Hold your baby in a position that will be comfortable, relaxed and secure – you may like to prop your arm on a cushion. Place your baby so that his or her body forms a straight line from your breast. That way, the baby's head doesn't have to turn in order to feed. Make sure that the baby is held high enough to reach your nipple easily.

The important thing is to get your baby 'latched on' (fixed on) to the breast properly. This will help to make sure your baby gets a good milk supply. It will also minimize problems such as breasts that are engorged with milk (because the milk is not flowing well) and nipple soreness.

1 The baby's mouth should be wide open before you present your breast for feeding. Bring your nipple close to his or her nose, and let the baby take it into the mouth. However, the nipple should be entirely within the baby's mouth and his or her jaws clamped on to your breast rather than on to the nipple itself.

2 Let the baby feed at one breast for as long as he or she wants. Then offer the other breast. If the baby doesn't want to continue feeding, offer this breast first next time around. Don't worry about having no idea when to stop – a baby will usually let you know when he or she has had enough milk.

Breastfeeding in the first few days

Tension is probably the biggest cause of initial breastfeeding problems, so try to relax and enjoy your baby as much as possible. Your breasts do not start to make milk until they are stimulated by a complex hormonal reaction that takes place after the birth. Before this happens, the breasts produce colostrum, a creamy, yellowish substance which you may have noticed leaking during the last few months of pregnancy.

In the first few days of your baby's life, you are feeding him or her colostrum. This gives valuable protection from bacterial infections and illnesses the mother has had in the past or has been immunized against. It cannot be artificially reproduced.

Expressing breast milk

There may be times when you would like the convenience of feeding your baby from a bottle, but you would still like to use your own milk. You may also be having problems with breastfeeding due to engorged breasts.

You can express milk from your breasts either by hand, or with a manual pump (see page 188), the latter method being much faster and easier. Always wash your hands before expressing milk, and make sure that any equipment is sterilized. With a manual pump, you simply fit the funnel over the areola of the breast so that it forms a good, tight seal. You then use a plunger or lever to express the milk. Expressed milk should be kept in a bottle with a tight-fitting lid and refrigerated until needed. Store it for up to a couple of days in a refrigerator, or for up to six months or so in a freezer.

BOTTLE-FEEDING

Many women find this more convenient than breastfeeding and bottle-feeding with formula milk is a good way of nourishing babies whose mothers cannot breastfeed. Formula milk can be made up from powders that are basically dried milk or can be bought in liquid form, the latter being more expensive. Other options include various organic formula products and soya products, for babies with a cow's milk allergy. Feeding your baby with formula milk can be more time-consuming than breastfeeding and does not have the same health benefits. However, there are various advantages to this method:

- Anyone can feed the baby, not just you. Your partner can share the feeding, which may help bonding between baby and father.
- If you need to return to work, bottle-feeding can be more convenient. It means that you can go out without the baby for longer periods.
- Bottle-feeding may be useful if you are recovering from a Caesarean or difficult delivery and if you are ill. It is also good for premature or sick babies who are too weak to suck.

What formula milk contains

- Water, but not enough, so your baby will need extra drinks of boiled water.
- Protein, but in too high a concentration, so it has to be diluted. This process lowers the calorie content of the feed, which is supplemented by lactose.
- Fat, which is less easily absorbed than breastmilk fat.
- Carbohydrate, but in insufficient quantity, so lactose has to be added.
- Vitamins and minerals, but not in the right amounts, so many formulas are enriched with extra vitamins and extra iron.

BURPING YOUR BABY

The aim of burping your baby – rubbing or patting his or her back – is to bring up any air that your baby may have swallowed during feeding, as trapped air can cause a baby some discomfort.

Trapped air is more common when babies are fed from a bottle because there is more opportunity for air to enter the baby's mouth. When babies are breastfeeding, their mouths are usually so closely locked onto the breast that little air can get in.

The two basic ways to burp babies are to sit them on your lap so that they are leaning forwards (they shouldn't bend at the waist) and are supported securely round their chest. Now pat gently on the back. Do not pat too firmly – this may make your baby regurgitate their feed. Another method is to hold your baby against your shoulder and rub their back gently, using upward strokes. Make sure that you have an old towel over your shoulder in case your baby brings up a little milk (known as possetting). Don't worry that there is something wrong if your baby does not burp – it simply means he or she had no need to do so.

Do not pat or rub too hard – go gently.

Preparing dried formula feeds

You should find clear instructions on the can or packet, and you must follow these carefully. Never add more powder than instructed in the hope of making the feed more nourishing, as this will give your baby too little water and too much protein and fat. Equally, don't add too little powder or the feed will not be nourishing enough. The water that you mix with the powder feed must be water that has been freshly boiled and allowed to cool slightly. Measure the water after it has boiled and cooled; if you do so before then you risk using too little water as you will have lost some through evaporation.

KEEPING CLEAN

All equipment associated with feeding must be kept thoroughly clean or sterilized, in order to reduce the risk of your baby catching any gastro-intestinal infection – newborns are very susceptible to such infections. Make sure that you always wash your hands before touching feeding equipment and giving the bottle to your baby. Also, always keep bottles of prepared formula feed in the refrigerator, but never for longer than 24 hours – prepare at the time if at all possible.

Methods of cleaning equipment are: placing in boiling water for at least five minutes (allow to cool before using); using a sterilizing tank and chemicals; using a steamer; using a microwave sterilizer. Before sterilizing equipment, wash the equipment in warm soapy water or a dishwasher. Make sure that everything is properly rinsed, and that teats are especially well cleaned.

When using a sterilizing tank, fill the tank half full with cold water and add a sterilizing tablet. When the tablet has dissolved, put in your equipment. Fill the bottles with water to keep them under the water and then fill the tank up with cold water.

A bottle-fed baby must be well supported at a slight angle with the head raised, so they can swallow and breathe easily without choking. Warm a bottle of formula milk in a bowl of warm water (not a microwave), splash a few drops on your inner wrist to see if it is tepid and unscrew the teat ring a little so the teat won't close up.

Any bottles and teats must always be thoroughly sterilized to reduce the risk of infection.

CLEANING BOTTLES AND TEATS

Using warm, soapy water, clean inside the bottle very thoroughly with a brush and then rub the teats. Many of the bottle-cleaning brushes available now have a special teat-cleaner on the end of the handle.

Make sure all traces of milk are removed.

Changing and bathing

Parents are often daunted by the idea of changing and bathing a baby, but if you are patient and allow yourself some trial and error, you should have few problems.

NAPPIES

There has never been such a wide range of nappy (diaper) options, so every parent can find something to suit:

- Disposables. Choose eco-friendly disposables rather than ordinary, standard types. Standard ones contain chemicals, especially in the absorbent gels used, that it is thought could be harmful to a baby. Disposal of these nappies causes problems for the environment.
- Fabric nappies. These reusable nappies are sold in a vast range of forms, from the classic terry towelling square to ready-shaped fabric nappies that close with integral fasteners (such as poppers) or with separate plastic fasteners (the modern equivalent of nappy pins). Many fabric nappies can be adjusted to fit a growing baby and you can use laundering services to clean them – such services tend to favour 'pre-folded' fabric nappies, now widely available.
- Liners. These fit right inside a fabric nappy to catch waste. Disposable liners that you simply flush away are very popular, and biodegradeable types are available. You can also buy washable fabric ones, which can be reused.
- Wraps and pants. These are reusable and fit over the top of nappies. The most natural option is a cotton wrap, with an inner waterproof layer, that closes with poppers or Velcro-type fastenings.
- All-in-ones. These are typically a cotton inner nappy permanently attached to a waterproof cover and fastened with poppers. The whole thing can be machine-washed and tumble-dried. These take some time to dry and seem costly as an initial outlay.

CHANGING AND CLEANING

Always check for redness or rashes. Nappy rash is common but quickly treated – try soothing calendula cream and homeopathic calendula powder. Never use talc on your baby (or on yourself), even unperfumed kinds, as it has been linked with possible harmful effects. Wash the baby often and change the nappy as often as necessary. Allow the baby to be without a nappy for short intervals each day, so that air can circulate – warm, damp areas can lead to rashes.

To clean your baby before putting on a new nappy, use cotton wool with lots of warm water or just a gentle, non-perfumed lotion (especially if he or she has a rash). Avoid soaps if possible, especially perfumed and coloured ones, and try to steer clear of disposable wipes, which strip skin of natural oils. Clean girls from front to back, to avoid spreading germs into the vagina or urethra. Do not separate the labia or clean inside. When cleaning a boy's penis and testicles, do not pull back the foreskin. Dry by patting gently, right into the folds, with a soft towel.

Top row, from left: all-in-one washable nappy (diaper) with integral pants, shaped fabric nappy, terry squares. Bottom row from left: washable waterproof over-pants, washable fabric nappy liner and plastic fasteners for some fabric nappies (instead of safety pins), biodegradeable disposable nappy. The Internet is a great source of companies offering natural, eco-friendly options.

Changing a terry nappy

The simplest type of fabric nappy (diaper) is the old-fashioned terry towelling square, which you will need to fold and fix to form a nappy yourself. The method shown is the 'kite' method, although there are many others.

1 Open up the square. Fold the sides in as shown (overlap these for a newborn, for extra absorbancy).

2 Now fold down the top edge and fold up the bottom edge, leaving a space in between.

3 Place a liner on top – either the disposable kind or a washable and reusable one (the latter is seen here).

4 Position your baby on top of the nappy. His or her waist should be aligned with the top edge of the folded square.

5 Bring the sides in and the bottom part up between the legs. Tuck the central panel into the corners of the side pieces. Fix with a modern 'pin'.

6 Now put a waterproof wrap or pants over the top of the nappy, to stop your baby from staining his or her clothes.

BATHING YOUR BABY

This is a good way to hold your baby in the bath, until he or she is able to sit up and play. Never leave a baby unattended in the bath – even for a minute and even if he or she is in a bath seat. Always check the temperature of the water before placing the baby in it. Do not let anyone who is not familiar with bathing children do this for you unless you are there, too.

1 Cradle the baby in your left arm as you test the temperature. (Use your right arm if left-handed.)

2 Support the baby's back, neck and head as you wash the hair with your right hand.

3 Hold under the left arm and bottom and lower the baby into the bath.

4 Continue holding under the arm as you wash with your right hand.

5 Lift the baby out. Wrap the head and body in a towel, and dry well.

Getting to know your baby

Just who is your new baby? What can they do, how do they relate to you and to the world around them, and how to they behave and develop in their first few weeks?

YOUR BABY'S REFLEXES

A baby is born with powerful basic reflexes, designed to protect them until they can make conscious movements. Some of these reflexes last for a day or two, others for a few months. The reflex that allows them to keep breathing involuntarily will stay with them throughout their life.

Grasping, foot-curling and stepping reflexes

Everyone knows just how tightly a baby's fingers grasp any adult finger that is offered – or any other object. A baby's full body weight can be supported by holding on to your fingers with both their hands. This reflex allows primates to cling to their mothers' fur. Another strong reflex is in the feet – a baby curls its soles if they are touched. If you hold a baby upright so the feet can touch a firm surface, another reflex emerges – your baby will make 'stepping' actions. This is not connected with learning to stand or walk.

The Moro reflex

When startled or held out in space, a newborn throws out their limbs as if trying to grab hold of something. They find this distressing, so try to hold your baby close to you.

IS MY BABY SMILING?

Most babies smile for the first time between five and six weeks, usually at their mother. However, very early smiles are often 'windy smiles' – simply a facial expression caused by wind. By 12 weeks the baby will smile when spoken to, and by 16 weeks he or she will laugh aloud. It is not until 20 weeks that babies smile at their own image in the mirror, and will be five to six months before a baby can express recognition and pleasure through smiling.

A baby's first smile is usually for his or her mother.

Sucking and swallowing reflexes

Another strong reflex in newborns is the sucking one, which is triggered when pressure is applied to their palate. Babies are also born with a good swallowing reflex – this is well developed because they have already been swallowing fluids while in their mother's uterus. The sucking and swallowing reflexes are vital survival tools, enabling a baby to feed the minute he or she is born. You'll also notice that, if you stroke a baby's cheek, they turn in that direction with their mouth open and waiting. This searching for a breast to feed on is known as the rooting reflex.

Blinking reflex

This protects a baby from bright light or eye damage – for example, babies automatically close their eyes if you touch their eyelids.

A newborn baby's sucking reflex is extremely strong, as is its swallowing reflex – both are vital for starting to feed as soon after birth as possible.

Talking to and cuddling your baby helps him or her to feel secure, and helps the senses to develop normally.

YOUR BABY'S SENSES

We now know quite a lot about how much babies see, hear and understand the world around them. In the days after birth, for example, we know that a mother and her baby are very sensitive to each other's smell and touch.

Smell, taste and touch

Newborn babies are highly receptive to smell and its related sense, taste. It is known that babies can smell their way to the mother's breast at birth. Babies quickly learn to distinguish the smell of their mother from that of other people in the first few weeks. They also like plenty of touch and closeness, and in the first few weeks their mouths are very sensitive touching tools.

Hearing and vision

Newborn babies have a strong sense of sound. It is through hearing that we learn language and acquire the ability to communicate with one another. Your baby starts this process early on: he or she learned to recognize the sound of your voice in the uterus some weeks before the birth. Once born, your baby will be able to distinguish your voice from that of other women very rapidly. Not much is known about how well babies hear in the first few months after birth. Paediatricians say that it is important that you talk to your baby from birth in order to help the development of speech and language. If the mother calls the baby by name from birth, he or she will usually respond by the age of one month.

Massage is a wonderful way of communicating through touch. As you massage, help to build a close relationship by maintaining eye contact.

> **" Talking to and cuddling your baby helps him or her to feel secure, and helps the senses to develop normally. "**

A baby's eyes open at about week 28 of the pregnancy. He or she can perceive light by this time and the pupils dilate in response. After birth, a baby can see what is just in front of him or her, but little else. At about two weeks, a baby recognizes its mother by sight. Newborn babies have a simple mental template of the human face. They search out and stare at human faces during their first two months, and so quickly become attracted to those who care for them in early life. Cradled in her mother's arms, he or she is at the perfect distance to see her face. Babies are still unable to focus on distant objects at this stage.

BEHAVIOUR AND MEMORY

Your baby will have a fascinating array of behaviour patterns. At first, many movements are controlled by the fact that he or she cannot support the weight of their head – putting the head to one side when lying on the back, for example. He or she will also have various crying patterns, with different root causes (see page 222), and will often sneeze and hiccup. Sneezing does not automatically mean a cold – bright light stimulates nerves in the nose, and sneezing will help to keep the nasal passages clear. Frequent hiccups are simply the result of sudden movements of the diaphragm muscle as the baby's breathing mechanisms develop. Spend lots of time interacting with your baby and you will soon start to learn what all of their expressions and cries mean.

How much memory does a newborn have? Newborns register a great deal of information, but have a limited ability to retain it. Only later, when a child starts to integrate a picture of the world into a coherent entity, using all of the five senses, can his or her memory begin to function fully. General comprehension and memory are not evident until around 16 weeks of age.

Coping with the early days

If you had your baby in hospital, you may stay in the maternity unit for anything between six hours to three days, and even up to ten days if there have been complications. When you get home, it may feel good to relax in your own environment once again. However, most women also feel overwhelmed at this point – partly due to the action of your hormones and partly because you are adjusting to the unfamiliar experience of being a parent. Mothers with older children are likely to experience this feeling too, and they may feel exhausted at the prospect of dealing with everybody's needs. These first weeks can be a demanding time. It may be reassuring to know that things settle down after about three months or so, but that can seem like a very long time.

Seek advice from your community midwife, health visitor or doctor if anything bothers you and make time to discuss things supportively with your partner. In the meantime, eat well (foods that are rich in vitamins B2 and B6, zinc and magnesium may help to normalize hormone levels), and try to get some fresh air every day – if possible, have a short walk with your partner and the baby so that you can enjoy being a family together.

RECOVERING FROM THE BIRTH

You may have to cope with various discomforts after the birth. If you have had an episiotomy or you have torn, your body will need time to heal. It may be helpful to take the homeopathic remedy arnica if there is any bruising but do not apply anything to the actual cut and sutures. Bathe

> **❝ You are likely to be unusually emotional. Give yourself time to get back to normal. ❞**

the area twice a day and dry with a warm (not hot) hairdryer since wetness will impede the healing process. If you have painful haemorrhoids, see your doctor. Eat plenty of high-fibre foods and apply a cold compress or soothing over-the-counter cream.

You are likely to be unusually emotional and fatigue will be a problem. Give yourself time to get back to normal and get plenty of rest. Try not to do too much, other than care for your baby – and let other people help out.

THE BABY BLUES

Most women experience the baby blues, in which they feel weepy for no obvious reason and experience a sense of helplessness. This usually happens around the fifth day after the delivery. If you feel awful, let someone know – your partner, a nurse, a doctor or whoever you find most approachable. These feelings will pass.

POSTNATAL DEPRESSION

A spell of the baby blues is normal for new mothers, and doesn't last long. It must not be confused with postnatal depression, however. Postnatal depression tends to occur later than baby blues, and the symptoms are those of classic depression. The mother may feel misery, fear and anger – directed at herself, her partner, her baby, or anyone else around her. Irritability, fatigue and sleeplessness are the hallmarks. The depression may not show itself until some months after the birth. Symptoms can include:

- Losing one's zest for life.
- Difficulty in sleeping.
- Waking early in the morning.
- Changes in appetite – eating more or less than usual.
- General feelings of apathy.
- Finding it hard to concentrate.
- Uncontrollable thoughts.
- Despair or suicidal feelings.

Yoga may be very beneficial in the early months after birth to get you back in shape and help you cope with the demands of parenthood. As the baby grows older, he or she will enjoy practising with you. Ask your doctor when he or she advises that you should start exercising.

Postnatal depression can be very debilitating. At its worst, the mother may harm herself or the baby. Immediate professional help, via the family doctor or the health visitor, is therefore very important if depression is making it difficult for you to function, or if you are having harmful thoughts about yourself or your baby. You will not be judged: depression is an illness and your doctor can help you to cope and to get better.

Women with mild depression may experience a sense of apathy or misery, as well as early-morning wakefulness or other symptoms. It is still important that you tell your health visitor or doctor about how you are feeling. Natural therapies such as acupuncture, aromatherapy or cranial osteopathy can often help to alleviate some of the symptoms of depression.

Simple tasks can feel overwhelming if you are suffering from depression. Ask your partner, friends or relatives for extra support – help with housework, for example.

SLEEP PATTERNS

The biggest problem for new parents is often lack of sleep – it is hard to function if you are deprived of rest. Understanding your baby's sleep may help you and your partner cope with interrupted nights. A newborn baby is awake for six to eight hours out of every 24, often for an hour or more at a time. Some babies are more wakeful

It is unlikely that your baby will feel sleepy when you do. This means that most parents need to devise a sleeping schedule that includes daytime naps.

SLEEPING SAFELY

The following measures should help to reduce the risk of sudden infant death syndrome (SIDS or cot death).
- Put a baby to sleep on its back, not the stomach.
- The baby must sleep in a well-ventilated room and not be too hot, but don't let a baby get too cold. The best room temperature is about 18°C (65°F).
- Keep a baby's head uncovered when it is sleeping.
- Arrange your baby and tuck in bedding so that bedding cannot be pulled up over its head (it should reach to shoulder level) and its feet are at the foot of the cot or pram.
- Choose a firm, flat, clean mattress with a waterproof covering and cover with a single sheet. Use sheets and lightweight blankets. Do not stifle with too much bedding or with duvets, quilts, baby nests, wedges, bedding rolls, pillows, fleeces or sheepskins, or any bedding with loose hairs.
- Avoid sharing your bed with your baby.
- Do not allow anyone to smoke near your baby or in the same room as your baby. Babies of smokers are more vulnerable to cot death than babies of non-smokers.
- Seek help promptly if you think your baby is unwell.

than others, The duration of sleep depends on a child's age and personality, the need for food, and also on the length of his or her daytime rests. At first, babies rarely sleep for longer than three to five hours at a time. However, by the age of four months most babies will sleep for six to ten hours at a time. They can also stay awake for several hours. Premature babies usually sleep for more than 16 hours per day, but within a year their sleep requirement will match that of full-term babies.

The main difficulty is that a baby's sleep patterns usually won't coincide with yours. Most adults like to sleep for about seven to nine hours every night, but a baby may wake up at 1 a.m. and then stay awake until just before dawn. Alternatively, the baby may sleep right through until 4 a.m. and then not sleep again for the remainder of the night. The only way to cope with this is to take extra naps in the day, and try to remain as calm as possible.

A baby needs to sleep in order to grow and mature. If your baby is tired but not sleepy, there are ways you can help him or her to drop off. Carrying a baby around in a sling may lull him or her to sleep – babies derive a sense of security from physical proximity and warmth. Rocking the baby and singing or playing music to him or her may also help. Some parents find that babies like 'white-noise' sounds such as that of a vacuum cleaner: you could try recording these sounds and playing it quietly if the baby won't settle.

Checklist of common problems

Some of the most common problems your baby may develop are dealt with below. Contact your health visitor or doctor if you have any worries about your baby's health. Note that the essential oil remedies mentioned should ideally only be used for babies over about two to three months old, as essential oils are very concentrated.

Crying Babies cry for many different reasons:
- Tiredness.
- Hunger.
- Need for physical reassurance.
- Boredom.
- Being too cold.
- Being too warm.
- Feeling uncomfortable (tight clothing etc).
- A full nappy (diaper).
- Being ill or in pain.

Make sure that the baby's obvious needs are catered for first. If the baby continues to cry after being fed and changed, try some of these: rocking the baby rhythmically, patting, stroking, caressing and smiling at him or her. You could also try soothing baby massage. If your baby cries a lot, try adding a herbal infusion to the baby's bath, such as chamomile, hops, lavender or lemon balm. Before you put him or her to bed, massage the feet and limbs with any of these herbal oils. You may wish to take him or her to a cranial osteopath (see page 225), particularly if the delivery was difficult. Sound sometimes solves the problem, so try playing music, singing to your baby, or playing a musical instrument yourself.

It is unwise to ignore a crying baby, however trying the constant crying may become. If you start to feel that you are at the end of your tether, put the baby in her cot or pram and telephone your health visitor, a relative or a friend to talk. Ask for help if you need it.

Colic Some babies experience bouts of painful intestinal cramp (colic), which usually occur from within a few days of birth up until about three months. The baby will howl, maybe for hours on end, drawing the knees up over the stomach. Colic typically occurs during the evening, with the baby being quite contented and well during the day. Be sure to feed the baby as slowly as possible. It may also help to give an aromatherapy massage using 1 drop Roman chamomile oil diluted in 150ml (5fl oz) almond oil towards the end of each afternoon. Fennel is the traditional herbal remedy for colic: before you feed the baby, try giving her a 25ml (1½ tbsp) infusion: add 1.5-2.5ml (¼-½ tsp) of the crushed herb to 100ml (7 tbsp) boiling water, leave for a few minutes, then strain. You can add the leftover infusion to the baby's bath. Homeopathic remedies include pulsatilla, nux vomica, aconite, dulcamara and bryonia, but seek the advice of a qualified homeopath.

Cradle cap A thick circle of dead skin may form on the scalp of a newborn baby. This will eventually clear up of its own accord. However, you can soften the scales so that they drop off more easily by using a massage oil such as almond, or blend 1 drop rose and 1 drop chamomile essential oil to 30ml (2 tbsp) almond oil. Massage very gently into the scalp for one to two days just before bedtime. The following morning shampoo with a natural baby shampoo and rinse with 7.5ml (1½ tsp) cider vinegar added to the water. Do not try to pick off the scales, as this can lead to infection.

Nappy rash One of the best ways to prevent nappy (diaper) rash is to allow the baby to be without a nappy as often as possible. You may also like to add one to two drops of chamomile or lavender oil, well-diluted in whole milk, to the baby's bath water. Jojoba oil is excellent for treating nappy rash: it leaves a fine waxy coating on the baby's skin, which moisturizes and soothes. Apply a little of the following blend when you change the nappy: 1 drop lavender and 1 drop rose or Roman chamomile to 30ml (2 tbsp) jojoba carrier oil. If the skin is very sore, use 10 per cent calendula (marigold) carrier oil in the blend. The homeopathic options include calendula or Rescue Remedy cream.

If your baby is colicky and cries for long periods, try to give yourself regular periods away from the house. Call on friends and relatives to help.

Calendula cream is very healing and may help to soothe the soreness of nappy rash. It is available from large pharmacists or health-food stores.

Colds and flu If your baby is sniffling or appears unwell, take his or her temperature. If it is raised, consult your family doctor without delay. If the temperature exceeds 38.5°C (101°F), seek emergency medical assistance. For mild symptoms, a warm, humid atmosphere loosens catarrh, while squirting a little breast milk into a baby's nostrils helps to dry the passages out.

Cough Again, a warm, humid atmosphere can help. If your baby's cough persists for more than a day or seems severe, seek immediate medical treatment.

Croup Croup often starts with the baby losing his or her voice and with the breathing sounding hoarse or croaky. This can lead to croup, which is characterized by spasms of coughing and difficulty in breathing. Croup sounds are not unlike the bark made by a sea lion. If your baby suffers from croup, try to relieve his or her breathing with steam. Boil a kettle and remove the lid so that the steam wafts over the baby. Light a vaporizer in the bedroom half an hour before baby's bedtime (any large pharmacy can supply one), with eucalyptus oil added for slightly older babies. Central heating should be kept as low as possible and the window should be open a little so that the air is less dry. If your baby's breathing continues to be laboured, speak to your family doctor (croup can sometimes be confused with whooping cough). If the breathing rapidly becomes worse, seek emergency medical treatment.

Diarrhoea and vomiting The main danger here is dehydration. Diarrhoea (in which the faeces are more liquid and frequent than normal) is not uncommon and may have various causes. As for vomiting, it is quite normal for babies to be sick after eating. If the vomiting or diarrhoea is mild and clears quickly, then help counteract

the conditions as follows: breastfed babies should be given short, very regular feeds, while bottle-fed babies will benefit from plenty of sips of plain, boiled and cooled water. If either condition persists, or is accompanied by other symptoms such as fever, then seek immediate medical treatment.

Constipation If your baby becomes constipated (straining but unable to pass stools), offer extra fluid. If bottle-feeding, ensure that you are making formulas up correctly. If the condition does not pass very quickly or other symptoms appear, then seek medical help.

Eye infection Bathe the eyes in cooled, boiled water, using a separate piece of clean cotton wool or tissue for each eye and wiping from the inner corner to the outer one (having washed your hands first). Breast milk can also be used, as it is anti-bacterial. Unless the condition is very mild and disappears rapidly, you should consult your health visitor or your family doctor.

DANGER SYMPTOMS
Seek emergency medical treatment if your baby or child exhibits any of these:
- Breathlessness or difficulty in breathing.
- Unexplained, abnormal drowsiness.
- Fever of 38.5°C (101°F) or more.
- Convulsions (fits).
- Any severe pain or obvious distress.
- Repeated or persistent vomiting, diarrhoea or constipation.
- Refusing food.
- Stiff neck, especially if combined with dislike of bright light.
- Severe headache.
- Impaired vision, especially with headache.

If a baby is hot, sponge the face with cool water.

Common Qs and As

Q: **My nipples don't stick out and I can't see how my baby will be able to feed. Is there anything that I can do?**

A: You will probably be fine. Health professionals used to recommend the use of nipple shields for inturned nipples. However, they rarely do nowadays because they know that the nipple is likely to become more defined once the milk comes in.

Usually the let-down reflex, which allows milk to be expressed from the breast, assists in the nipple becoming more prominent. Otherwise, you may find it helpful to splash very cold water over the breast, or even hold ice cubes against it for a minute or two, to help the nipple out.

Q: **My bust is tiny (30 AA). Will I be able to make enough milk for my baby?**

A: Don't worry – the size of the breast is not relevant, and you almost certainly will be able to feed your baby. Start off by feeding every two hours or so, as this helps to establish a good flow.

Many women believe that they are not making enough milk to meet their baby's needs, and this is often the reason for a specialist hospital referral. However, paediatricians often find that the baby is thriving, and weight checks show that weight gain is on course. The only problem is that the mother thinks she is not providing enough milk.

Rest assured that you will soon know about it if your baby feels hungry or undernourished. Talk to your midwife if you think that this is the case.

Q: **My breasts become engorged at the wrong time. When they are full, my baby doesn't seem that interested in feeding. Then, when she is hungry, there doesn't seem to be enough to satisfy her. What is going on?**

A: This does happen in the early days while you and the baby are getting used to one another. It may take as long as several weeks for a harmonious pattern to develop. So, do not despair.

Ask your family doctor, community midwife or health visitor for an appointment to see a breastfeeding counsellor if the situation continues. Difficulties in breastfeeding are often a problem of technique – the mother's or the baby's.

Q: **I had a very difficult birth and wasn't able to breastfeed or hold my baby for the first few weeks. You hear so much about the importance of bonding in the first days, and I feel I have failed her. How can I make it up to her?**

A: There is no need to feel that you have failed your baby in any way. There have obviously been very good reasons why you and your baby were unable to be together for the first few weeks of her life. This often happens with premature babies and with ill babies, when the baby is whisked away to an intensive baby care unit, usually at a central teaching hospital, while the mother is left in the local hospital where she delivered.

As for making it up to her, smiles, cuddles, laughing and feeding – and even changing her nappies with love and care – will all help to bring about the bonding process. Your baby will not remember the first few weeks, but she will respond to all your love now. Just be positive and enjoy her.

Q: **How does everyone else cope with fatigue? I feel as if I am sleepwalking.**

A: The best advice is to take each day as it comes. When you are really tired, you just have to go with the flow. Take every opportunity you can to sleep, and if you can't sleep, rest.

Make as few plans as possible, and don't worry if you do not achieve something that you set out to do. If you have the option, don't go back to work until you feel on top of things.

Q: **My newborn baby is often sick when he is in the car. How can I prevent this?**

A: First of all, consider whether you are rushing to get out of the house. If so, slow down. Be sure that you leave home in a calm and unflurried state with plenty of time to allow you to reach your destination. This helps to reduce anxiety in you, which would readily transmit itself to your baby.

Feed your baby at least an hour before you want to take him or her out in the car. It is also worth considering whether your baby has had enough sleep when they first get in the car – take him or her out for a trial run when you know they are rested.

How smoothly you drive and at what speed will have a bearing on how well your baby travels. Keep your speed down, avoid jerky manoeuvres and don't attempt to overtake.

If the problem continues, there are herbal and homeopathic options with which to treat carsickness. However, it is much better to try to treat the cause rather than the symptoms, particularly since your baby is so young.

Q: **We have both a dog and a cat. Should we be worried about having them around a newborn baby?**

A: Be very careful and take no risks. Dogs do suffer from jealousy, and have been known to attack with absolutely no warning. Cats may also react unpredictably. Do not leave your baby alone with the dog or cat, and keep the door to your baby's room shut while she is sleeping. Basically, if a pet shows signs of undue aggression towards others, then it may be a problem. If you are at all worried about either pet's behaviour, then regrettably the safest course of action would be to re-home him or her.

Q: **Quite a few of my friends and some of the other women in my antenatal group have taken their new babies to see a cranial osteopath. What is this?**

A: Some people take their newborn baby to a cranial osteopath to check and treat any birth trauma, especially to the head and neck. Treatment consists of the practitioner placing his or her hands on the baby's body and identifying any areas of restriction or tension. Gentle stroking is used to release these. It can be a very effective therapy for babies, particularly in treating sleeping problems.

Cranial osteopathy is a branch of osteopathy, and so practitioners have been through rigorous training. Be sure that anyone you take your baby to see is suitably qualified and experienced in dealing with young babies.

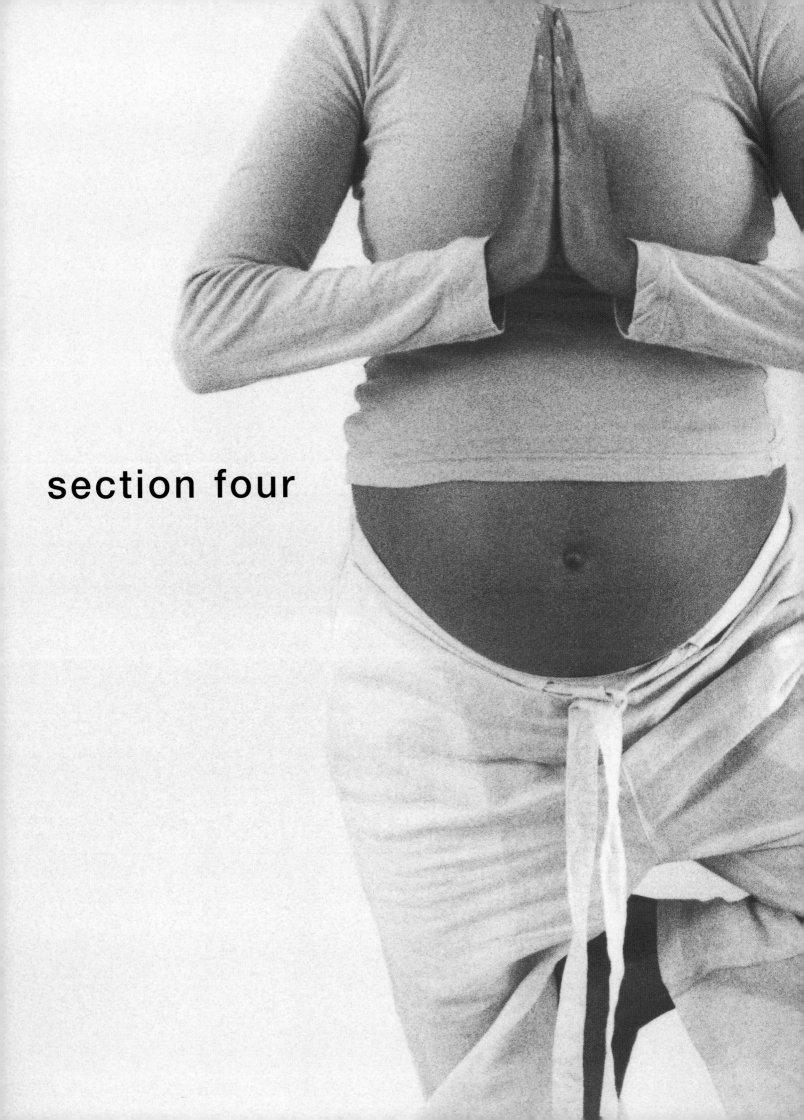

section four

natural healing therapies

Natural remedies may aid conception, alleviate ailments in pregnancy and speed recovery after the birth. However, they should be used with caution: many therapies need to be adapted for pregnant women, and others are not suitable in the first weeks. It is important to seek out a qualified practitioner who is used to working with pregnant women. Always tell the therapist if you are trying to conceive or are pregnant. Tell your doctor about any therapy you are receiving, and about any recommendations made to you.

Herbalism

Many plants have therapeutic properties, which can be used to improve health and treat illness. Researchers are currently substantiating many of the claims made for herbal remedies. For the mother-to-be, herbs can offer support in all kinds of ways, from alleviating morning sickness to easing varicose veins.

Many modern medicines are derived from plants. Science has made it possible to isolate the active ingredients or recreate entirely synthetic versions. So, pharmaceutical drugs are now far removed from their natural origins. By contrast, herbal remedies use parts of the whole plant – roots, seeds, petals or leaves. Herbalists say that the subtle interaction of all the herb's ingredients promotes healing in a holistic (whole body) way rather than merely attacking a single symptom or disease as many laboratory-produced drugs do.

HERBAL MEDICINE AND PREGNANCY

Women have long used herbal remedies to alleviate the discomforts of pregnancy, prepare the body for childbirth, and aid recovery afterwards. Herbalists say that remedies can also be used to enhance fertility.

Herbal medicines are usually gentler than chemical ones, but this is not always the case. It is important to bear in mind that herbal remedies can have powerful effects. This is very important during pregnancy, when many herbs should not be used. It is not a good idea to self-prescribe herbal remedies, particularly if you are trying to conceive or are pregnant. See a qualified medical herbalist for advice.

SEEING A HERBALIST

When you see a herbalist, a medical history will be taken and you will be given a physical examination. You should tell your practitioner about any drugs you are taking since they may interact badly with natural remedies; for the same reason, tell your doctor about any remedies you are given. A medical herbalist will advise you on your diet and lifestyle

as well as prescribing remedies for your individual needs. You will usually have at least one follow-up appointment; often several sessions will be necessary.

SELF-HELP HERBAL REMEDIES

A few herbs are gentle enough to be used in infusion form during pregnancy. In the first trimester, ginger tea may alleviate morning sickness and aid the digestion. Later on, dandelion, meadowsweet, lime flower and nettle can be helpful. Drink no more than three cups of herbal tea a day.

Herbal ointments, compresses and poultices can ease symptoms relating to pregnancy, birth and breastfeeding. For example, calendula cream is often recommended for cracked nipples, and witch hazel can help promote healing of the perineum. Some plants are used whole: cabbage leaves are often used to soothe sore breasts.

Fennel is a good remedy for indigestion, but like many herbs it can be harmful if taken in large quantities during pregnancy.

HERBS NOT TO USE IN PREGNANCY

• angelica	• golden seal	• poke root
• barberry	• greater	• rhubarb
• black	celandine	• rosemary
cohosh	• juniper	• rue
• bloodroot	• liferoot	• saffron
• buckthorn	• male fern	• sage
• celery	• mandrake	• southernwood
• cinchona	• mistletoe	• tansy
• cinnamon	• mugwort	• thuja
• cottonroot	• nutmeg	• thyme
• feverfew	• pennyroyal	• wormwood

Homeopathy
This gentle therapy can help with many of the physical symptoms and difficult emotions experienced while trying to conceive and during pregnancy. The remedies are derived from natural substances, and aim to stimulate the body's capacity for healing and restore well-being.

Homeopathy is based on the idea that 'like cures like': so a substance that causes illness can also be used to cure it. The remedies have been so diluted that only the merest trace of the active ingredient remains. In this state, they are far too weak to cause harm, but homeopaths believe that the minute dose can promote self-healing and cure the very symptoms that it may cause if taken in large amounts. Some doctors are sceptical about homeopathic remedies, but others accept that they can have good results. Some have trained in this therapy and offer it to patients as an adjunct to orthodox medical care.

Homeopathic remedies are considered very safe in pregnancy. They can help to relieve many ailments, such as morning sickness, and to speed recovery after the birth. Self-help remedies are available from many pharmacies, but it can be difficult to choose exactly the right one for you. For this reason, it is much better to consult a homeopath.

SEEING A HOMEOPATH
A homeopath will take a full personal and medical history during the first session, which can last two hours. People are often surprised by the number and type of questions they are asked. However, the homeopath needs to build up a picture of your habits and preferences as well as your mental, physical and emotional make-up. This information enables him or her to assess your 'constitutional type'.

Homeopaths consider both the patient's constitution and symptoms when choosing from the 2000 remedies at their disposal. You will be given instructions on how to take the remedies, and may also be given advice about your diet and lifestyle. A follow-up appointment is usually arranged; often several sessions are necessary.

EFFECTIVE HOMEOPATHY
- See a homeopath who is experienced in treating pregnant women; tell him or her if you are pregnant or are trying to conceive.
- Follow the homeopath's instructions when taking the remedy: peppermint, coffee and tea can nullify the effect, and you should avoid drinking or eating for 15 minutes after taking a remedy.
- Contact your homeopath if your symptoms worsen (this may be part of the healing process).
- Tell your doctor about any remedies you take, and report any unusual symptoms.

Flower remedies are a useful 'instant cure', and can be used to help resolve uncomfortable emotions, such as self-doubt, anxiety or low spirits.

BACH FLOWER REMEDIES
The Bach Flower Remedies are homeopathic remedies preserved in grape alcohol. Plant based, they are designed to help with negative feelings or states of mind. The most popular is Rescue Remedy, which is used for panic, tearfulness or shock. The remedies are available from health-food shops and pharmacies, and are usually self-prescribed.

To take a flower remedy, place a few drops in a glass of water and sip. Repeat several times a day if you are struggling with a recurring emotion. Flower remedies are preserved in alcohol, but you take only a tiny amount so they are safe for use in pregnancy. See your doctor if you are at all unsure about whether or not you should use them.

Aromatherapy

Aromatherapists use aromatic oils extracted from herbs and flowers to promote well-being. Certain oils have a wonderfully relaxing effect, which is very helpful throughout pregnancy. Others can help to relieve conditions such as the indigestion that is common in pregnancy, or lift spirits during labour.

Aromatherapy oils have wonderful aromas, and they are very pleasurable to use. They can be a gentle and effective way of boosting general health and treating minor ailments.

We do not know exactly how essential oils work, but it is thought that the scents trigger a reaction in smell receptors in the nostrils, which send messages to the brain. When the oils are used in massage, they also penetrate the skin and have a direct effect on the nerve endings here.

Some of the oils have proven medicinal qualities: tea tree, for example, is an antiseptic, antifungal and antibacterial agent, while chamomile has antispasmodic and antidepressant properties. Lavender is one of the most versatile oils: it helps with stress, insomnia, migraine and headaches, and it can also promote healing after a burn.

BENEFITS OF AROMATHERAPY

Aromatherapy is believed to be most helpful in treating long-term conditions, or recurring illnesses. Practitioners say that it can help to alleviate stress and related problems, including depression, headaches and insomnia. It may also relieve the pain of long-term conditions such as arthritis and may help skin problems such as eczema.

Most people find that aromatherapy's main benefit is relaxation. It can also help to induce general feelings of well-being, reduce fatigue and relieve backache.

In pregnancy, essential oils can be used to help the circulation, and so reduce the likelihood of varicose veins and haemorrhoids. Aromatherapy massage helps to

One of the gentlest ways to use essential oils is to heat them in a vaporizer. Their scent will fill a room and have an uplifting or relaxing effect upon everyone in it.

OILS TO AVOID IN PREGNANCY	
• basil	• myrrh
• cedarwood	• nutmeg
• cinnamon bark	• oregano
• clary sage	• parsley
• cypress	• peppermint
• fennel	• rosemary
• hyssop	• sage
• juniper	• savory
• marjoram	• thyme

maintain the elasticity of the skin, thus helping to prevent stretchmarks. Minor ailments such as constipation and heartburn may also be helped by essential oils.

However, many essential oils are not suitable for use during pregnancy, because they may stimulate the uterus, causing miscarriage. Never use an oil unless you have checked that it is safe in pregnancy; the oils listed in the box above should definitely be avoided. It may be safest to avoid using essential oils entirely in the first trimester; see page 124 for good oils to use in the second trimester.

SEEING AN AROMATHERAPIST

Aromatherapists are usually trained masseurs. During the first session, a practitioner will ask you about your medical history and any problems you are experiencing. You should say if you are trying to conceive, or are already pregnant. If this is the case, it is probably best to see an aromatherapist who regularly works with conceiving or pregnant women.

The therapist will select which oils to use, and ask you to smell them to check that you like the aromas. Up to five oils may be used, and they will be blended in a carrier, such as almond oil. You will be asked to undress and lie on a massage couch. The therapist will then massage your whole body, smoothing the oils into your skin. The massage usually lasts an hour, and you should be given a few minutes to rest at the end. Your therapist may give you advice on using oils at home.

SELF-HELP AROMATHERAPY

Essential oils are widely available, and they can easily be used at home to enhance general well-being. To treat particular disorders (in conjunction with conventional medical treatment), you may need to consult a professional aromatherapist. The following methods can be used for self-help at home.

BATHS

Aromatherapy baths are wonderfully relaxing, and can help to ease tension, and relieve backache and aching muscles. A warm bath with a soothing oil such as Roman chamomile before bedtime can promote restful sleep. Medicinal oils such as sandalwood and lavender can be used to ease cystitis and thrush (if pregnant, use only after 16 weeks).

Mix four to six drops of essential oil with a carrier oil or whole milk, then add to a full bath (not to running water). Lie back in the bath and breathe deeply, for 10-15 minutes.

FOOT AND HAND BATHS

An aromatic footbath can be a relaxing end to the day. You can also use a hand or foot bath to treat localized aches and pains, foot problems and swelling.

Mix eight to ten drops of essential oil in a carrier, then add to a large bowl of hand-hot water. Soak the feet or hands for 10-15 minutes; have a boiled kettle to hand so that you can top up with more hot water. Dry thoroughly. Smooth diluted essential oils over the skin, then wrap in a towel for 15 minutes, for a superb moisturizing treatment.

MASSAGE

Self-massage is a great way of applying essential oils, and can help with stress, skin complaints and fluid retention. It is often recommended in later pregnancy as a way of preventing stretchmarks. An essential oil should always be well-diluted in a vegetable oil, such as jojoba, sesame or almond: use a dilution of one drop per 5ml (1 tsp) base oil (or per 10ml (2 tsp) if you are pregnant).

COMPRESSES

Aromatherapy compresses can be used as to treat bruises, varicose veins, haemorrhoids, sprains, burns and scalds: lavender is often a good oil to use here. Use a warm

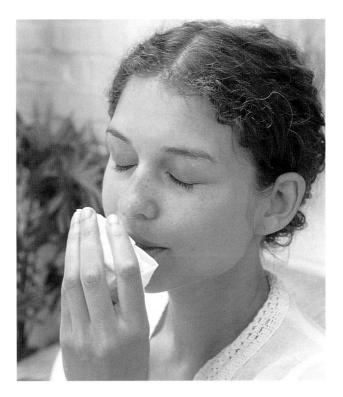

For instant relief, put a couple of drops of essential oil on a tissue and inhale. Tea tree is good for easing cold symptoms; sandalwood may alleviate anxiety.

compress for aching and pain, and a cold one if there is any heat or swelling. Dilute about eight drops of essential oil in a carrier, then add to a bowl of warm or ice-cold water. Drop in a small towel or flannel and soak for a few moments. Wring it out and hold over the affected area.

INHALATION

Another good way of treating stress, insomnia and colds is by inhalation. The simplest method is to put two drops of essential oil on to a tissue, and inhale. Slip a tissue with Roman chamomile on it under your pillowcase at night if you are finding it hard to sleep. For a steam inhalation, put five drops of essential oil into a bowl of hot water. Cover your head and bowl with a towel, and breathe (eyes closed).

A footbath is a lovely treat at the end of the day: add your favourite essential oils to warm water, then relax. Try ginger and mandarin for a warming, reviving combination.

SAFE AROMATHERAPY

- Never apply an essential oil directly to your skin – always dilute it in a carrier first: use one drop per 5ml (1 tsp) carrier; one drop per 10 ml (2 tsp) if you are pregnant.
- Only use oils that you know to be safe – if you are not sure, check with a professional aromatherapist.
- Do a patch test before use: apply diluted oil to a small area on the inside of your wrist, then wait 24 hours. If you have no reaction, the oil is safe. Women may be more sensitive when pregnant, so it is a good idea to repeat a patch test at this time.

Massage
Touch has been used to enhance health for thousands of years and is a powerful way of giving comfort and relieving pain: we instinctively hug a friend in distress or rub an aching limb. Massage is a leading touch therapy that can be especially helpful as a pain-relief tool in the delivery room.

The term 'massage' covers many different therapies. On the one hand, there is purely physical Western massage, which works on the muscles. On the other, there are forms of Eastern pressure massage, which seek to enhance energy flow along invisible pathways in the body. These include shiatsu and acupressure. Massage techniques also form an important element of therapies such as osteopathy, aromatherapy and reflexology.

SWEDISH MASSAGE
In the West, most therapists practise Swedish massage. This system was devised by a Swedish gymnast, Per Henrik Ling, in the late 18th century. The techniques include:
- **Stroking** (effleurage) to relax. Firmer strokes are used to stimulate the circulation and release muscular tension.
- **Kneading** (petrissage) which soothes tense muscles and increases blood flow to particular areas. It can be used to relax deep muscles, such as those of the shoulders.
- **Friction** in which small, circular movements are made with the pads of the thumbs. It is used to break down areas of muscular spasm.
- **Percussion** in which fast, rhythmic movements are performed with the sides of the hands on fleshy parts of the body. It should be avoided during pregnancy.

RECEIVING A MASSAGE
To receive a Swedish massage, you'll be asked to undress and lie on a special couch. However, you can keep your underwear on if you wish. Towels will be placed over any areas of your body not being massaged. The therapist will usually massage your whole body, but may spend longer on some areas and leave out others. He or she will use oil or cream to prevent any dragging of the skin. The session typically lasts an hour, and you will usually be left to relax for a few minutes at the end.

Benefits of Swedish massage
There has been a great deal of research into massage, and most doctors accept that it promotes general good health. In pregnancy, it is good for backache and joint pain, and its relaxing effects mean it can help with anxiety, depression, blood pressure and digestive problems, as well as stress-related complaints such as headaches or insomnia. Stroking the lower back during labour can help to soothe pain and aid relaxation.

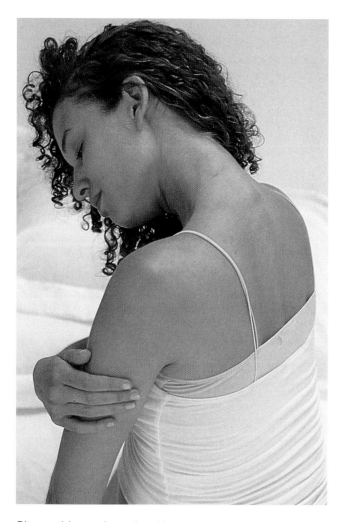

Pleasurable touch on the skin encourages the body to release endorphins, natural pain-killing chemicals. These help to induce feelings of happiness and well-being, and are one reason why massage can be helpful during labour.

Effective massage in pregnancy
Check with your doctor or midwife before having massage in pregnancy. Seek out a therapist who is experienced in treating pregnant women.
- Always tell the therapist that you are pregnant.
- You should not have deep pressure on the abdomen or lower back.
- Varicose veins, bruises or lumps must not be massaged.
- Do not have a massage if you have an infection or fever or if you feel unwell.
- Drink plenty of water and avoid strenuous activity afterwards. If possible, rest.

Shiatsu

The term shiatsu is Japanese for 'finger pressure'. Practitioners work to stimulate pressure points associated with the vital organs, in order to encourage a good flow of chi (energy) around the body and promote better health. Uses in pregnancy include dealing with backache and raised blood pressure, and pain-relief during labour.

Many Japanese people undergo regular shiatsu treatment, sometimes as often as once a week. They believe that it can help to prevent illness as well as detect and treat any symptoms early on. Shiatsu is a holistic system of healing, meaning that the whole person – mind, body and spirit – is treated at once. However, it can also be used to treat problems such as back pain, digestive problems, insomnia, depression, migraine and toothache, and to help strengthen the immune system.

Shiatsu should generally be kept simple and non-specific during the first three months of pregnancy, when all the baby's organ systems are developing. To be safe, you should see a practitioner who specializes in working with pregnant women. A shiatsu practitioner can attend the birth to help with pain relief, or can teach the father or another birth assistant some simple pain-relief techniques with which to support the mother during her labour.

SEEING A PRACTITIONER

At the first consultation, a shiatsu practitioner should take a detailed medical and lifestyle history from you. He or she will take your pulses: there are six at each wrist, each associated with a vital organ. He or she may also feel your abdomen, which can give clues to problems elsewhere. The sound of your voice, your appearance and posture will also be observed.

To receive treatment, you keep your clothes on and lie on a mat on the floor. The practitioner will apply pressure to points all over the body using a variety of techniques. Sometimes the bulb of the thumb is used, sometimes the fingertips, and sometimes the palm or the heel of the hand. An elbow may also be used or perhaps a forearm or a knee. The practitioner may also perform gentle stretching or rocking movements.

How hard the therapist applies pressure depends on many things, including the part of the body being treated, how you react and whether you require a tonic or a sedating effect. Pressure is applied for a few seconds at a time and is repeated several times at each spot.

You can learn how to apply finger pressure at home after learning the techniques from a trained shiatsu practitioner.

Shiatsu practitioners often use finger pressure (above) to activate an energy point, but they also use the whole hand, the forearm (below), the elbows or the feet.

Acupuncture

Practised for centuries in China as a means of promoting good health and treating illness, acupuncture is now widely available in the West, and most doctors accept that it has positive effects. Acupuncture can help with fertility problems and with many pregnancy-related disorders.

Acupuncture is based on the idea that chi (energy) flows along invisible pathways – known as meridians – in the body. When this energy flows freely, good health and well-being are maintained. Illness and emotional upset are said to be a result of blockages or imbalances in the circulation of this energy.

In acupuncture, fine needles are inserted into certain points on the meridians to correct imbalances and improve the flow of chi. Acupuncture is usually practised holistically, so its ultimate aim is to bring the body back to its natural state of equilibrium. However, it can be used to treat specific complaints, such as back pain and digestion problems.

PREGNANCY AND ACUPUNCTURE

Acupuncture can relieve many pregnancy-related ailments, including morning sickness, constipation and poor circulation. It may also help with fertility problems or recurrent miscarriage. It is very important that you tell your practitioner that you are pregnant or trying to conceive, since some points should not be stimulated in that case. For this reason, it is best to choose a qualified practitioner who is experienced in working with pregnant women.

SEEING AN ACUPUNCTURIST

On your first visit, a full medical and personal history will be taken: your practitioner will ask you many questions about, for example, your appetite, bowel movements, sleep and energy levels. Your pulses will be taken and your tongue will be checked. Your practitioner will also observe other details, such as the sound of your voice and the colour of your skin.

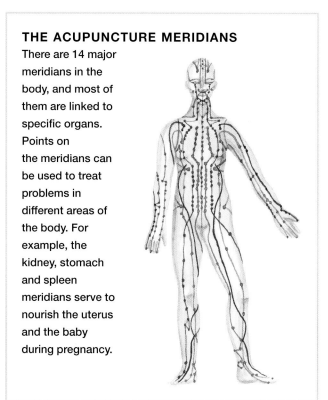

THE ACUPUNCTURE MERIDIANS

There are 14 major meridians in the body, and most of them are linked to specific organs. Points on the meridians can be used to treat problems in different areas of the body. For example, the kidney, stomach and spleen meridians serve to nourish the uterus and the baby during pregnancy.

You lie on a massage couch to receive treatment. The acupuncturist will insert needles into different points on your body – this is swift and painless. Sometimes, the needles will be left in place for several minutes.

Most people have weekly or fortnightly sessions to start with, but you may need only occasional sessions once treatment has been established.

OTHER ACUPUNCTURE TECHNIQUES

Finger pressure can be used instead of needles to stimulate acupoints. Acupressure is less invasive than needling, and it can be used for self-help. Some acupuncturists will advise you and your partner on which points to stimulate during labour.

Another technique is moxibustion, where the herb moxa (mugwort) is burned on energy points. This can exert a profoundly soothing effect.

You may feel a slight tingling when an acupuncture needle is inserted, but it should not hurt.

Reflexology

Reflexologists believe that every body part is linked by an energy pathway to a specific point on the foot, and that finger pressure on the feet can detect and treat health problems. A range of pregnancy-related problems can be tackled, from backache to relieving pubic joint discomfort prior to the birth.

Reflexology is good for promoting general well-being and relaxation. It can also help alleviate complaints such as back pain, digestive problems and constipation. Some midwives use the techniques to promote regular contractions and for pain relief during labour. One study found that reflexology could reduce a woman's need for pain relief, and cut the length of labour by as much as half.

Many women enjoy reflexology during pregnancy, but it should be used only after the first 12 weeks. Some areas – the heels, Achilles tendons and ankles – should not be worked on at all because this can induce contractions. For this reason, it is important to see a practitioner who understands the needs of pregnant women.

SEEING A REFLEXOLOGIST

On your first visit, your practitioner will ask about your medical history, symptoms, diet, lifestyle and any other therapies you are receiving. You will be asked to take off your footwear and sit on a chair or couch. The reflexologist will massage your feet to relax them – which can be deeply pleasurable. After the initial massage, every area of your foot will be pressed and massaged in turn.

Some areas may feel very sensitive – this is said to be a sign of imbalance. Tender points will receive extra massage

WHAT THE DOCTORS SAY

Many doctors accept that reflexology can have a deeply relaxing effect. This may be the result of pressure on the nerve endings, of which there are more than 7000 in the feet. In addition, massage helps to stimulate the circulation of blood, which improves the delivery of oxygen and nutrients to different areas of the body.

If you are having reflexology treatment, you should let your doctor know. It is also important that you continue to report any unusual symptoms.

in order to stimulate energy flow to the corresponding area of the body. This can sometimes be painful, but tenderness should ease as the massage continues. The reflexologist will adjust the pressure, depending on your sensitivity.

Your reflexologist may show you some techniques that you can practise at home. The hands also contain a 'map' of the body, and these are often recommended for self-help because they are easier to treat than the feet.

Like most complementary therapists, reflexologists seek to help the body to heal itself. Regular sessions are often recommended in order to maintain well-being.

FOOT REFLEXES

Reflexologists work systematically round the foot, and they always treat both feet. Tender or sensitive points may receive extra massage to encourage healing in the related part of the body.

RIGHT FOOT

lymph nodes and lymph drainage
ear
shoulder
lung
liver
gall bladder
ascending colon
appendix

LEFT FOOT

top of head
back of head
pituitary gland
thyroid gland
eyes
trachea
spine
stomach
pancreas
kidneys
small intestine
rectum/anus
bladder
sciatic nerve

lymph nodes and lymph drainage
ear
shoulder
lung
heart
spleen
transverse colon
descending colon
sigmoid colon

Osteopathy

Osteopaths believe that good health depends on the proper functioning of our muscles and joints. They use manipulation and massage to correct imbalances caused by injury, poor posture and stress. Their approach can be especially helpful in easing the digestive problems often experienced in pregnancy.

Most people see an osteopath because of backache, but the therapy can also help with other physical problems, such as headaches, digestive disorders and breathing difficulties. Osteopathy is safe in pregnancy, but you should be sure to choose a qualified practitioner with experience in treating pregnant women: osteopathic techniques can be dangerous if performed by an untrained practitioner.

You should always tell your osteopath that you are pregnant, or if you are trying to conceive, and let your doctor know that you are having treatment. Some doctors will be able to recommend an osteopath to you.

WHAT TO EXPECT

An osteopath will take a full medical and lifestyle history on your first visit, and he or she will also give you a physical examination. People are usually asked to undress to their underwear so that the osteopath can observe the body's framework.

The practitioner will use gentle touch – palpation – to detect any areas of weakness or strain in your body. You may be asked to perform simple exercises while standing, sitting and lying on a couch so that your osteopath can check your posture, muscle tone and breathing technique. Sometimes other medical tests – such as blood tests – will be carried out to help with diagnosis.

CRANIAL OSTEOPATHY

Some osteopaths practise cranial osteopathy. This gentle technique focuses on the delicate manipulation of the bones of the skull in order to improve the circulation of blood and fluid in the head. It is said to help many of the same conditions as conventional osteopathy, and it is often used to help babies who are suffering from sleeplessness, colic or birth trauma.

In cranial-sacral therapy, subtle pressure is applied to the head and the base of the spine. Therapists are aiming to regulate the flow of cerebrospinal fluid, which affects the whole nervous system and thus the functioning of the body. Many people find this therapy deeply relaxing, and it can help with insomnia, backache and headaches.

Doctors tend to be more sceptical of these gentle techniques than of conventional osteopathy, but many patients report good results. Some cranial-sacral therapists may not have undergone the rigorous training of an osteopath. Seek treatment only from qualified osteopaths or chiropractors with experience in dealing with pregnant women and babies.

You lie on a massage couch for treatment. The osteopath will then carry out a series of manipulations, which are tailored to your individual needs. The techniques used include massage, limb stretches and sharp thrusts. You may hear a clicking sound as a joint slips back into alignment, but you should not feel any pain.

The first session can last an hour but subsequent treatments are usually 20-30 minutes long. Most people need several sessions, and you may also be given instructions on exercises to do at home.

Pregnant women are often advised to have regular sessions to help them adjust to changes in their posture as the baby grows. This is a good way of preventing and treating lower back pain. Some osteopaths say that regular treatment during pregnancy can help to make the birth easier.

Many people are nervous of the clicking sound that occurs when an osteopath pops a joint back into place. However, this should not be painful. Treatment also includes gentle massage and stretches, which are very relaxing.

Chiropractic
Chiropractors use their hands to work on the spine, believing that a well-aligned spine is vital in maintaining good health because it supports the rest of the body and houses the central nervous system. Its main use for pregnant women is to ease back problems caused by carrying a growing baby.

Chiropractic is mainly used to help with back and neck problems. Gentle manipulation of the spine is performed to improve posture, and to correct any kinks caused by injury or stress. Regular sessions of chiropractic can help pregnant women to adjust their posture so that they cope better with the strain of carrying a growing baby. It may also alleviate pelvic problems and make childbirth easier.

Chiropractics say that working on the spine can also help seemingly unrelated problems. This is because nerve pathways branch off the spine at different levels and travel to all areas of the body. Distortions in the spine can affect nerve function, and may therefore be the cause of problems elsewhere. Fatigue, indigestion, constipation and headaches may all be helped by chiropractic treatment.

SEEING A CHIROPRACTOR
Your first session will focus mainly on the diagnosis of your problem. A full medical history will be taken and you will also be asked questions about your work, lifestyle and diet, and any exercise that you do.

You will be asked to undress to your underwear so that the chiropractor can observe your closely. If you feel embarrassed, you may be able to wear a gown. The chiropractor will observe your posture as you sit, stand and

THE ORTHODOX VIEW
Chiropractic is widely accepted as a useful technique for many back problems. However, many doctors are sceptical about claims that it can help with problems such as digestive disorders.

OTHER FORMS OF CHIROPRACTIC THERAPY
Practitioners of McTimoney or McTimoney-Corley chiropractic use many of the same techniques as conventional chiropractors, but they tend to work in a more gentle way.

McTimoney chiropractors agree that the distortions in the spine are the principle cause of ill health but they think that all other joints should be treated as well. They examine and work on the whole musculoskeletal system in each treatment session. McTimoney-Corley chiropractic is different again: practitioners manipulate the vertebrae using their fingertips, and they do not practise the more vigorous techniques of chiropractic. They emphasize the importance of self-help exercises.

lie down, and you will be asked to perform some simple exercises. The chiropractor may check the mobility of your joints by asking you to perform a few stretches. He or she will then examine your spine to detect any misalignments or areas of stiffness, as well as the source of any pain you may have. Other checks, such as blood pressure or reflex tests, may also be performed.

You will be asked to lie on a massage couch for treatment. The chiropractor will use a variety of techniques to realign the vertebrae: these include gentle stretches, precise thrusts and massage. You may ache or feel rather stiff afterwards, but the treatment should not hurt.

Most people need several sessions of chiropractic, but you may start to see some improvement in your condition after just one treatment.

Chiropractors are able to treat much more than just back problems. For example, regular headaches and bouts of indigestion may also be relieved by releasing built-up tension in the spine.

The Alexander technique

In this therapy, gentle posture-improving exercises show clients how to stand, sit and move. This eases pressure on muscles and joints and is held to relieve all kinds of mental and physical problems, the main one in pregnancy being back strain from carrying a heavy 'bump'.

As children, we have naturally good posture. However, as we grow up we tend to develop bad habits: we may slouch or cross our legs when we sit, stand with our weight pushed on to one leg, and twist the back when lifting. Our mental state, too, can affect our posture: when stressed we may lift the shoulders and hold them in a state of tension, for example, and the problem may be compounded by poor sitting technique and by working at a computer.

Eventually, these habits, known as 'patterns of misuse', become ingrained. Poor posture becomes the norm, and we no longer notice when we are placing the body under strain. Over time, poor posture causes damage to our muscles and joints, and our digestive, respiratory and circulatory systems may also be affected.

HOW THE ALEXANDER TECHNIQUE WORKS

The Alexander technique is a way of training people to become aware of bad habits, so that they can start to stand and move in a naturally better way. It emphasizes aligning the head with the spine, so that the neck remains free of strain. The technique is best taught on a one-to-one basis. During the first session, you will be asked to adopt various positions and perform simple movements, while the teacher observes how you stand, sit and move.

You will be asked to lie down, and the teacher will make subtle adjustments to your limbs, head, pelvis and so on, so that you can experience good posture for yourself.

During the classes, the teacher will show you how to perform a whole range of everyday tasks in the Alexander way – such as answering the telephone, getting in and out

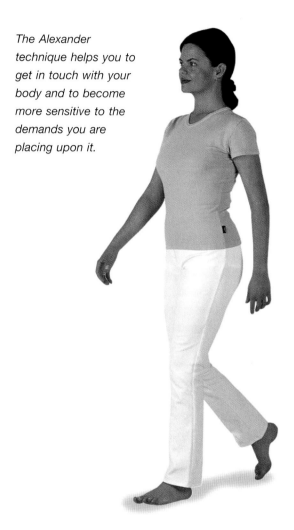

The Alexander technique helps you to get in touch with your body and to become more sensitive to the demands you are placing upon it.

of a chair, writing a letter, answering the phone, carrying a bag, and walking. The lessons will combine gentle manipulations with verbal instructions. The aim is to build your awareness of how to move correctly – called 'thought in action'. Eventually, you will be able to bring this awareness into daily life, and maintain good posture.

Sessions are usually given once or twice a week for several months; thereafter top-up sessions may be needed.

HOW IT HELPS

The Alexander technique is accepted as an effective way of treating many back and neck problems. Practitioners say that posture work can also help people to become more resistant to stress. Other conditions that may be helped by the technique include depression, anxiety, headaches, high blood pressure, infertility, breathing problems, fatigue, arthritis, back pain and digestive disorders.

PREGNANCY AND THE ALEXANDER TECHNIQUE

The Alexander technique can help pregnant women adapt to their changing shape as the baby grows. This may prevent the backache that is commonly associated with pregnancy.

It will also help you to prepare for the birth. The Alexander technique teaches women to stay upright during labour – in a squatting position – so that the force of gravity can assist the baby's passage. An Alexander teacher will help you to learn how to cope with contractions without tensing the body. This can make childbirth easier, since tension increases pain.

Pilates

This is an effective form of body conditioning, which also develops mental awareness and an effective breathing technique. Some Pilates exercises are similar to yoga postures, but they are repeated to create a flowing sequence. Like yoga, Pilates can help alleviate back pain and other problems common in pregnancy.

Pilates aims to bring the body back to its natural alignment. The exercises encourage you to work to your maximum capability, without placing undue strain on the body. As a result, regular practice helps to improve your posture and flexibility, as well as toning the muscles. Pilates is particularly good for developing 'core' strength in the lower back and abdomen. It aims to work the mind as well as the body, and many practitioners find it deeply relaxing.

Pilates was originally developed in the First World War as a means of helping injured soldiers regain their mobility. It is still often recommended as a form of rehabilitation. Teachers say that almost anyone can practise Pilates because the exercises involved can be adapted to suit the individual's needs.

Pilates is safe for pregnant women because it uses carefully controlled movements and encourages you to work within your body's limitations. Advocates say that it can help to reduce backache, ease delivery and hasten recovery after the birth. However, it is important that the exercises are done correctly. Seek out a specialist qualified teacher who regularly works with pregnant women.

LEARNING PILATES

There are many books on Pilates, but it is best to learn the exercise from a qualified and experienced instructor. Pilates can be learned on a one-to-one basis or in a small class.

Some exercises are practised on a mat and others are done on specialized apparatus. The teacher demonstrates the exercises, and then guides the students through each series of movements. You should receive individual attention, even in a group class, and be shown how to adapt exercises where necessary. Blocks and supports may be used to help you to do this.

Classes usually last an hour. However, once you have learned the techniques, mat exercises can be done at home. Pilates teachers say that it is important to practise three or four times a week in order to obtain the most benefit from this therapy.

SAFE PILATES

- If you are pregnant and new to Pilates, do not start classes until after the first trimester. Try to find special pregnancy classes. Otherwise, go for individual instruction with an experienced teacher.
- Do not push your body further than is comfortable: you will build up flexibility and strength with practice.
- If you feel uncomfortable at any point, stop and rest.
- Do not do any exercises that require you to lie flat on your back after 30 weeks.
- Build up slowly – it will take time for you to increase your flexibility and strength.

Many Pilates exercises are seemingly easy stretches like this one. When done correctly, they quickly build strength and muscle tone.

CHOOSING A TEACHER

Anyone can call themselves a Pilates teacher – even if they have had just a few days' training. It is important that you check that your teacher has completed a reputable training course and that he or she has been practising Pilates for several years. All Pilates teachers should have insurance.

Yoga

Doctors and midwives now commonly recommend yoga to pregnant women. This ancient form of exercise is known to foster general good health and improve posture and flexibility. It can also help to prevent or relieve common ailments such as backache, constipation and headaches.

Yoga is proven to help people relax, which makes it highly beneficial for women who are trying to conceive or who are already pregnant. Relaxation helps to improve the flow of blood, and so increases the supply of oxygen and nutrients to the baby. Yoga relaxation and breathing techniques can be very helpful during labour. A regular practice can help to strengthen the body and loosen up the pelvis in preparation for the birth; it can also aid recovery afterwards.

Yoga has been practised for thousands of years in India and is now widely taught in the West. Most yoga practised by Westerners is a form of hatha yoga. This means that it involves physical postures (asanas) as well as breath-control techniques, meditation and relaxation exercises. General classes are usually advertised simply as hatha yoga. There are also some very particular styles, such as Iyengar, which emphasizes precise alignment of the body.

Certain yoga poses, such as the spinal twists and headstands, should be avoided in pregnancy: so it is best to attend a class aimed specifically at pregnant women. Antenatal yoga classes are available in many areas for women in their second and third trimesters.

If you are pregnant and want to take up yoga for the first time, it is best to wait until you are past the 12-week mark before starting classes. If you already practise a regular, well-established yoga routine, it should be safe to continue in the first trimester, as long as you work gently and avoid unsuitable postures. However, tell your teacher that you are pregnant so that he or she can help you to practise safely.

CHOOSING A YOGA TEACHER

Anyone can teach yoga, and standards do vary. Before committing to a class, ask your yoga teacher about his or her experience and training – reputable teachers should be happy to discuss this. Your teacher should also be insured. Pregnant women should only attend 'yoga for pregnancy' classes.

Many yoga asanas need to be adapted for pregnancy. This woman is doing modified dog pose; the standard position would place a strain on her uterus.

YOUR YOGA PRACTICE

In yoga, everyone works to his or her own capacity. So, although a class of students may be shown the same exercise, they may perform it in many different ways. Some people are flexible and can get into advanced postures quite easily; others are very stiff and need to work with a simplified version of the pose.

It is important that you do not push yourself any further than you are naturally able to go. With practice, your body will become stronger and more flexible. In many yoga classes, specialist equipment is available to help you work with the postures.

This is a version of shoulder-stand that is suitable for pregnancy. It helps blood to drain from the legs and may help to prevent varicose veins if done daily.

YOUR YOGA CLASS

Yoga classes can vary widely, depending on the form being taught and the particular teacher's training and interest. They usually last 1–1½ hours. Generally, you will start with easy postures, which serve to warm up the body, and then move on to more advanced ones. Usually, sitting, standing, reclining and some inversions (adapted if you are pregnant) will be covered.

The teacher will demonstrate each posture, then talk the class through the series of movements needed to get into it. He or she will also explain and demonstrate simplified versions of the postures where necessary. You may be given individual attention – and sometimes gentle physical

Gentle lifts can help to extend the spine and release tension in the lower back. Place a flat cushion or block under your head for comfort.

adjustment – in order to improve your alignment. All the postures should be done on a non-slip mat.

The class will end with simple breathing exercises and relaxation. It is very important that you complete the relaxation since it gives the body a chance to cool down. It also helps to calm the mind. People often like to cover themselves with a light blanket for this part of the class.

Yoga is most effective if you do it regularly. Your teacher will give you advice on which postures to do at home.

GETTING THE MOST FROM YOGA

- Always tell your yoga teacher that you are pregnant. Mention any health problems that you have.
- Do not eat or drink a large amount of water for an hour before the class; avoid eating a large meal in the three hours beforehand.
- Wear loose, comfortable clothing – a T-shirt and light tracksuit pants are ideal. You should always do the poses in bare feet, but you can put socks on for the relaxation if you wish.
- If you are practising at home, make sure that any postures you do are suitable for pregnancy. Do not do any postures that involve lying flat on your back after 30 weeks.
- Never strain or over-extend your body.
- Breathe freely: do not hold your breath when getting in or out of a posture.
- If you feel faint or uncomfortable, stop and rest on your left side for a few minutes.
- Always end a yoga session with at least ten minutes of relaxation time.

You'll need to adapt the relaxation pose in later months, when you should not lie flat on your back. Lie on your side, or place a bean bag in front of you and relax into it.

T'ai chi

The gentleness of t'ai chi exercise makes it ideal in pregnancy. It is a stylized form of martial art, performed in a controlled way so that you look as if you are dancing in slow motion. Regular practice is said to promote good health, strength, flexibility, balance and the breath control that is vital during labour.

T'ai chi is based on the idea that our well-being depends on the circulation of energy through invisible channels (meridians) in the body – the same theory that is behind acupuncture. The movements combine with breathing techniques to enhance this energy flow.

T'ai chi can be done by anyone. It improves posture and balance and also helps to keep the joints flexible. Researchers have found that it can lower blood pressure and improve breathing technique. Once learned, it is very relaxing, and can be an effective method of relieving stress.

The practice of T'ai chi can be beneficial for women who are trying to conceive or who are already pregnant, especially because it is such a calming influence and a gentle type of exercise. It may help with ailments such as backache, breathing problems, digestive problems and constipation. Its ability to develop physical and mental control can be of immense benefit when it comes to labour and birth. You should seek out a t'ai chi teacher who is used to dealing with pregnant women, as some stances may not be suitable.

LEARNING T'AI CHI

There are many aspects to t'ai chi, so it is difficult to learn more than the basics from a book or video. It is taught in classes of up to 30 people, but you can also learn it on a one-to-one basis. There are several forms of t'ai chi. The type most commonly taught in the West is Yang style, short form. This consists of 24 linked movements, which take about five minutes to perform.

Learning the movements properly takes time – you may spend a whole class on only one or two of them. The teacher will demonstrate each movement and then talk the class through it. There are many things to bear in mind, including the position of your hands, your leg movements, posture and breathing.

Only when each movement has been practised many times can you start to synchronize all the different elements. T'ai chi masters say that it takes years of practice to perform the movements perfectly. The movements are linked together to create a single flowing sequence. You practise the same sequence every day. This element of repetition, as well as the need to focus mind and body, make t'ai chi deeply relaxing, so that it is commonly described as 'meditation in motion'.

A t'ai chi class usually lasts an hour. Wear comfortable clothing that does not restrict your movements. Ideally, you should wear flat shoes with flexible soles (t'ai chi shoes are sold in Chinese supermarkets), but you can also do t'ai chi in bare feet. Most teachers will ask you to practise at home as well as attend classes – a daily practice session achieves the greatest benefits.

T'ai chi trains the mind as well as the body. You have to concentrate on your posture in order to keep your movements smooth and co-ordinated.

SAFE T'AI CHI

Few people suffer ill effects from practising t'ai chi. However, it is important to tell your teacher that you are pregnant, and to mention any health problems.

One problem associated with t'ai chi practice is sore knees, caused by incorrect posture. To avoid this, do not move the knee further forwards than your toes, nor allow it to collapse inwards or outwards.

Meditation

This is a form of mental exercise that can lead to greater inner harmony and awareness, making it the ideal way to relax and deal with the stresses of conception and pregnancy. It developed as a spiritual practice, but you do not have to subscribe to any particular philosophy to enjoy its benefits.

Many doctors believe that relaxation is an important part of general health care, and recommend meditation to their patients. Research has shown that regular meditation can reverse the effects of stress and help to alleviate ailments such as insomnia and digestive problems.

Meditation can soothe the emotions and help people to gain a wider perspective. Spending a few minutes each day in quiet contemplation can help women to cope with the disappointments that can be part of trying to conceive, as well as the challenges of pregnancy and new motherhood.

PRACTISING MEDITATION

Meditation practices vary, but they can often involve concentrating on a single object. The simplest way of practising meditation is probably to focus on your own breathing. You can also choose to focus on a physical object such as a flower or a candle flame, or on a sound that you repeat over and over again (known as a mantra). These concentration practices help to still the mind and have a relaxing effect on the body.

LEARNING MEDITATION

You can learn basic meditative techniques from a book or tape, and there are some simple exercises to try in this book. Most people find that it is much easier to learn and to concentrate when they are in a group. An experienced teacher will be able to answer any questions that you have.

Classes vary widely and it is important that you choose one you feel comfortable with. Talk to the teacher beforehand about what is involved.

SAFETY POINT

Check with your doctor before starting meditation if you have suffered from any form of psychiatric illness in the past. Sometimes meditation can bring up disturbing thoughts and images.

VISUALIZATION

This is a form of meditation that involves picturing an object, a happy event or a relaxing, beautiful scene in your mind's eye. It is a recognized technique for self-help and is much used by sportsmen with an athletic goal or achievement in mind.

Visualization can be used to promote well-being; in pregnancy, it may be helpful for easing anxiety and promoting bonding. For example, you can imagine your baby developing healthy and strong, or visualize healing pink or golden light surrounding you and your child. It can also be a good way of preparing for the birth, by imagining the birth canal opening and expanding.

Meditation takes time to learn – like, for example, mastering a musical instrument. However, its advocates say that perserverance can bring life-long benefits. Some people find that they prefer to practise meditation in conjunction with an alternative practice based on physical movement, such as yoga or t'ai chi.

Meditation is best learned from an experienced practitioner. Classes vary widely: some may be based on Buddhist, Hindu, Christian or New Age philosophies; others may simply focus on relaxation in general.

Hypnotherapy

Hypnotherapists work by inducing a relaxed, trance-like state in their clients – a state in which clients are highly receptive to any suggestions, including suggestions for self-healing. This can be particularly helpful in dealing with the hopes and fears surrounding conception and childbirth.

Practitioners say hypnopsis can be used to help a person overcome addiction, combat anxiety, dispel a phobia or release negative states of mind, such as lack of confidence. It works by implanting positive suggestions that will help the person change ways of thinking or behaviour patterns that are contributing to their difficulties.

Hypnosis can be an effective way of relieving chronic pain and alleviating the symptoms of stress. The therapy usually works best if the subject is taught to use the techniques for self-hypnosis to control his or her symptoms.

Hypnotherapy is relaxing, and it may help some women who are trying to conceive. Practitioners say that they can help women to prepare for childbirth, particularly if they are fearful or anxious about the labour. Some hypnotherapists may attend the birth to assist with pain relief.

Hypnotherapy does not work for everyone, but nine out of ten people can apparently achieve a trance-like state. Practitioners maintain that it is impossible to hypnotize a person who does not wish it, claiming that the mind can always repel an unwanted hypnotic suggestion, although many people would dispute this. It is very important to find a reputable and experienced practitioner. Your doctor may be able to recommend somebody to you.

SEEING A HYPNOTHERAPIST

Hypnotherapy usually requires several sessions to show results. During the first session, the practitioner will discuss your reasons for seeking treatment and will take a full medical history, including any current mental or physical symptoms you may be experiencing. You should have an opportunity to ask about how hypnotherapy works and about the effects it may have on you.

SAFE HYPNOSIS

There has been considerable research into hypnotherapy, and many doctors believe that it can be helpful. However, they stress it should be used as an adjunct to medical treatment, not as a substitute.

Choose a serious, qualified practitioner you trust, and check that he or she belongs to a reputable professional association. You should not have hypnosis if you suffer from epilepsy or if you have suffered severe depression in the past.

Self-hypnosis is a gentle healing technique that can help you to manage anxiety and stress-related symptoms. Some women find it a helpful way of preparing for childbirth.

You may sit on a comfortable chair or lie down for treatment. The practitioner then induces a trance by talking to you in a slow, soothing voice. You may be asked to look at a pendulum or a spot on a wall to help you relax. Imagery is often used: for example, you may be asked to picture yourself walking down a staircase. When people go into a trance, they usually feel deeply relaxed, but they are still aware of what is happening around them.

The practitioner will ask you questions in an attempt to discover the cause of the problem – sometimes deep-rooted anxieties and fears can be uncovered. He or she will also seek to implant positive thoughts or instructions that will help you to use the power of your mind to manage your particular problem.

At the end of the session, you will be slowly brought back to full consciousness. There should be an opportunity for you to discuss what has happened at this point. Most hypnotherapists will give you advice on using self-hypnosis and will ask you to practise the techniques in between sessions.

Reiki

This form of hands-on healing was developed by a Japanese scholar, Dr. Mikao Usui. It is based on the idea that there is a life-force energy – *rei* means 'universal' and *ki* (like *chi*) means 'life force' – that we can access for healing. This gentle therapy is often used to relieve mild depression during and after pregnancy.

Practitioners of reiki say that they act as channels for the healing energy (ki/chi) that flows through the universe and all things in it. In the course of a treatment, they lay their hands on or just above a person's body, so that this energy can be directed to wherever it is most needed. Neither the practitioner nor the person being treated need know exactly what the problem is in order for the healing to work.

BENEFITS

Many people find reiki deeply relaxing, and it may be helpful for stress, anxiety, depression and minor ailments such as backache or constipation. Most doctors are sceptical about the claims made for reiki, but usually see it as harmless so long as it is not used as a substitute for medical treatment. It is quite safe in pregnancy.

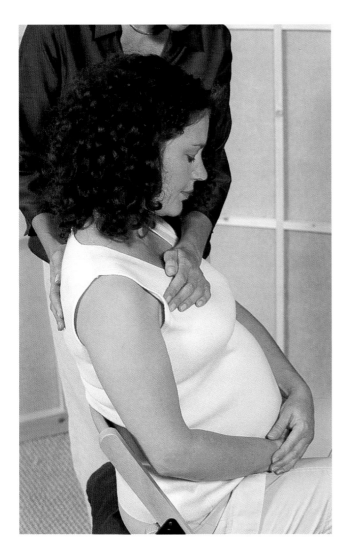

SAFE REIKI
- Choose a well-established reiki practitioner.
- Avoid practitioners who promise miracle cures or dramatic transformations.
- Continue to report any symptoms to your doctor.

HAVING A REIKI TREATMENT

Reiki sessions take about an hour. You lie fully clothed on a massage couch. If you are pregnant, it may be more comfortable to sit in a chair. In any case, you should not lie flat on your back after 30 weeks.

The practitioner will place his or her hands on different parts of your body for several minutes at a time. Twelve basic positions are used: four on the head, four on the back and four on the front. These are said to relate to different centres of energy in the body.

You may feel a sensation of tingling or heat emanating from the practitioner's hands. This is said to be a sign of the healing energy being drawn into your body, and it can feel very pleasurable. After a treatment, some people feel relaxed and sleepy; others feel energized. Practitioners recommend that you go home and rest afterwards. Regular sessions are usually recommended to maintain well-being.

SELF-TREATMENT AND TRAINING

Reiki practitioners believe that everyone has the capacity to access life-force energy and use it for healing. You can learn basic reiki in a weekend; the course usually includes instruction on using your hands for healing, ethical guidelines and 'attunement', a ceremony in which your healing channels are said to be cleared. After the course, you can practise healing on yourself and those close to you.

Practitioners have usually done further training: however, this is not regulated in any way, and can involve no more than a weekend workshop. Anyone can set up as a reiki therapist, and so it may be wise to find a practitioner who has completed the longer, more rigorous training that confers the accreditation of Master reiki teacher.

During a reiki session, healing energy is transmitted through the hands of the practitioner and into the recipient. It is a non-invasive therapy, and you remain clothed to receive treatment.

Feng shui

The Chinese art of feng shui is based on the idea that a life-force exists within everything and that buildings and rooms also contain this force. Feng shui aims to direct this energy to bring us spiritual and material benefits. One of the uses for parents-to-be is to create an harmonious nursery for their baby.

Feng shui is the art of arranging your home in order to harness positive energy, and using it to improve your health, relationships, career, fertility or other aspects of your life.

There are different schools of feng shui. The traditional form incorporates Chinese astrology and the use of a special compass (the lo pan). Some practitioners use a tool called a bagua to determine which areas of your home relate to different aspects of your life. Many Western practitioners work intuitively, preferring to sense which areas of your home are lacking in chi (energy).

Some aspects of feng shui can be used for self-help. However, much of the theory is complicated and using a practitioner is recommended if you want to ensure that your home is organized according to feng shui principles.

It is a good idea to talk to a practitioner on the 'phone before arranging a consultation. As with any complementary therapy, choose someone you feel comfortable with, in order to benefit fully from the advice given.

WHAT A CONSULTATION INVOLVES

A feng shui practitioner will usually visit your home, but some practitioners work by post, using a floor plan. You should mention any difficulties you have experienced since living there – such as relationship or fertility problems.

During the visit, the practitioner will assess the surrounding environment to see whether there are negative influences: these could include a large tree that casts a shadow on your home, or a prison or hospital nearby.

Each room will be assessed to determine whether it has a positive or negative influence on your life. Some aspects

of feng shui may seem strange: for example, it is considered to be bad luck to place your bed so that your feet face the doorway. Others may feel like common sense: feng shui says that your home should be clutter-free.

The practitioner may suggest that you use the rooms differently – sometimes people are recommended to site their bedroom elsewhere. You will be advised on the arrangement of the furniture, the decoration and lighting and the placement of any ornaments and pictures. A written report is usually sent, so that you can consider these recommendations at your leisure.

FENG SHUI SELF-HELP

- Keep doorways and outside pathways clear, to encourage chi into your home. Clean windows regularly.
- Repair or discard broken or damaged items.
- Remove clutter so that chi can circulate freely.
- Leave space around each item of furniture, and do not store anything underneath.
- Brighten up a dull corner with a lamp or colourful picture.

A bright and airy room like this one is said to be full of positive chi. However, the sharp edge of the sloping roof would be considered inauspicious. A feng shui practitioner may recommend 'cures' to counteract any bad luck that this could bring.

Colour therapy and crystal healing

Therapists say that colours and crystals give out positive vibrations that can have a beneficial effect on the mind and body. For the parent-to-be, they offer a pleasant way to deal with fluctuating moods and to promote a calm state of well-being.

COLOUR THERAPY

Colour therapists vary widely in what they believe and how they work: some draw on Western psychological research; others adhere to Eastern mysticism. All of them believe that colours transmit healing vibrations, and that these vibrations can be used to treat illness and improve well-being. Colour is an important aspect of feng shui, and some complementary therapists use elements of colour therapy in their work.

Most doctors are sceptical about the health claims made by colour therapists, but research has shown that colours can have a powerful effect on our mood. For example, blue can be very calming, while yellow can help to enhance learning ability. You can use the characteristics of colour for self-help – for example, by decorating a room in a particular hue – or you can consult a therapist for specific treatment.

Colours and their qualities
- **Red** is the colour of vitality, creativity and passion.
- **Yellow** lifts the spirits and promotes mental clarity.
- **Orange** increases your sense of happiness and joy.
- **Green** works to harmonize, balance and heal.
- **Violet** is associated with self-esteem and also with self-empowerment.
- **Pink** can be soothing, loving and supportive.
- **Blue** helps to quieten the mind and promote restful sleep.
- **Turquoise** serves to cleanse, calm and purify.

Seeing a colour therapist

Colour therapists work in a variety of different ways. Some may diagnose your problem by 'sensing' what colours you need; others ask clients carry out a simple exercise, such as ranking a set of colour cards in order of preference.

You may be asked to lie draped in coloured silks or to sit in front of a machine that directs coloured light at you. The therapist may advise you on visualization and meditation techniques, and may suggest that you wear particular colours and include foods of the same hue in your diet.

COMPLEMENTARY HEALING
Colour therapy or crystal healing may help some people with stress-related conditions and emotional problems. However, you should still report any symptoms to your doctor. Avoid practitioners who offer miracle cures.

If you suffer from anxiety, a colour therapist may recommend you wear soothing blue.

The crystal chrysocolla can be placed over the throat chakra to promote good communication – essential for coping with the many challenges of pregnancy, childbirth and parenthood.

CRYSTAL HEALING

Crystals are often used in feng shui, and healers say that they can be used to help a wide range of symptoms and emotional disturbances. If you visit a crystal healer, several crystals may be placed on different parts of your body – often over the body's energy centres (chakras) – to encourage healing. You may also be given a crystal to wear, carry or place in your home. These are some of the crystals used to foster well-being:
- **Amethyst** encourages peace and tranquillity and can help to promote restful sleep.
- **Rose quartz** has gentle, loving qualities and is associated with the heart.
- **Jade** soothes the emotion and promotes balance. It is said to encourage healing and recovery.
- **Coral** is a protective stone that may be used to ward off any negative energy.
- **Garnet** lifts the spirits and is a source of positive energy. It is associated with sexuality and fertility.
- **Smoky quartz** is said to be good for mood swings.

Which therapy?

Therapies

Here is a guide to which therapies may help certain conditions. You may need to experiment to find what works best for you. Always get a diagnosis and any necessary treatment from your family doctor.

Conditions

Condition	Herbalism page 228	Homeopathy page 229	Aromatherapy pages 230–231	Massage page 232	Shiatsu page 233	Acupuncture page 234	Reflexology page 235	Osteopathy page 236	Chiropractic page 237	Alexander technique page 238	Pilates page 239	Yoga pages 240–241	T'ai Chi page 242	Meditation page 243	Hypnotherapy page 244	Reiki page 245
Anxiety/Stress	●	●	●	●	●	●	●				●	●	●	●	●	●
Backache		●	●	●	●	●	●	●	●	●	●	●				●
Bleeding gums	●	●														
Breastfeeding problems	●	●				●										●
Breathlessness						●		●	●	●	●	●	●			
Conception difficulties	●	●	●			●	●						●			●
Constipation	●	●	●	●	●	●	●	●	●		●	●	●			
Cramps	●	●	●	●	●	●					●	●				
Cystitis	●	●			●	●										
Dizziness	●	●		●	●	●		●	●	●						
Fatigue	●	●	●	●	●	●	●			●	●	●	●	●	●	●
Flatulence	●	●	●	●	●	●					●					
Haemorrhoids	●	●	●	●	●	●	●	●	●							
Heartburn	●	●				●	●	●	●				●			
Incontinence, urinary	●	●				●					●					
Insomnia	●	●	●	●	●	●					●	●		●	●	●
Labour	●	●	●	●		●	●				●				●	
Milk, insufficient supply of	●	●	●													
Morning sickness	●	●			●	●					●		●	●	●	
Oedema	●	●	●	●	●	●					●					
Pelvic discomfort			●			●		●	●	●	●					
Perineal discomfort (postnatal)	●	●	●													
Postnatal depression	●	●	●	●		●	●				●					
Stretchmarks	●	●	●	●												
Sweating	●	●	●								●					
Thrush	●	●	●			●										
Urination (frequent)	●	●									●					
Varicose veins	●	●	●		●						●					

Glossary

Amniocentesis This is a specialized test that involves taking fluid from the amniotic cavity (amnion). The amnion is the inner sac that surrounds the baby in the uterus. The cells contained within the fluid can be analysed and also grown in a tissue culture. Together the results provide information about chromosomal defects, the sex of the baby, inherited disorders, and open neural tube defects. *See pages 114-147.*

Amniotic fluid The fluid contained within the amnion. *See* **Amniocentesis**.

Antenatal This means before birth.

AIH Process in which the woman is inseminated with her partner's sperm by means of a syringe while she is ovulating. *See pages 62-77.*

Baby blues *see* **postnatal depression**.

Birth plan With the help of the hospital antenatal unit you will be invited to draw up a birth plan, which states all your wishes for the management of your labour and delivery.

Braxton Hicks contractions Painless contractions of the uterus that occur throughout pregnancy and more noticeably during the last trimester of pregnancy, when they may be mistaken for the contractions that signify impending birth.

Breaking of the waters The membranes surrounding the baby in the uterus rupture painlessly at the onset of labour, producing a gush of 'water'. The waters refer to the liquid contained within the membranes that surround the baby. Once the waters have broken, hospital admission or bed rest is advisable, since the baby is now no longer protected from infection or from any impact.

Caesarean A Caesarean section is performed by making an incision along the bikini line and lifting out the baby. This surgery is performed either with general anaesthetic or with an epidural.
An **emergency** Caesarean is performed when it becomes clear to medical staff that the baby cannot be born naturally and the need becomes urgent to deliver the baby quickly. An **elective** Caesarean is one in which the need for a Caesarean has been decided in advance.

Chorionic villus sampling This is a non-routine test carried out to detect fetal abnormality, and it is usually carried out at 9-10 weeks. A narrow tube is passed into the uterus, either through the vagina or through the abdomen, to the outer sac surrounding the baby, known as the chorion. A sample of the floating tendrils of the chorion, the villi, is sucked into the tube and analysed for information about the baby's genes. Ultrasound is used throughout the procedure to locate precisely the chorion and the villi. The test carries a risk of miscarriage.

Colostrum A milky fluid high in protein, minerals, vitamins and nitrogen, which precedes the flow of breast milk for two or three days after delivery. Colostrum also contains antibodies that bolster the baby's immune system, helping to fight infection.

Dilation The cervix gradually opens (dilates) to allow the baby's head to pass into the birth canal, and into the world.

Donor insemination *See pages 62-77.*

Eclampsia *see* **pre-eclampsia**.

Ectopic pregnancy The fertilized egg implants not in the uterus but elsewhere in the abdomen or Fallopian tubes. Symptoms include bleeding and abdominal pain, sometimes severe, and pain in the shoulder. Immediate hospital admission is required.

Egg donation *See pages 62-77.*

Embryo The fertilized egg that eventually becomes the developing baby is known as the embryo for the first eight weeks of life. After that it is known as a fetus, until birth.

Endorphins The feel-good hormones that are released during exercise (and lovemaking) and continue to make us feel good and relieve pain for some time after the exercise itself has stopped.

Engagement The engagement of the baby's head in the upper part of the woman's pelvis. This usually occurs after the 36th week. (The pressure exerted by the baby's head is one of the factors that makes women need to urinate frequently in pregnancy.)

Epidural Local anaesthetic is injected into the epidural space between the spinal cord and the backbone of the lumbar region to provide total pain relief during labour and/or during a Caesarean. The baby is less likely to be affected by epidural than by pethidine or general anaesthetic.

Episiotomy A surgical incision is made into the perineum (between the vagina and the anus) towards the end of the second stage of labour before the baby is born. The cut is made to relieve pressure on the muscle of the perineum, to prevent tearing of the muscle, to help the baby out, and if a forceps or ventouse delivery needs to be done.

Fertile period The woman's fertile period lasts for a few days around ovulation. Ovulation itself takes place 14 days before the expected next period. This is not the same as saying it takes place 14 days after the last period because women's menstrual cycles vary in length very considerably. They can sometimes be as short as 21 days or as long as 38 days rather than the standard 28.

Fetoscopy This procedure involves a microscope camera being inserted into the uterus through the abdomen in much the same way as amniocentesis so that the fetus can be photographed. By sampling tissue it may be possible to diagnose several blood and skin diseases that the test amniocentesis cannot. In some centres, certain fetal conditions can be treated before delivery by means of a fetoscopy. *See pages 114-147.*

Fetus *see* **embryo**.

Follicle-stimulating hormone *see* **reproductive hormones**.

Forceps A pair of forceps looks like a pair of tongs or a pair of spoons. If there is a delay in the second stage of labour, they are passed up through the vagina and gently applied either side of the baby's head so that the baby can be drawn gently and slowly down the birth canal and delivered quickly. They are used when it can been seen that the baby needs some assistance, but that a Caesarean can still be avoided.

Gas and air Method of pain relief used during labour. The woman breathes in nitrous oxide and oxygen through a mouthpiece.

Genetic counselling Genetics is the science of heredity. Genetic counselling is offered to those couples who fail to conceive, who have repeated miscarriages or who have genetic disorders in their family medical histories.

GIFT (Gamete intra-Fallopian transfer) *See pages 62-77.*

ICSI (Intra-cytoplasm sperm injection) *See pages 62-77.*

In-vitro fertilization *See pages 62-77.*

Incompatibility Some women's bodies repel their partner's sperm. Some sperm is attacked by antibodies, which may be produced by either man or woman. This biochemical incompatibility may be resolved by one of the methods of assisted fertility described in the chapter on delayed conception, *pages 62-77.*

Induction Labour can be induced artificially in hospital if it has become apparent that the baby needs to be born without delay but there is no sign of labour contractions starting. The three possible methods of induction include rupturing the membranes, administering pessaries and the use of a drip.

IUI (Intrauterine insemination)
See pages 62-77.

Laparoscopy A laparoscopy is a procedure in which a narrow tube with a telescopic eyepiece is inserted through a cut in the mother's abdomen. Light is transmitted along a cable within the tube and through the window at the top of the tube, enabling the surgeon to see into the abdomen and identify any problems or abnormalities that may be preventing conception. The procedure is carried out under general anaesthetic.

Luteinizing hormone *see* **reproductive hormones**.

Meconium The faeces within the baby's rectum, meconium is composed of cellular debris, vernix and some lanugo, and is greenish-black in colour. If it is passed while the fetus is still in the uterus and under stress, it may discolour the amniotic fluid. The fluid's colour is carefully observed, therefore, when the waters break in order to detect any sign of meconium stain. If there is, this can signify fetal distress, necessitating the delivery of the baby without delay.

Miscarriage This is the lay (non-medical) term for the spontaneous loss of a pregnancy. A large percentage of pregnancies are lost, often for no known reason, sometimes before the woman even knows that she is pregnant. The medical term for miscarriage is spontaneous abortion.

Morning sickness Nausea and vomiting during pregnancy, commonly in the first trimester and commonly in the mornings, can occur throughout pregnancy and at any time of day. They are caused by hormonal changes, disturbing the normal metabolism of the body, by vascular changes leading to large variations in blood pressure; by upset to the digestive system caused by changes in the rates of secretion in the stomach and small intestine; and by psychological changes, which can produce anxiety.

Motility Sperm gain the ability to move (known as motility) by means of a process that is not yet fully understood. Sperm cannot swim. They are transported by muscular contractions through the man's reproductive system and, when they enter or are propelled into the woman's reproductive system, they continue to be transported.

Neonatal The period of four weeks immediately after the baby's delivery. A neonate is a newborn baby up to the age of four weeks.

Nuchal fold ultrasound The nuchal fold ultrasound is also sometimes known as the nuchal fold, the nuchal translucency test or the translucency scan. This is carried out at 11 to 14 weeks and is used to detect Down's syndrome cases. The procedure is as for a routine ultrasound, but the operator concentrates on getting a good image of the

fetus's neck on the screen and measures a layer of fluid at the back of the neck. The thicker this layer is, the greater the chance the baby will have Down's syndrome. The chance or risk is expressed as a probability such as a one in 10,000 chance or a one in 100 chance.

Oestrogen This describes a number of hormones produced by the ovaries and the adrenal gland. During pregnancy, the placenta also produces oestrogen. The oestrogen hormones are responsible for the development of the female breasts and genitals at puberty and they also play a part in controlling the menstrual cycle. In pregnancy the hormones stimulate the growth of the uterus and breast tissue. *See also* **reproductive hormones**.

Pethidine A method of pain relief used in labour, this is an anaesthetic given by injection which lasts for three to four hours. It gives better pain relief than gas and air but is not as effective as an epidural.

Placenta The placenta is located within the uterus and to it is attached the fetus through the umbilical cord. The placenta provides the fetus with nutrients from the mother, eliminates fetal waste products and enables the fetus to breathe.

Postnatal depression Baby blues are common in new mothers. They may occur within five days of the birth and most women quickly recover from this temporary hormonal slump. Postnatal depression usually occurs later, even months after the birth. The mother's misery, fear and anger may be directed at herself, her baby or both. Irritability, fatigue and sleeplessness are characteristic. Professional help is needed. *See also pages 208-225.*

Pre-eclampsia This is the precursor to the very serious condition of convulsions in pregnancy, known as eclampsia. It is characterized by the development of high blood pressure, swelling (especially of the face, ankles, and wrists), and by the appearance of protein in the urine. Urgent referral to hospital is required.

Progesterone One of the female hormones, progesterone is produced by the corpus luteum in the ovary, to a lesser extent by the adrenal gland, and in pregnancy by the placenta. It is responsible for building up the endometrium in the uterus, which feeds the developing embryo in the early days of pregnancy. Progesterone stimulates the growth of the glandular, milk-producing tissue and helps smooth muscle to relax. *See also* **reproductive hormones**.

Pudendal nerve block Type of local anaesthetic injection used in labour, which numbs the perineum, vagina and vulva prior to short, second stage labour procedures, such as forceps delivery and ventouse.

Reproductive hormones The menstrual cycle is controlled by the reproductive hormones, FSH (follicle-stimulating hormone) and LH (luteinizing hormone), which are released by the brain and which stimulate the ovaries to produce the female sex hormones, oestrogen and progesterone.

Show The first thing to happen at the beginning of labour is the appearance of a mucus plug from the vagina. This is known as a show of mucus and it is sometimes tinged with blood, which gives it a pinkish appearance. This is followed by the breaking of the waters, when hospital admission or bed rest are advised.

Sperm count This is the number of sperm in any one ejaculate of semen. A low sperm count is a well-known cause of infertility.

Stillbirth The death at or before the birth of the baby after 24 weeks' gestation. The term perinatal death, which doctors often use, includes stillbirth and the death of a baby in the first week of life.

TENS Transcutaneous Electrical Nerve Stimulation is a form of pain relief used during labour in which electrode pads discharging an electrical stimulus are placed on the woman's back. The woman controls the amount of electrical input with a hand-held control. Some women find it effective, while others do not.

Termination This is the medical or surgical ending of a pregnancy, which may be done for medical or social reasons. It is commonly known as abortion.

Triple alphafetoprotein (AFP) test Simple, safe and reliable blood test, taken between weeks 15 and 18, that yields information about the baby's health and development. *See pages 114-147.*

Ultrasound This enables the fetus to be viewed in the uterus, providing useful information about the baby's health and development at different stages from week seven of gestation.

Umbilical cord This connects the fetus to the placenta, from which it derives nourishment. After the baby has been delivered, the cord is clamped and cut. The umbilical stump remains protruding from the baby's navel, then shrivels and eventually falls off towards the end of the first week of life.

Ventouse suction Also known as vacuum extraction, this is a last-minute medical assistance with delivery, which is carried out when the baby is in difficulties. A small cup is passed up the vagina and attached by suction to the baby's head, suction being induced by means of a small hand pump. The cup is then gently pulled to help the baby down the birth canal.

ZIFT (Zygote intra-Fallopian transfer)
See pages 62-77.

Useful addresses and websites

UNITED KINGDOM

Foresight, The Association for the Promotion of Preconceptual Care
28 The Paddock
Godalming
Surrey GU7 1XD
tel: 01483 427839
www.foresight-preconception.org.uk

The Human Fertilisation and Embryology Authority
Paxton House
30 Artillery Lane
London E1 7LS
tel: 020 7377 5077
www.hfea.gov.uk/ForPatients

Infertility Network UK
Charter House
43 St Leonard's Road
Bexhill-on-Sea
East Sussex TN40 1JA
tel: 01424 732361
www.child.org.uk

Miscarriage Association
Clayton Hospital
Northgate, Wakefield
West Yorkshire WF1 3JS
tel: 01924 200799
www.the-ma.org.uk

The Multiple Births Foundation
Queen Charlotte's and Chelsea Hospital
Du Cane Road
London W12 0HS
tel: 020 8383 3519
www.multiplebirths.org.uk

National Childbirth Trust
Alexander House
Oldham Terrace
Acton, London W3 6NH
tel: 0870 4448707
breastfeeding support line:
0870 4448707
www.nctpregnancyandbabycare.com

Relate (relationship counselling)
Herbert Gray College
Little Church Street
Rugby, Warwickshire CV21 3AP
tel: 01788 573241
Helpline: 0845 1304010
www.relate.org.uk

Royal College of Obstetricians and Gynaecologists
27 Sussex Place
London NW1
tel: 020 7772 6200
www.rcog.org.uk

Complementary Therapies

The British Register of Complementary Practitioners (BRCP)
Institute for Complementary Medicine
PO Box 194
London SE16 7QZ
tel: 020 7237 5165
www.icmedicine.co.uk

ACUPUNCTURE
The British Acupuncture Council
63 Jeddo Road
London W12 9HQ
tel: 020 8735 0400
www.acupuncture.org.uk

ALEXANDER TECHNIQUE
The Society of Teachers of the Alexander Technique
1st Floor, Linton House
Highgate Entrance
39-51 Highgate Road
London NW5 1RS
tel: 0845 230 7828
www.stat.org.uk

AROMATHERAPY
The International Federation of Aromatherapists
182 Chiswick High Road
London W4 1PP
tel: 020 8742 2605
www.ifaroma.org

BACH FLOWER REMEDIES
Bach Centre
Mount Vernon
Sotwell, Wallingford
Oxon OX10 0PZ
tel: 01491 834678
www.bachcentre.com

CHIROPRACTIC
General Chiropractic Council
44 Wicklow Street
London WC1X 9HL
Tel: 0207 713 5155
www.gcc-uk.org

HERBALISM
The National Institute of Medical Herbalists
56 Longbrook Street
Exeter EX4 6AH
tel: 01392 426022
www.nimh.org.uk

HOMEOPATHY
The British Homeopathic Association
Hahnemann House
29 Park Street West
Luton LU1 3BE
tel: 0870 4443950
www.trusthomeopathy.org

HYPNOTHERAPY
The British Hypnotherapy Association
67 Upper Berkeley Street
London W1H 7QX
tel: 020 7723 4443
www.hypnotherapy-association.org

MASSAGE
The London College of Massage
5 Newman Passage
London W1T 1EH
tel: 020 7323 3574
www.massagelondon.com

MEDITATION
The School of Meditation
158 Holland Park Avenue
London W11 4UH
tel: 020 7603 6116
www.schoolofmeditation.org

OSTEOPATHY
The General Osteopathic Council
Osteopathy House
176 Tower Bridge Road
London SE1 3LU
tel: 020 7357 6655
www.osteopathy.org.uk

REFLEXOLOGY
Association of Reflexologists
27 Old Gloucester Street
London WC1N 3XX
tel: 0870 5673320
www.aor.org.uk

YOGA
British Wheel of Yoga
25 Jermyn Street
Sleaford, Lincolnshire NG34 7RU
tel: 01529 306851
www.bwy.org.uk

Iyengar Yoga Institute
223a Randolph Avenue
London W9 1NL
tel: 020 7624 3080
www.iyi.org.uk

UNITED STATES

The American College of Obstetricians and Gynecologists
409 12th Street NW
Washington DC 200024-2188
tel: 202 638 5577
www.acog.org

National Association of Childbearing Centers
3123 Gottschall Road
Perkiomenville PA 18074
tel: 215 234 8068
www.birthcenters.org

National Women's Health Network
514 10th Street NW
Washington DC 20004
tel: 202 347 1140
www.womenshealthnetwork.org

Resolve (fertility problems)
1310 Broadway
Somerville MA 02144-1779
tel: 617 623 0744
www.resolvemn.org

Complementary Therapies

American Holistic Medical Association
12101 Menaul Blvd., NE, Suite C
Albuquerque NM 87112
tel: 505 292 7788
www.holisticmedicine.org

ACUPUNCTURE
American Association of Oriental Medicine
5530 Wisconsin Avenue
Suite 1210, Chevy Chase MD 20815
tel: 301 941 1064
www.aaom.org

CHIROPRACTIC
American Chiropractic Association
1701 Clarendon Boulevard
Arlington VA 22209
tel: 800 986 4636
www.amerchiro.org

HERBALISM
American Herbalists Guild
1931 Gaddis Road
Canton GA 30115
tel: 770 751 6021
www.americanherbalistsguild.com

HOMEOPATHY
National Center for Homeopathy
801 North Fairfax Street
Suite 306, Alexandria VA 22314
tel: 703 548 7790
www.homeopathic.org

HYPNOTHERAPY
American Institute of Hypnotherapy
1805 E Garry Avenue
Suite 100, Santa Ana CA 92705
tel: 714 261 6400
www.aih.cc

MASSAGE
American Massage Therapy Association
1701 820 Davis Street
Suite 100, Evanston IL 60201
tel: 847 864 0123
www.amtamassage.org

OSTEOPATHY
American Osteopathic Association
142 East Ontario Street
Chicago IL 60611
tel: 312 202 8000
www.osteopathic.org

REFLEXOLOGY
International Institute of Reflexology
PO Box 12642
St Petersburg FL 33733
tel: 813 343 4811
www.reflexology-usa.net

YOGA
International Association of Yoga Therapists
PO Box 426
Manton CA 96059
tel: 530 474 5700
www.yrec.org

CANADA

Canadian Examining Board of Health
Care Practitioners Inc
658 Danforth Avenue
Suite 204, Toronto
Ontario M4J 5B9
www.canadianexaminingboard.com

Infertility Network
160 Pickering Street
Toronto, Ontario M4E 3J7
tel: 416 690 8015
www.infertilitynetwork.org

Canadian Women's Health Network
Suite 203, 419 Graham Avenue
Winnipeg, Manitoba R3C 0M3
tel: 204 942 5500
www.cwhn.ca

AUSTRALIA

Australian Complementary Health Association
247 Flinders Lane
Melbourne, Vic 3000
Tel: (03) 9650 5327 Fax (03) 9650 8404
www.diversity.org.au

Fertility Society of Australia
61 Danks Street
Port Melbourne, Vic 3207
tel: 03 9645 6349
www.fsa.au.com

Australian Women's Health Network
www.awhn.org.au

NEW ZEALAND

The New Zealand Health Information Network
PO Box 337
Christchurch 8015
tel: 03 980 4646
www.nzhealth.net.nz

New Zealand Infertility Society
PO Box 34151
Birkenhead, Auckland
tel: 0800 333 306
www.nzinfertility.org.nz

SOUTH AFRICA

www.childbirth.co.za
www.activebirth.co.za

African Health Anthology
www.nisc.co.za

INTERNATIONAL WEBSITES

www.pregnancy.com
www.activebirthcentre.com
www.homebirth.org.uk
www.mothers35plus.co.uk

Further Reading and Acknowledgements

FURTHER READING

Janet Balaskas, Yehudi Gordon *The Encyclopedia of Pregnancy and Birth* (Little Brown and Co, London, 1992)

Belinda Barnes and Suzanne Gail Bradley/in association with Foresight, the Association for the Promotion of Preconceptual Care *Planning for a Healthy Baby* (Vermilion, London, 1994 and by Random House in Australia, New Zealand and South Africa)

Hilary Boyd *Working Woman's Pregnancy* (Mitchell Beazley, London, 2001)

Nikki Bradford *The Miraculous World of Your Unborn Baby* (Salamander, London, 1998 and by Contemporary Books, a division of the McGraw-Hill Companies, USA, 1998)

Dr Sarah Brewer *Pregnancy the Natural Way* (Souvenir Press, London, 1999)

Miranda Castro *Homeopathy for Pregnancy, Birth and Your Baby's First Year* (St Martin's Press, New York, 1992)

Anne Charlish *Your Natural Baby: Complementary Therapies for the First Three Years* (National, Australia, 1996)

Anne Charlish *Your Natural Pregnancy: A Guide to Complementary Therapies* (Boxtree, London, 1995)

Kaz Cooke *The Rough Guide to Pregnancy and Birth* (Rough Guides, London, 2001. Also published as *Up the Duff* by Penguin, Australia)

Glade B Curtis, MD, FACOG *Your Pregnancy Over 30* (Element, Dorset, 1998)

Alison England *Aromatherapy and Massage for Mother and Baby* (Vermilion, London; Random House in Australia, NZ, South Africa, 1999)

Françoise Barbira Freedman and Doriel Hall *Yoga for Pregnancy and Mother's First Year* (Lorenz Books, London, 2003)

Marilyn Glenville *Natural Solutions to Infertility* (Piatkus, London, 2000)

Harriet Griffey *How to Get Pregnant* (Bloomsbury, London, 1997)

Charles B Inlander and Karla Morales *Take this Book to the Obstetrician with You* (St Martin's Press, New York, 1998)

Maggie Jones *Infertility: Modern Treatments and the Issues They Raise* (Piatkus, London, 1991)

Sally Keeble: *Conceiving Your Baby: How Medicine Can Help* (Cedar/Mandarin, London, 1995)

Dr Mary Ann Lumsden et al *Royal College of Obstetricians and Gynaecologists/Complete Women's Health* (Thorsons, London, 2000)

Dr Jane MacDougall *Pregnancy Week-by-Week* (HarperCollins, New York and London, 1997)

Alison Mackonochie and Sara Lewis *Practical Encyclopedia of Pregnancy, Babycare and Nutrition for Babies and Toddlers* (Lorenz Books, London, 2003)

Vivien Marx *The Semen Book* (Free Association Books, London, 2001)

Anne McIntyre *The Herbal for Mother & Child* (Thorsons, London, 1992)

Dr. Ann Robinson *The Which? Guide to Women's Health* (Which? Books, London, 1999)

Peter Saunders *Your Pregnancy Month-by-Month* (Hodder & Stoughton, 1996)

Sherman J Silber, MD *How to Get Pregnant with The New Technology* (Warner Books, USA, 1998)

Allan Templeton et al *Management of Infertility for the MRCOG and Beyond* (RCOG Press, London, 2000)

Rosalind Widdowson *Yoga for Pregnancy* (Creative Publishing International, Minnesota, for USA/Canada; by Octopus, London, 2001)

Mari Winsor with Mark Laska *The Pilates Pregnancy* (Perseus Publishing, Cambridge, Massachusetts, 2001)

Professor Robert Winston, MB, BS, FRCOG *Getting Pregnant: The Complete Guide to Fertility and Infertility* (Pan, London, Sydney and Auckland, 1989)

Professor Robert Winston, MB, BS, FRCOG *Infertility: A Sympathetic Approach* (Martin Dunitz, London, 1986)

ACKNOWLEDGEMENTS

Anne Charlish:
I am grateful to Mr Donald Gibb, to Professor Gedis Grudzinskas and Patricia Roberts for their assistance over many years on the subjects of pregnancy and birth. I am grateful to Mr Malcolm Whitehead for his insights into the menopause and premature menopause. Lastly, I am greatly indebted to Professor Robert Winston for his tireless research and illuminating publications into the complex subject of fertility.

Publisher:
The Publishers are grateful to the following picture libraries for permission to reproduce the photographs listed below in this book (all those not listed below are © Anness Publishing Ltd): t=top; b=bottom; c=centre; l=left; r=right

Science Photo Library:
p47 tl /BSIP, Chassenet; p62 /BSIP, HARDAS; p69 bl and br /James King-Holmes; p72 br /Alexander Tsiaras; p73 tl /James King-Holmes; p87 tr P. Saada/Eurelios; p106 b /Ruth Jenkinson/MIDIRS; p119 tl /Neil Bromhall; p137 tr /Faye Norman; p142 b /Hank Morgan; p153 t /GE Medical Systems; p169 bl /Ian Hooton; p170 b /Ruth Jenkinson/MIDIRS; p181 tl /Mark Clarke; p183 t /Petit Format; p195 tr /Ruth Jenkinson/MIDIRS; p200 /Tracy Dominey; p201 br /Hank Morgan; p202 tr /Mark de Fraeye; p210 /Simon Fraser; p211 bl /BSIP, Astier; p212 tr /BSIP, Astier; p218 bl /BSIP, Astier; p234 br /Mark Thomas

Corbis:
p45 bl /Larry Williams; p49 /Norbert Schaefer; p51 cr /Royalty-free; p55 tr /Royalty-free; p71 t Corbis only; p109 t /Tom and Dee Ann McCarthy; p115 tr /Angela Wood; p115 br /Larry Williams and Associates; p151 tr /Larry Williams; p179 br /Douglas Kirkland; p186 b /Mug Shots; p199 br /Larry Williams; p208 Corbis only; p211 tr /Ariel Skelley; p221 /Susan Solie Patterson

The publishers would also like to thank:
MOT Models agency; Pregnant Pause Agency; the Warehouse studio (location setting); Bridget Baker for advice; Bonieventure Bagalue for assisting photographer Alistair Hughes; Sue Duckworth for helping with props; *Born* in Bristol for nappies and advice; Chris Bernstein for the index; Doriel Hall and Françoise Freedman for use of material, which we have adapted, on yoga and massage (mainly pp58/9, 100/1, 132/3, 162/3, 164/5 and 166/7).

Index

This edition is published by
Lorenz Books

Lorenz Books is an imprint of
Anness Publishing Ltd
Hermes House
88–89 Blackfriars Road
London SE1 8HA
tel. 020 7401 2077
fax 020 7633 9499
www.lorenzbooks.com
info@anness.com

© Anness Publishing Ltd 2004

UK agent: The Manning
Partnership Ltd
tel. 01225 478444
fax 01225 478440
sales@manning-partnership.co.uk

UK distributor: Grantham Book
Services Ltd; tel. 01476 541080
fax 01476 541061
orders@gbs.tbs-ltd.co.uk

North American agent/distributor:
National Book Network
tel. 301 459 3366
fax 301 429 5746
www.nbnbooks.com

Australian agent/distributor:
Pan Macmillan Australia
tel. 1300 135 113; fax 1300 135 103
customer.service@macmillan.com.au

New Zealand agent/distributor:
David Bateman Ltd
tel. (09) 415 7664; fax (09) 415 8892

Publisher Joanna Lorenz
Editorial Director Helen Sudell
Project Editor Ann Kay
Copy Editor Kim Davies
Designer Lisa Tai
Special photography
    Alistair Hughes
Illustrations Sam Elmhurst
Production Wanda Burrows